Health Reforms Across the World

The Experience of Twelve Small and Medium-sized Nations with Changing Their Healthcare Systems

Health Reforms Across the World

The Experience of Twelve Small and Medium-sized Nations with Changing Their Healthcare Systems

edited by

Kieke Okma
McGill University, Canada & Catholic University, Leuven, Belgium

Tim Tenbensel
University of Auckland, New Zealand

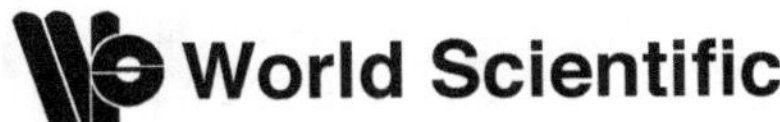

NEW JERSEY · LONDON · SINGAPORE · BEIJING · SHANGHAI · HONG KONG · TAIPEI · CHENNAI

Published by

World Scientific Publishing Co. Pte. Ltd.

5 Toh Tuck Link, Singapore 596224

USA office: 27 Warren Street, Suite 401-402, Hackensack, NJ 07601

UK office: 57 Shelton Street, Covent Garden, London WC2H 9HE

British Library Cataloguing-in-Publication Data
A catalogue record for this book is available from the British Library.

First published 2020 (hardcover)
Reprinted 2022 (in paperback edition)
ISBN 978-981-125-224-2 (pbk)

HEALTH REFORMS ACROSS THE WORLD
The Experience of Twelve Small and Medium-sized Nations with
Changing Their Healthcare Systems

ISBN 978-981-120-891-1

For any available supplementary material, please visit
https://www.worldscientific.com/worldscibooks/10.1142/11515#t=suppl

Typeset by Stallion Press
Email: enquiries@stallionpress.com

Contents

Introduction

Kieke Okma and Tim Tenbensel

What is this book about?

This book presents a diagnosis of the health reforms in 12 small- and mid-sized nations.[1,2] The countries span the globe, hailing from Africa, Latin America, Asia, Oceania and the Middle East, to Eastern and Western Europe. The study seeks to contribute to cross-national policy learning based on structured multi-country research.

At first glance, these countries do not have much in common. They are located on different continents and vary greatly in size, population numbers, ethnicity and historical backgrounds. Some are member states of the Organization for Economic Co-Operation and Development

---

[1] This book is a follow-up study of *Six Countries, Six Reform Models: The Healthcare Reform Experience of Israel, the Netherlands, New Zealand, Singapore, Switzerland and Taiwan* of 2010.

[2] One question we have not addressed extensively in this book is what counts as a small or medium country. Most international comparative studies focus on the world's largest countries: the United States, the United Kingdom, Canada, Germany, France, Japan and sometimes other OECD member states (if only because of the availability of statistical data). We use the term small and medium-sized to indicate countries that clearly do not belong to that group as they have (much) smaller populations. Harold Wilensky (2002) argued that rather than actual size in terms of population or geographic area, it is the complexity of administration that matters. However, there is another feature of policy-making in small countries worth noting: the small size of the market and policy arena creates strong barriers for exit. There is often personal overlap in functions (e.g., board membership of hospitals or health insurance agencies combined with political functions), and the major players in the health policy arena often know each other personally.

(OECD), others not. They vary in cultural orientations and economic circumstances, with very different styles of socio-economic and fiscal policy-making. In that sense, this study represents a "most different system design" (Marmor 1988) under a common analytical approach.

However, the 12 countries have some important features in common. They are all small to mid-size democracies with open economies. They share the general policy goal of broadening access to good quality healthcare while restraining public expenditure. Over time, they faced similar fiscal strains (with the notable exception of Singapore and perhaps Taiwan), growing and changing demand for medical services, and shifting views of the role of the state in society. Moreover, all have discussed a similar range of reform options, and sought to increase access to healthcare services by either expanding (public and private) health insurance or tax-based health financing.

Another shared feature of this group of countries is that they did not just discuss policy options, but actually undertook major reforms during the last decades of the 20th century and early 21st century. Public dissatisfaction with existing arrangements, combined with the availability of feasible policy options and political willingness to act, created windows of opportunity for major change. In several cases—illustrating the need to carefully distinguish policies as intention or plan versus actual, implemented change—the ultimate outcomes of the reforms differed substantially from the initial proposals. Finally, and perhaps most importantly, the cases selected are somewhat "under the radar": they are not usually included in comparative international studies (even while there has been a recent surge in interest in the experience of Switzerland and Holland; see e.g., Herzlinger and Parra 2004; Reinhardt 2004; Leu et al. 2009).

Despite the abovementioned similarities in policy goals, policy options and pressures for change, we did not find a dominant pattern of overall institutional or policy convergence in the health reforms. The central questions this book seeks to address are therefore: Why have the 12 countries, facing similar pressures to restructure their healthcare systems, with similar options for government action and almost identical goals, chosen such very different reform pathways? What caused a window of opportunity for change? What did they do? What happened after the implementation of reform legislation?

This introductory chapter of the book addresses some of the methodological issues of international comparison. It presents the major analytical frameworks used throughout the book and summarizes the main findings.

The five regional sections of this book analyze the reform experiences of two African nations: Ghana and Tanzania; two in Latin America: Chile and Ecuador; two in Western Europe: the Netherlands and Switzerland; three in Eastern Europe and the Middle East: the Czech Republic, Slovenia and Israel; and three nations in Asia and Oceania: New Zealand, Singapore and Taiwan. Each chapter presents a brief overview of the historical development of the national healthcare system and the country's current arrangements for the financing, contracting and payment, ownership and administration of healthcare. The chapters analyze the external and internal pressures for change, the discussion of policy options, the process of implementation, as well as the oft-neglected but almost universal post-reform adjustments. The regional sections also contain maps depicting graphic representations of selected data on population, income, health spending and some data regarding the health status of the nations discussed in that section. These data come from the Appendix that presents statistical data on the countries' size, population and economic growth, income levels, health, healthcare and healthcare spending, and notes major similarities and differences between the 12 nations. The final chapter of this book discusses both the empirical findings and the theoretical conclusions on the comparative methodology of this study.

The study is a truly collaborative international undertaking. The authors have all lived and worked in one or more of the 12 countries, combining academic and administrative backgrounds with personal experience. They brought together a unique degree of in-depth knowledge that allowed for more detailed findings than studies based solely on aggregate data of international organizations like the World Health Organization, World Bank or OECD.

Our study confirms the need to collaborate across countries and disciplines. As Richard Rose (1993) concluded, no individual researcher can do a systematic study of change and non-change in, say, more than three or four countries at this depth of understanding and detail. Furthermore, the study confirms the need to pay more attention to small- and medium-sized countries that are currently under the radar. The vast majority of comparative research in the field focuses on big countries, with the United States, Canada and the United Kingdom as the usual suspects, and sometimes France, Germany, Japan and Australia. There is far less research on the experience of small- and mid-sized countries, while in fact the vast majority of the world's populations (outside of China and India) live in this category. To fill this gap, many more studies are needed. This research aims to take a step into that direction.

Analytical Approaches

Harold Lasswell's famous book *Politics: Who Gets What, When, How* (1936) summarizes the essential questions of public policy. In healthcare, those translate into a wide range of public activities like the provision and financing of public health services, research and medical education, the regulation of health professionals, the protection of patients and the general public and the protection of family income against insurmountable costs of illness by spreading medical expenditure across the population.

The mechanisms to spread the costs of healthcare (or "risk pooling") vary, but usually require public action to define the populations who have access to certain plans. Such regulation extends to the entitlements under public coverage, the mandatory contributions of social health insurance and other financial conditions and the administration and monitoring of the system. Private markets pool risks, too, only on a more limited scale. Insured with private plans face premiums that reflect their actuarial risk (i.e., expected future costs): the higher the risk, the higher the premium.[3] People with certain medical conditions like chronic illness or disabilities

---

[3]This volume labels the income-related payments for social health insurance contributions, and flat-rate (nominal) payments for private insurance "premiums" following the OECD in Paris.

("pre-existing conditions") may be denied coverage altogether. The premiums of private insurance are based on segmentation of the insured into smaller, more or less homogenous groups. Public health insurance, in contrast, creates wider risk pools. It accepts insured regardless of their medical conditions and charges contributions based on ability to pay. The community-rated payments in social health insurance ignore the actuarial risk of the individuals, but spread the financial burden across wider populations via general taxation or income-related contributions for mandated insurance. It aims to provide access to medical treatment to all who need care, without undue financial barriers.

Most industrialized countries share underlying principles and goals in health policy (even if somewhat rhetorically at times): universal (or near-universal) access to good quality healthcare, and solidarity in sharing the financial burden of medical treatment (OECD 1992, 1994).[4] With a growing public share in healthcare financing, improving efficiency and cost control have become major concerns for governments, too. Many nations

---

[4] In health policy, the term "solidarity"—often but perhaps mistakenly taken as equity—translates into quite divergent arrangements. In a narrow (most commonly used and least questioned) sense, it means that everybody has access to essential medical services, when needed, without undue financial barriers. Here, solidarity refers to the fair sharing of the financial burden of medical treatment. The measure for equity is usually taken as a share of income; thus, proportional tax is seen as equal, but out-of-pocket payments and (community-rated) flat premiums as regressive, because higher income groups pay a lower percentage of their income than low-income families. The early European sick funds charged all their members the same flat-rate contribution amounts, and offered the same medical services to all. In the mid-20th century that changed to income-related contributions. Until recently, all members of one particular sick fund in Germany paid the same contribution rates (but the rates differed between the funds). The community-rated contributions served as an equalization mechanism between the members, not between the funds. In contrast (until 2006), all Dutch sick fund members paid the same income-dependent contribution, plus a modest flat-rate premium per person. The British NHS gets most of its financing from general taxation; the degree of equity thus depends on the redistributive workings of the tax system. Those financing mechanisms had quite different distributional effects, even while the general population perceived them as fair or equitable.

also regard patient satisfaction, patient choice and the professional autonomy of physicians as important goals.[5]

Nonetheless, there is wide variety in the financing mechanisms of healthcare. Canada, Australia, Italy, New Zealand, the United Kingdom, Spain and Scandinavian countries, for example, generate most of their healthcare financing out of general taxation. In lower-income nations, out-of-pocket spending often constitutes a major share. As illustrated in this volume, several countries engaged in efforts to increase the share of general taxation or social insurance in recent decades (sometimes subsidized by foreign development aid). In Austria, Belgium, France and Germany, mandatory social health insurance is the main funding source, supplemented by private coverage. The Netherlands and Switzerland moved from a mix of public and private health insurance to a population-wide mandate to acquire insurance (see the respective chapters in this volume). In all countries, patients pay for some healthcare out of their own pockets, or take out private insurance to cover those costs. Governments often mitigate the effects of user fees by exempting certain groups, or limiting the amounts families pay annually, rather than setting limits on how much reimbursement families can receive each year, as is common in private health insurance.

The variations in financing and contracting models are rooted in country-specific historical developments. Two particular events in Europe played a crucial role. The first was the introduction of German social health insurance by Chancellor Otto von Bismarck in 1883.[6] This

---

[5] For most patients, in most countries, consumer choice in healthcare refers to their ability to see a provider of their own choice. In modern-day health policy-making, however, the term often refers to the option to sign up with a health insurance or health plan of one's own choice. Paradoxically, increased choice of plan often restricts the choice of provider. When insurers can selectively contract, their insured may find that their particular plan has no contract with, say, their long-standing family physician or dentist.

[6] This peaked the interest of policy elites across the globe. Several countries in Europe—and some in Latin America and Asia—followed the German example of state-sponsored (but not state-administered), mandatory social insurance to protect the families of industrial workers against the financial risks of illness, disability, unemployment and old age. The unique feature of the Bismarckian scheme of 1883 was that it was built on the existing 19th century mutual societies (or sick funds), which themselves had very old historical roots, tracing back

6

legislation required industrial workers (and their dependents) to become members of a sick fund. That meant that sick funds had more stable revenue streams and could create wider risk pools. In the 20th century, they gained influence as core actors in the public policy arena, sharing the responsibility for social policy-making, but also facing more and more governmental regulation.

The second major innovation in the financing of healthcare was the establishment of Britain's National Health Service (NHS) in 1948, paid out of general taxation (Klein 2006).[7] The NHS extended the German insurance model by providing coverage to the entire population. While the NHS nationalized hospitals, family physicians retained the status of independent practitioners.[8]

---

to the Middle Ages (De Swaan 1988). Bismarck did not replace those sick funds, but mandated membership for certain categories of workers. The sick funds (commonly but somewhat mistakenly labeled sickness funds; the literal translation of the original German term *Krankenkasse* means fund of—and for—the sick) remained legally independent, risk-bearing insurers. Both labor unions, as workers' representatives, and employers participated on the boards. Each fund set its own premium, shared on a 50–50 basis between workers and employers, by law, since 1883. The funds also offered modest amounts of income replacement in case of illness, disability or death of the family breadwinner. They owned clinics and employed physicians to provide healthcare to their members.

[7] In 1943, an expert committee headed by William Beveridge proposed a new model for British social security after the War. It advocated extending access to healthcare to the entire population, paid out of general taxation, with nationalized health facilities (Klein 2006). The war itself had created a window of opportunity: for the first time in history, social classes met in times of duress. They had shared underground shelters during air raids, for example, and were ready to acknowledge that everybody needed healthcare, regardless of income or background. The Beveridge report argued that additional investments in hospitals and other services would only be temporary: those would help the wounded war veterans and disabled workers return to the labor force as soon as possible. The nationalization of hospitals gave government the say over (and financial responsibility for) hospital capacity. In the post-war decades, the NHS became very popular. It did deliver on its promise of universal healthcare, albeit in a frugal way. There were some concerns about costs; but, as noted by Pierson (1994), it had created its own constituencies, that actively defended its almost untouchable position for decades.

[8] Almost 10 years before the start of the British NHS in 1948, hospital care in New Zealand had already become a universal entitlement for the entire population, paid out of general taxation.

The two models spread across the globe in the 20th century. Several countries in Western Europe, Asia and Latin America followed the German example and implemented income protection schemes for certain societal groups (e.g., disability, health and unemployment benefits for civil servants or industrial workers). Others followed the population-wide NHS model. It was only after the Second World War, however, that nations in Western Europe and North America embraced the full range of modern welfare state arrangements, including pensions, disability and unemployment benefits, sick pay, child support and health insurance.

By the end of the 20th century, healthcare financing became hybridized as more and more countries incorporated elements of both models, combining employment-based social insurance with tax-based universal schemes. This hybridization had important consequences for efforts to group countries into categories (see below).

There was strong popular support for the expansion of the state-sponsored schemes in the decades after World War II. That changed rather suddenly in the mid-1970s. A confluence of economic, demographic and ideological factors contributed to reshaping the notion of the welfare state as a solution for social problems to that of an economic burden and a cause of economic stagnation (Timmins 1995; Wilensky 2002). The economic stagflation following the oil crises of the 1970s, with persistent and high levels of unemployment, meant that state incomes stagnated or declined while public spending continued to grow. Moreover, at the end of the post-war baby boom demographers realized they had to revise earlier demographic projections downwards (and estimates of future pension expenditures upwards).

In addition, ideological views on the role of state had changed. Critics on both the left and the right of the political spectrum agreed that state powers had become too broad, too dominant and too intrusive in the lives of individuals. Rising consumerism, growing dissatisfaction over fiscal burdens, disappointment in the results of public programs and patient advocacy groups claiming a stronger voice in the allocation and organization of healthcare all added to the pressures for change.

Governments were thus prompted to look elsewhere for new (if often untested) ideas and solutions: "no one wants to be caught wearing yesterdays' ideas," Klein (1995) once observed. This search fueled a rapid proliferation of cross-national studies in the field of health policy, in the 1980s and 1990s. The majority of those comparative studies, however, consisted of collections of descriptive case studies based on aggregate national statistics. They often lacked a common vocabulary or focus, and suffered from poorly defined terms (Marmor et al. 2003). The studies frequently used terms like "health reform," "managed competition" or "consumer-driven healthcare," but rarely defined these in any operational way.[9] Many comparative studies claimed to analyze processes of health reform across the globe, but few paid attention to what it was, conceptually, that they sought to explain (Rose 1993).

Another common mistake is the assumption that policy as stated, in formal government documents or law, is the same as policy actually implemented (Palmer and Short 1989). As we will show, for a variety of reasons, the ultimate outcome of reform often differs greatly from original policy intentions and statements. Faced with public discontentment over (intended or unintended) results, governments often feel pressured to adjust their policies.

In this contribution, we take health reform as major shifts both in the decision-making power over the allocation of resources and the financial risks. Such shifts include, among others, the abolishment (or reinstatement) of selective contracting with providers, changes in the authority over capital investments and expansion or contraction of insurance entitlements. The shift can also include (new) restrictions over medical decision-making by practice guidelines and other rules. Furthermore, decision-making power and financial risks can shift between national,

---

[9] "Governance" is another example of a conceptually fuzzy term that traveled from government to the corporate sector, and back again to the public sector (Okma 2002). During this migration, it shed its neutral meaning of administration and took on a normative connotation under the label "good governance" and later, stewardship. In this contribution, we take governance in a neutral sense: (public or private) administration of health services and health insurance.

regional and local governments, or between governments, health insurers, and individual patients and insured.

The main focus of this study is on changes in health insurance and medical care, including prescription drugs and medical aids. The dividing line between medical care and related social services (e.g., long-term care for the elderly or handicapped) is not always clear, and countries have different cultural views of what counts as healthcare. Another limitation of this study is its main focus on health policies aimed to protect family incomes against the financial risks of illness and to improve the organization of healthcare. With this focus, it pays less attention to the wider range of policies that predominantly or exclusively aim to improve the health of the population (e.g., by improving road safety, food quality, consumer protection or lifestyle behaviors).

The study combines analytical categories from economic theory with concepts from political science. The economic terms describe the basic constituent elements of healthcare systems: the financing, contracting and provision of health services (see the Appendix for the explanation of the "house model" of healthcare). According to the OECD (1992, 1994), it is possible to describe any given healthcare system in terms of a country-specific mix of public and private financing, contracting and modes of providing medical services. The major financing sources for healthcare are general taxation (general revenues, earmarked taxes and tax expenditure), public and private insurance, direct patient payments (co-payments, coinsurance, deductibles and uninsured services) and voluntary contributions. For some low-income countries, external aid can be a major source as well.

There are three basic contracting models in healthcare. The first is the integrated model with the financing and ownership of services under the same (public or private) responsibility. The best-known example is the original British NHS of 1948. The NHS provided healthcare for all, largely paid out of general taxation, in state-owned hospitals (and private practices of general practitioners). The second model is the contracting model, where government agencies or other third-party payers (e.g., the administrative agencies of social health insurance or private health insurers) negotiate long-term contracts with healthcare providers (e.g., the annual negotiations between regional German sick funds and representatives of hospitals and medical professionals). The third contracting model, common in private insurance, is that of reimbursement, where the patient first pays his provider and then seeks reimbursement from his insurance.

On the provision side, the ownership and management of health services can be public, private (both for profit and not-for-profit) or—common in most countries—a mix of those.[10] Moreover, as noted earlier, there are country-specific mixes of formal and informal care, traditional and modern medicine and medically related social services.

Obviously, the combination of those three core elements: financing, contracting (including the payment modes) and ownership, largely determines the allocation of financial risks and decision-making power over the main players in healthcare. For example, the risk-rated premiums of private insurance expose low-income families to higher risks than social insurance (particularly as income levels generally correlate with health status: the lower the income, the poorer the health of population groups). Social insurance, with income-related contributions and without exclusions, reduces such financial risks for families. As another example, tax financing and government ownership make for strong government influence whereas private financing (private insurance and direct patient payments) combined with legally independent providers entails stronger decision-making power for both insurers and providers (as in Switzerland or the Netherlands). This is true even while governments can—and often do—impose rules to protect patients or safeguard the quality of and access to healthcare, for example, by requiring insurers to include certain benefits like contraceptive care, mental health or home care in their coverage.

Another analytical approach used in this volume focuses on the changing behavior of the actors in the policy arena: governments, patients,

---

[10] Private provision in Europe generally includes non-government actors, both for-profit and non-profits. In contrast, in North America, the term "private" usually refers to investor-owned providers.

providers, insurers and others. Hirschman (1970), for example, sees two classic mechanisms for consumers to express their dissatisfaction with given arrangements: exit or voice. Exit is the base for consumer sovereignty and plays a crucial role in economic traffic. If consumers do not like the price-quality ratio of a given product (and if there is sufficient competition on the market), they may simply exit and look elsewhere, thus forcing companies (or governments) to adjust and improve the quality of their goods and services. Exit, as an indicator, does not provide management or government with much information as to what is wrong. Customers do not have an interest in improving the product or service, just in finding a better one somewhere else. For many customers—especially in healthcare—exit is costly and difficult to put into practice (healthcare is mostly a local service industry, and most people do not move to another part of the country to get better healthcare). Voice seems to be a better alternative, but it also comes with costs. It requires a critical number of participants to start collective action. Different political regimes allow for different degrees of voice (military dictatorships and authoritarian regimes commonly suppress or eliminate opposing voices altogether). Voice thus can be not only costly but sometimes dangerous. Traditionally, economists assumed that there is a trade-off between choice and exit, but Hirschman also argued that the two mechanisms actually complement each other. He found situations where exit mechanisms worked better when consumers could also express their voice, and vice versa.

The abovementioned economic terms help to characterize certain features of healthcare systems. They do not explain the causes or effects of policy change, however. In trying to understand why countries have embarked on particular reform paths, we have to look not only at the external and internal pressures for change, but also at the structural features of social policy-making that enable politicians and other policy entrepreneurs to change the system.

We therefore borrowed terms from political science serve to analyze the workings of the healthcare system and the behavior of the main actors in the health policy arena: governments, patients and insured, health insurers, healthcare providers and others. Klein and Marmor (2006) argued that

12

the main elements affecting public policy-making fall under three broad headings: ideas, interests and institutions. These terms refer to underlying ideas or beliefs, organized stakeholders in society, and political institutions that shape social policy in all countries.

Douglas and Wildavsky (1982) highlighted three clusters of ideas (or dominant cultural orientations) in welfare states: hierarchical collectivism, competitive individualism and sectarianism. The fiscal and social policy of northwestern European countries proceeds from the fundamental commitment to principles of solidarity and equality. They have collectivist traditions, with strong bureaucracies to implement policy. In some countries, in particular Germany and the Netherlands, those bureaucracies engage in semi-permanent neo-corporatist consultations with organized stakeholders. The United States, in contrast, is often depicted as a more liberal welfare state, with strong emphasis on individual competition, individual rights and responsibilities, weak collectivism and an outspoken streak of sectarianism.

Another set of labels relevant to the interaction between governments and interest groups are the (semi-)pluralist, (semi-)corporatist and exclusionary modes of social policy-making (Labra 2007). While pluralism corresponds with the individualistic orientation, and the corporatist institutions with the hierarchical collectivist tradition, the exclusionary policy mode highlights the power of central government. For example, a military dictatorship or strong centralized state power can exclude certain groups from decision-making in social policy. We will come across examples of all of those orientations and policy styles in this book.

It would be an error, however, to take such orientations as precise representations of particular countries or policy-making styles. General models do not cover countries on a one-to-one basis. Different styles of governance exist side by side, and as we will show, there are—sometimes dramatic—shifts in emphasis from one style to another over time. Another important point to note is that styles of governance are not identical to policy outcomes. Underlying values and dominant orientations do make certain policy outcomes more likely than others, however. Thus, values affect policy; conversely, policies reshape and strengthen values (Marmor et al. 2006). For example, the British NHS and Canada's medicare have become important symbols of solidarity in the United Kingdom and in Canada. In both countries, politicians do not want to be seen undermining the universal coverage.

Theories of historical institutionalism and path dependency (Immergut 1992; Pierson 1994) emphasize that major change in social policy is rare; it only occurs in specific circumstances as institutional legacies and popular support for existing policy arrangements create powerful barriers to change. In fact, this study presents several instances of windows of opportunity for change. Such opportunities occur, according to Kingdon (1984), at the confluence of three, more or less independent streams: the problem stream (a general sense of urgency or feeling that a major problem requires action), the policy stream (the availability of acceptable and feasible policy solutions based on the gradual accumulation of knowledge and perspectives among specialists) and the politics stream (fueled by certain political events such as a change of administration). Policy entrepreneurs, Kingdon adds, are like surfers waiting for the next big wave and the policy window offers them an opportunity to push their pet solutions. Like a wave, the (policy) window of opportunity may disappear, thus timing is important for success in presenting and implementing major policy change.

The Swiss, Israeli and Dutch health policy arenas all reflect, to different degrees, features of neo-corporatist policy-making where governments share the responsibility for social policy with organized interests (Lijphart 1968). New Zealand, in contrast, has a legacy of Westminster politics where the majority party in power can play winner-takes-all politics.

Carolyn Tuohy's book *Remaking Policy* (2018) mentions four types of health reform strategies: blueprint, big bang, mosaic and incremental change. It locates the Dutch reform as a blueprint. In fact, as argued in the chapter about Holland, the Dutch health reforms started out as a blueprint in 1987 but became much more incremental (and incoherent) over time. Likewise, Israel's big bang reforms petered out to become more gradual. New Zealand experimented with new regional models of administration, but also saw a shift from big bang towards more incremental change with the creation of coalition governments in the 1990s, which required more consensual policy-making. The Dutch, Israeli and New Zealand cases also illustrate the difficulty in categorizing or labeling health systems or health policies into fixed categories. Of all the cases of this study, Singapore and Taiwan appear least bound by ideology or labels, preferring a pragmatic approach.

The country chapters in this volume apply combinations of the above economic and public policy approaches to describe and analyze the shaping and outcomes of national health reform experiences.

Main Findings

The case studies of this volume confirm that, indeed—and not surprising for scholars of public policy—national values, institutions and interests all play an important role in the shaping and outcomes of health policy.

The seemingly common experience in external and internal pressures (fiscal pressures, demographic, epidemiological and ideological change), similarity in reform goals (universal access, fairness in distribution of the financial burden, improved efficiency, cost control, consumer choice) and means (changes in public and private financing, regulation, administration) can easily lead to generalized assumptions of (global) convergence (of institutions or policies; see e.g., O'Connor 2007). The health politics and health policies of the 12 nations of this study did not converge in one common direction, however. In fact, the countries' reform directions and processes of implementation diverged extensively. Each nation implemented change within the restraints of existing national institutions, culture and political boundaries. Only a few countries systematically studied experiences abroad in search of new policy directions; but, in many cases, countries borrowed reform concepts from others without much reflection.

The 12 cases reveal a remarkable variety of reform activity, ranging from efforts to develop universal coverage in the African nations and in Ecuador, adjustments of the public–private mix of health insurance in Chile, new procedures to assess the social insurance entitlements of Israel, changes in the regional governance models in New Zealand, quasi-privatized schemes in Switzerland and the Netherlands, a complex mix of insurance schemes and individual savings schemes in Singapore and the implementation of nation-wide social health insurance in Taiwan.

The speed of change in the health reform processes varied as well. In some countries, notably in New Zealand, Singapore and Taiwan, governments were able to implement major change relatively rapidly. Others, facing strong opposition from organized stakeholders, had to adjust, delay or even abandon part or all of their reform efforts. The introduction of market competition commonly went hand-in-hand with increased government control.

One important finding concerned the level of analysis. The last two decades have seen a proliferation of studies that aimed to group countries into certain categories. For example, Esping-Anderson's widely quoted book *Three Worlds of Welfare* (1990) distinguishes three categories of welfare states: the liberal welfare state, with frugal levels of income protection and means-tested, targeted services (e.g., the United Kingdom and the United States); the social democratic state, with high levels of income protection and tight central control (e.g., the Scandinavian countries); and the functionally decentralized consensual, corporatist state (e.g., Germany and the Netherlands). The latter refers to countries where governments share the responsibility for social policy with organized interests.

Such categorization assumes that the ideal models share features that determine certain patterns of policy-making and help explain developments and outcomes of their social policy. Over time, however, systems have changed shape, borrowed from others, and become hybridized, by combining Bismarckian employment-based income protection schemes with population-wide arrangements. In some areas (most notably, pensions and healthcare), states have commonly assumed more responsibility for income protection than in other areas (such as housing or education). With such hybridization, efforts to group countries in pre-set categories have become problematic (Goodin et al. 1999).

At the level of specific programs and policies rather than at the national level, however, we saw more similarity across nations. For example, several countries with public financing experimented with the separation of the provision from healthcare financing. Almost everywhere there have been shifts in payment for medical care in hospitals, for example, from general budgets based on historic costs to per diem and then, to case-based payments. Many countries are moving towards mixed payment models for independent practitioners that combine fees for service with some form of capitation, specific payment for certain services, and in some cases, pay for performance. Importantly, almost everywhere, purchaser–provider splits and efforts to change payment methods took (much) more time than originally envisioned (and often failed to bring the hoped-for efficiency gains).

Despite the market rhetoric and stated policy to reduce the role of the state in healthcare, governments continued to use their budget control powers to restrain healthcare expenditure almost everywhere. Governments commonly softened the effects of market competition by imposing restrictions on healthcare insurers and providers. In a way, the experience has been one of bounded privatization: while shifting risks and decision-making power to non-state actors, governments kept their regulatory role by mandating certain entitlements in the coverage of private health insurance, for example, or forcing private insurance to accept everyone seeking insurance, or imposing national fee schedules for health services and quality norms for both publicly and privately funded healthcare.

As noted earlier, this book presents the country chapters by region. It starts with the two African nations, Ghana and Tanzania, followed by two countries from Latin America, Chile and Ecuador. Then it moves to the European Continent with two examples from Western Europe, the Netherlands and Switzerland, followed by three cases from Eastern Europe and the Middle East: the Czech Republic, Slovenia and Israel. The last regional chapter includes New Zealand, Singapore and Taiwan. This book thus starts with countries that, as we found, are not often included in international comparative studies—if only because they are not covered by the OECD database. As the reader will see, however, there are surprising commonalities in the experience of the framing and implementation of health reforms across the globe, even while we found little or no common convergence of the overall health reforms.

References

De Swaan, A. 1988. *In Care of The State: Health Care, Education and Welfare in Europe and the USA in the Modern Age.* Oxford: Unity Press.

Douglas, M. and A. Wildavsky. 1982. *Risk and Culture.* Berkeley: University of California Press.

Esping-Anderson, G. 1990. *The Three Worlds of Welfare Capitalism.* Cambridge: Polity Press.

Goodin, R., B. Heady, R. Muffels, and H-J. Dirven. 1999. *The Real Worlds of Welfare Capitalism.* Cambridge: Cambridge University Press.

Herzlinger, R.E. and R. Parsa-Parsi. 2004. "Consumer-driven health care: lessons from Switzerland." *JAMA,* 292(10): 1213–1220.

Hirschman, A.O. 1970. *Exit, Voice and Loyalty. Responses to Decline in Firms, Organizations, and States.* Cambridge: Harvard University Press.

Kingdon, J.W. 1984. *Agendas, Alternatives, and Public Policies.* New York: Longman.

Klein, R. 2006. *The New Politics of the NHS* (5th ed.). Harlow, UK: Longman Group.

Klein, R. February 23–25, 1995. *Learning from Others: Shall the Last Be the First Markets? Four Country Conference on Healthcare Reforms and Healthcare Policies in the United States, Canada, Germany and the Netherlands.* Rijswijk: Ministry of Health, Welfare and Sport.

Klein, R. and T.R. Marmor. 2006. "Reflections on Policy Analysis: Putting It Together Again." *The Oxford Handbook of Political Science.* R. Goodin (ed.). Oxford: Oxford University Press: 982–912.

Labra, M.E. 2007. "Modes of Health Policy Making and Medical Interests in Chile in the 20th Century. Updated English version of Labra, M.E. 2000." "Padrões de Formulação de Políticas de Saúde no Chile no Século XX." *DADOS-Revista de Ciências Sociais,* 43(1): 153–182.

Lasswell, H. 1936. *Politics: Who Gets What, When, How* (2nd ed.). Cleveland: World Publishing.

Leu, R.E., F.H. Rutten, W. Brouwer, et al. January 16, 2009. "The Swiss and Dutch Health Insurance Systems: Universal Coverage and Regulated Competetive Insurance Markets." *Health Policy, Health Reference and*

Perform Improvement (Vol. 104). Washington, DC: The Commonwealth Fund.

Lijphart, A. 1968. *Verzuiling, pacificatie en kentering in de Nederlandse politiek* [Pillarization, Pacification and Change in Dutch Politics]. Amsterdam: J.H. de Bussy.

Marmor, T.R., K.G.H. Okma, and S.R. Lathan. 2006. "Values, Institutions and Health Politics. Comparative Perspectives." *Soziologie der Gesundheit. Koelner Zeitschrift fur Soziologie und Sozialpsychologie,* 46: 383–405.

Marmor, T.R., R. Freeman, and K.G.H. Okma. 2003. "Comparative perspectives and policy learning in the world of healthcare." *J Compar Policy Anal,* 7(4): 331–348.

O'Connor, J. 2007. "Convergence of European Welfare States: Convergence of What?" *Investigating Welfare State Change. The 'Dependent Variable Problem' in Comparative Analysis.* J. Clasen and N.A. Siegel (eds.). Cheltenham, UK: Edward Elger.

OECD. 1992. *The Reform of Health Care, A Comparative Analysis of Seven OECD Countries.* Health Reform Studies (2). Paris: Organisation for Economic Co-Operation and Development.

OECD. 1994. *The Reform of Health Care, a Review of Seventeen OECD Countries, Health Reform Studies No. 5.* Paris: Organisation for Economic Co-Operation and Development.

Okma, K.G.H. May 2002. "What is the best public-private model for Canadian healthcare?" *Policy Matters,* 3(6), Montreal: Canadian Institute for Research on Public Policy.

Okma, K.G.H. and L. Crivelli. 2010. *Six Countries, Six Reform Models: The Healthcare Reform Experience of Israel, the Netherlands, New Zealand, Singapore, Switzerland and Taiwan.* Singapore: World Scientific.

Pierson, P. 1994. *Dismantling the Welfare State? Reagan, Thatcher and the Politics of Retrenchment.* Cambridge: Cambridge University Press.

Reinhardt, U.E. 2004. "The Swiss health system: regulated competition without managed care." *JAMA* 292(10): 1277–1231.

Rose, R. 1993. *Lesson-Drawing in Public Policy. A Guide to Learning across Time and Space.* Chatham, NJ: Chatham House Publishers.

Timmins, N. 1995. *The Five Giants, a Biography of the Welfare State*. London: Fontana Press.

Tuohy, C.H. 2018. *Remaking Policy. Scale, Pace and Strategy in Healthcare Reforms*. Toronto: University of Toronto Press.

Wilensky, H.L. 2002. *Rich Democracies, Political Economy, Public Policy, and Performance*. Berkeley: University of California Press.

Section I

Healthcare Reforms in Africa: Ghana and Tanzania

This regional section discusses the health reforms of two sub-Saharan nations: Ghana and Tanzania, located respectively on the west and east coasts of the continent. The section also contains maps that present some core data on population, income level, health spending and health status of the populations. Those data are based on the Appendix of this volume.

Many African nations still bear traces of their colonial legacies: national borders crosscutting traditional tribal areas, economies largely based on primary commodities, a small formal employment sector and weak fiscal and administrative capacities resulting in low tax revenues. Many countries also face the double burden of high population growth and epidemiological transitions, which result in the combination of high levels of "old" diseases (e.g., malaria, river blindness and tuberculosis) and "new" ones (obesity, diabetes and other chronic illness). Most nations are still young, gaining independence only after the 1960s. They commonly feature unstable political regimes, widespread fraud, corruption and a lack of civic society organizations. These features all create barriers for the development of nation-wide health insurance, which require trust, administrative experience, a stable fiscal environment, and active support from stakeholders. Some of the poorest African countries depend heavily on foreign aid for specific health programs. Such external financing often resulted in silos, or fragmentation into disease-specific programs, and undue external interference in the shaping of domestic health policy.

Despite those legacies, many sub-Saharan African countries have made substantial progress in terms of education levels, income and the health of their populations. Infant and maternal mortality dropped by more than 20 percent in 18 countries, and average life expectancy increased by at least five years in 10 cases between 1990 and 2007. At the same time, the HIV/AIDS epidemic, among other contagious diseases and manmade disasters, caused a drop in average life expectancy in other sub-Saharan nations.

In many African nations, at the time of post-colonial independence, healthcare was free for all, financed out of general taxation—at least on paper. However, low tax revenues resulted in chronic underfunding, poor quality of services and a lack of basic facilities, essential medicines and qualified staff. Another common feature was the dominant emphasis of hospital-based medical care in urban areas over primary services for rural populations. This meant that many people did not have access to modern medical care and remained dependent on traditional healers and out-of-pocket payments.

By the late 20th century, in an effort to diversify healthcare financing away from government taxes, both governments and non-government organizations initiated new forms of local community-based insurance, often with the financial support of external donor organizations. The experience with those local schemes later served as a base for developing proposals for population-wide health insurance. At first, international organizations like the World Bank were hesitant to support these efforts, but the debate over the Millennium Development Goals fueled interest in the loftier ambition of population-wide universal health coverage (UHC).

The experiences of Ghana and Tanzania illustrate the challenges in realizing this policy goal. These trials are not unique to the African continent; as we will see in this volume, countries in Latin America and Eastern Europe have faced similar issues when they sought to (re-)establish healthcare financing arrangements that safeguard universal access for their population without undue financial barriers.

Map 1. Africa Ghana and Tanzania: Population, Income per Capita and Health Expenditure, 1960–2015.

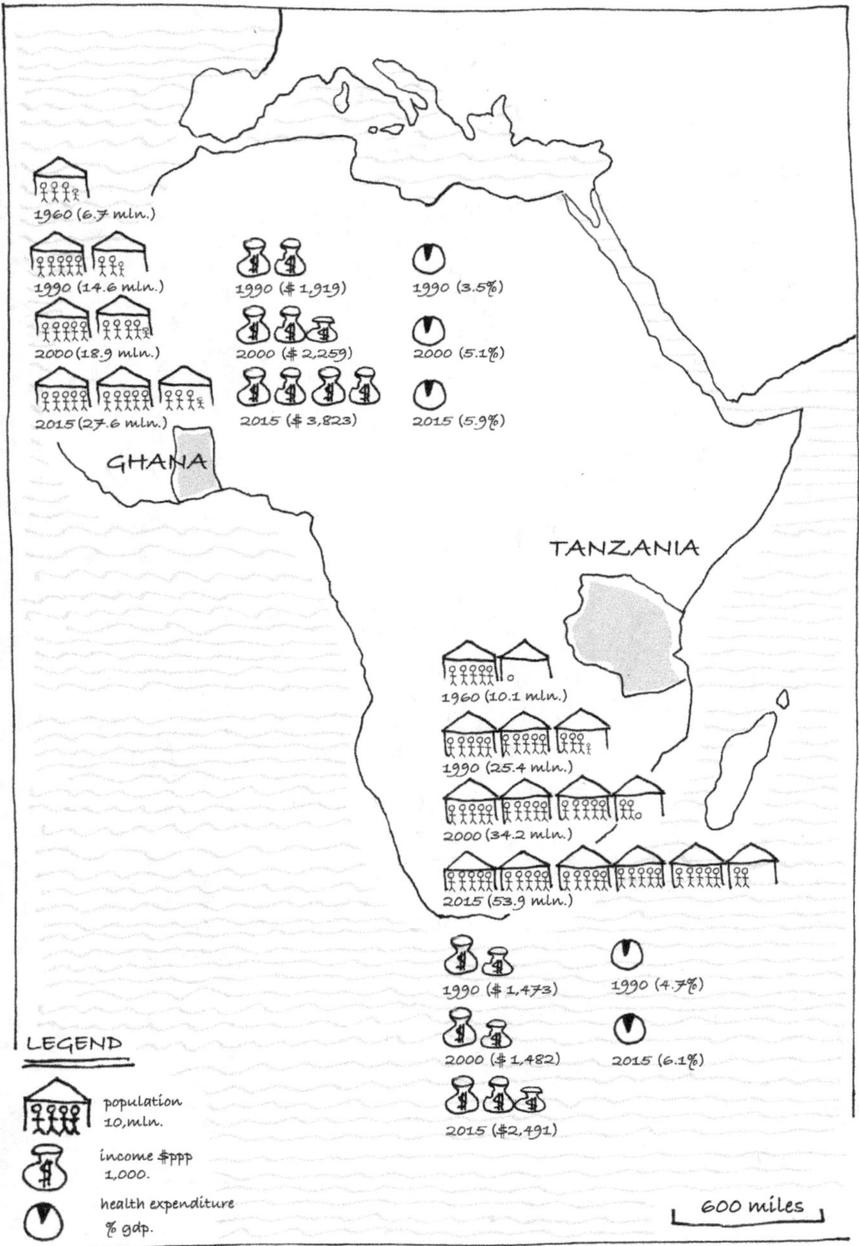

Map 2.   Africa Ghana and Tanzania: Physicians, Infant Mortality and Life Expectancy.

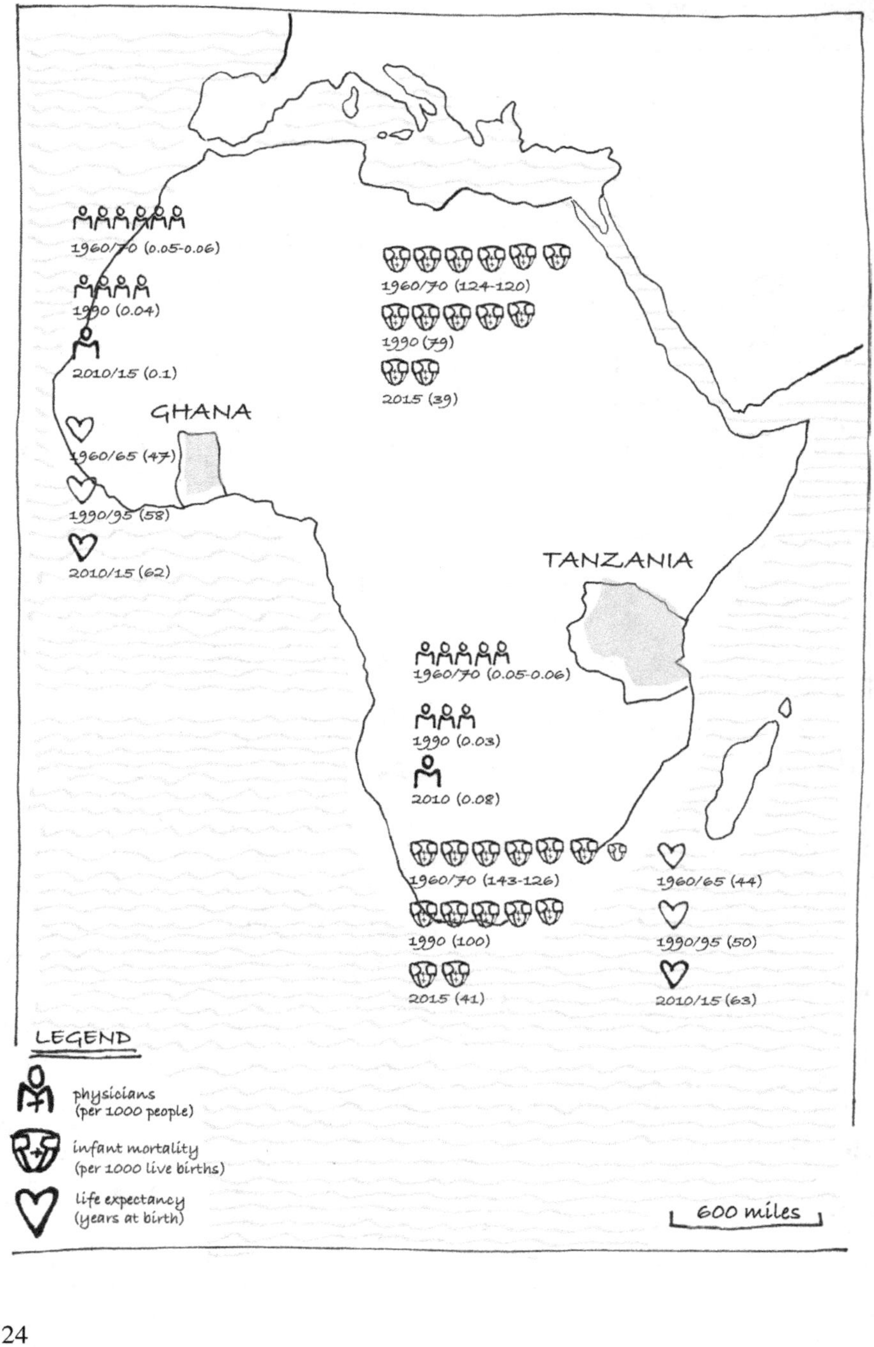

Chapter 1

Healthcare Financing Reforms: Ghana's National Health Insurance

Adam Fusheini

Introduction

This chapter examines the evolution and development of health policy and healthcare reforms in Ghana over the last two decades with a focus on the National Health Insurance (NHI).[1] The NHI was adopted in 2003 with the passage of Act 650 by Parliament (later replaced by Act 852 of 2012). The overall goal of the NHI was to achieve universal health coverage (UHC) within five years of implementation. The NHI aimed to make healthcare affordable to all by removing out-of-pocket payment at the point of service, and to achieve equity of access based on patients' needs rather than ability to pay (Agyepong and Adjei 2008; Witter and Garshong 2009; Sakyi et al. 2012; Fusheini 2016).

The chapter begins with a brief profile of Ghana. It then explores the key details of Ghana's health system including the NHI, the historical development of the healthcare system since Ghana's independence in 1957 and the factors and processes that led to the adoption of the NHI in 2003. Then it addresses the implementation, challenges and further developments of the NHI and ends with a conclusion. In sum, the chapter illustrates how the need for change arose, and how this got pushed through the

---

[1]The NHI also goes under the name National Health Insurance Scheme (NHIS). In this chapter, we will use the term NHI.

25

policy, politics and bureaucratic lacunae. In doing so, we show that Ghana's health system development and reform trajectory is not so much "the product of one, logical policy-making experience" but rather "the manifestations of many years of historical developments" (Katuu 2018; Mayes 2004).

Brief Profile of Ghana

The Republic of Ghana is located centrally on the West African coast (see the following map). Ghana's neighbors are three French-speaking countries: Togo to the east, Burkina Faso to the north and northwest, and Côte d'Ivoire to the west. The Gulf of Guinea on the south forms a coastline extending 350 miles (Fusheini 2013).

Ghana was the first sub-Saharan African nation to gain independence from Britain in 1957. Ghana is a lower middle-income country (LMIC), with a population of about 29.6 million in 2018 (World Bank 2018b). The gross domestic product (GDP) was approximately $47.3 billion or $1,640 per person in 2017 (World Bank 2018c). The proportion of the population defined as poor was about 24 percent in 2012 (Kotoh et al. 2018; GSS 2014), or 7 million people. The economic growth rate was estimated at 8.1 percent in 2017 (Myjoyonline 2018). Total health spending was about 5.9 percent of GDP, almost $80 per capita in 2015 (WorldBank 2018a, b, c).

Ghana is a unitary constitutional Republic with a multi-party democracy and a hybrid presidential system.[2] The government includes an executive president elected for four years with a maximum of two terms, a Parliament elected every four years and an independent judiciary branch. There is also a vibrant private media. The unitary constitutional Republic has 10 administrative regions: Western, Central, Greater Accra, Volta, Eastern, Ashanti, Brong Ahafo, Northern, Upper East and Upper West. The referendum of December 2018 approved the creation of six additional

---

[2]The system is a hybrid as it blends the American presidential with the British parliamentary system. The president is popularly elected but half of the ministers come from the Parliament, a feature of the British system.

regions. The regions are further subdivided into 170 districts (local government areas). The districts are responsible for implementing resource allocation and administration of national policies on a local level. This includes 170 districts with health directorates or management teams.

The Republic of Ghana, Administrative Divisions, 2010.

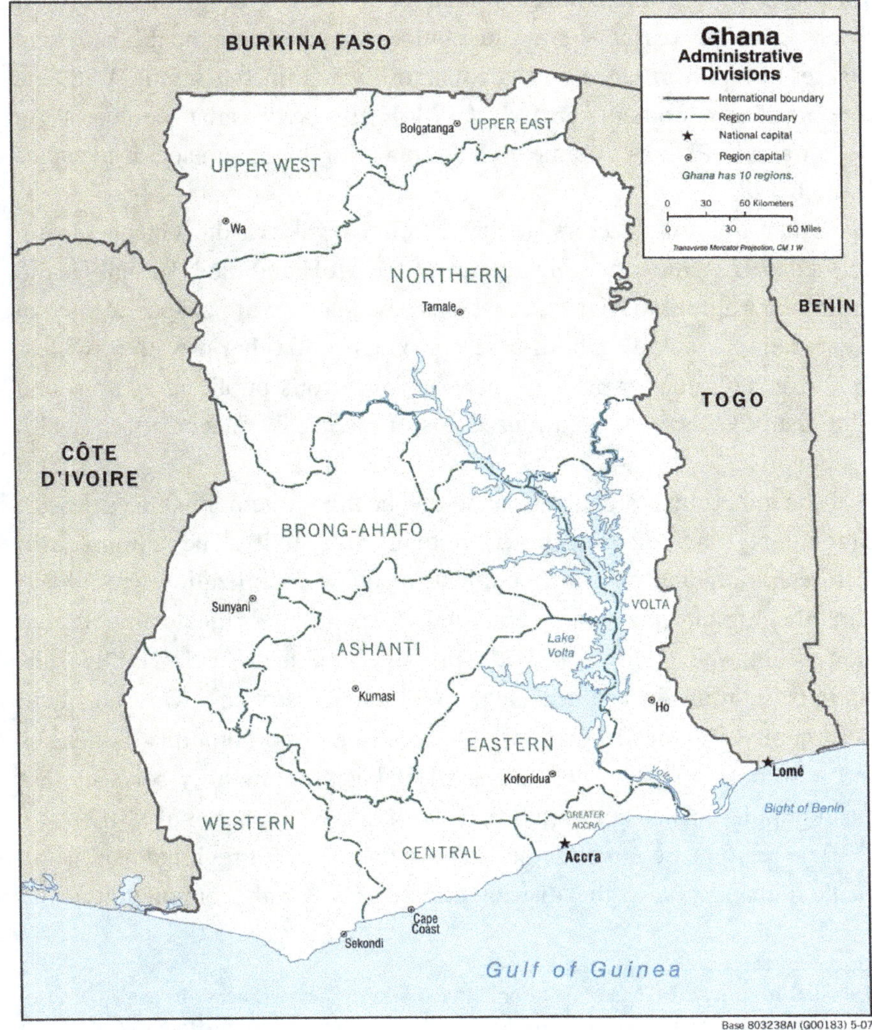

Source: Cartoko 2010.

Key Features of Ghana's Health System

Ghana's healthcare features a three-level (national, regional and district) administrative architecture.[3] At the national level, the Ministry of Health (MoH) is in charge of sector-wide policy development, as well as financing, regulation, monitoring and evaluation. It provides overall policy directions, institutional development, coordination of the activities of other agencies, partners and stakeholders involved in healthcare, and ensures the performance and accountability within the sector. With the support of development partners, the MoH also devises the Medium Term Development Plan as a framework for planning by health sector agencies and others.

Other important actors at the national level are the Ghana Health Service (GHS), the executing agency of the MoH and the National Health Insurance Authority (NHIA), as well as a wide range of non-governmental organizations, including faith-based providers and other private providers (both for- and not-for-profit). There are numerous public regulatory and administrative entities at various levels of the highly decentralized health system.

The functional organization of the health system is at five levels: national, regional, district, sub-district and community. The national level features policy and plan development, resource mobilization and allocation; the regions provide operational oversight, technical support and monitoring; the districts provide primary healthcare (PHC); the sub-districts administer health centers and clinic services while resident Community Health Officers (CHOs) assisted by community structures and a volunteer system are in charge of basic community services that reach populations of between 3,000 and 4,500 (Schieber et al. 2012).

The regional health directorates have oversight for regional health and medical matters, and the district directorates for the organization and

---

[3] Detailed histories of Ghana health policy and service development are available elsewhere (see e.g., Aikins and Koram 2017; Arhinful 2003; Van den Boom et al. 2008; Kuganab-Lem 2007).

delivery of PHC. Regional health management teams (RHMTs) take charge of strategy translation, and oversight over district teams and the provision of secondary services, while district teams (DHMTs) are responsible for providing PHC, first referral and community-level services. While health policy-making, planning and provision are largely decentralized, the MoH and the GHS still have a great deal of authority (Vecchione and Parkhurst 2016).

Financing Healthcare in Ghana

The government and its development partners, as well as Ghanaian households are the major healthcare finance sources. The main revenues of the MoH are public budget transfers. The revenues of the NHIA consist of contributions for the NHI and special levies on pension payments into the Social Security and National Insurance Trust (SSNIT). Ghana's development partners support the MoH, NHIA and individual health facilities through grants, technical assistance and concessional and commercial loans. Household contributions (apart from taxation) include NHI contributions and out-of-pocket spending (OOPS) at the point of care (Wang et al. 2017). The public revenues include the health budget allocation, targeted revenues for NHI and local government revenues. The NHI was established as the pivotal financing channel for the health sector (RVO.nl 2015). The NHIA administers the National Health Insurance Fund (NHIF). NHIF's revenues consist of a mix of tax subsidy, members' contributions and other income (GoG 2012; Fusheini et al. 2017b; Osei-Akoto and Adamba 2017; Carbone 2011):

— A health insurance levy of 2.5 percent on top of the existing value-added tax (VAT) on goods and services
— 2.5 percent of the formal sector workers' 18.5 percent contribution towards retirement benefits to the Social Security and Pension Scheme Fund, taken from the SSNIT
— Annual NHI payments by informal sector workers (non-contributors to the Pension Fund);

— Parliamentary allocations to the NHIF
— Investment income of the NHIF
— Grants, donations, gifts and any other voluntary contributions to the NHIF
— Fees charged by the NHIA in the performance of its functions
— Money accruing under section 198 of the Insurance Act of 2006.

Informal sector workers and formal sector employees who do not contribute to SSNIT have to pay between GH¢22 and GH¢48 (about $5 to $10) each year. In practice, however, everybody pays the minimum amount (Kotoh et al. 2018). Many insured are exempt from paying: people classified as poor or indigent; adults over 70 and children under 18; contributors to the SSNIT and its pensioners. Other exemptions apply to women in need of prenatal, childbirth and postpartum care; people with mental disorders; and persons categorized as physically or mentally disabled or in need of social welfare support (GoG 2012; Osei-Akoto and Adamba 2017).

The main revenue sources of the NHI consisted of health insurance levies (61.0 percent); investment income (17.0 percent); SSNIT contributions (15.6 percent); premium payments (3.8 percent); budget support (2.3 percent) and other income (0.2 percent) in 2009 (NHIA 2009). This mix reflected the combined features of a classical social health insurance (SHI) and a tax-based system (Witter and Garshong 2009; Carbone 2011).

Total spending of the NHIF went up from GH¢3.3 billion ($680.6 million), or about 6.4 percent of GDP, when the NHIS began operation in 2005, to GH¢4.7 billion ($964.7 million) in 2010—a 42-percent increase (GoG 2015). This change was, however, not reflected in total health expenditure as a percentage of GDP due to the rebasing of the GDP in 2006. Thus, the increment in the size of the national economy did not match that of health expenditure (GoG 2013). Table 1 presents more detailed data on the changing composition of health expenditure between 2005 and 2015.

Table 1 shows how total health spending, as a share of GDP, rose from 6.3 to 6.5 between 2005 and 2010, but declined to 5.9 in 2015. The share

Table 1. Financing Ghana's Healthcare, 2005–2015

Health Financing	2005	2010	2015
Current health expenditure (CHE) as a share of GDP (percent)	6.3	6.5	5.9
CHE per capita ($)	51.2	85.5	79.6
CHE per capita ($ PPP)	232.6	195.4	249.3
Government health expenditure (GGHE-D) as a share of CHE (percent)	30.0	39.9	34.9
Private health expenditure (PVT-D) as a share of CHE (percent)	55.7	49.8	39.5
External health expenditure (EXT) as share of CHE (percent)	14.3	10.2	25.6
GGHE-D as a share of general government expenditure (GGE; percent)	10.0	10.1	7.1
GGHE-D per capita in ($)	15.4	34.2	27.8
GGHE-D per capita ($ PPP)	69.8	78.0	87.1
PVT-D per capita ($)	28.6	42.6	31.4
PVT-D per capita ($ PPP)	129.6	97.4	98.4
EXT per capita ($)	7.3	8.7	20.4
EXT per capita ($ PPP)	33.2	20.0	63.8
Out-of-pocket expenditure (OOPs) as share of CHE (percent)	49.8	43.9	36.1
Out-of-pocket expenditure (OOPs) per capita ($)	25.5	37.6	28.7
Out-of-pocket expenditure (OOPs) per capita ($ PPP)	115.7	85.8	90.0

Source: WHO/AFRO 2018.

of public funding increased between 2005 and 2010, but then dropped again slightly. Out-of-pocket spending as a share of CHE has decreased since 2005, since the implementation of the NHI. EXT went up sharply, even while Ghana became a LMIC with less access to external donor finance. The economic challenges that also affected the NHI, however, required more foreign aid to sustain any gains made.

Provision of Healthcare Services

Ghana's pluralistic healthcare includes a mixture of public, private, non-governmental and traditional medicine. Since independence, the missionary or faith-based providers have remained the second largest provider of healthcare services after the public sector (Aikins and Koram 2017). Other providers include Islamic, quasi-governmental and private organizations (Aikins and Koram 2017). Traditional medicine, which preceded the establishment of biomedical facilities in the colonial era, has grown in numerical and symbolic strength (ibidem). The Traditional Medicine Practice Act (Act 575) of 2000 offered traditional medicine greater recognition and access to public finance. That expanded its role, particularly in rural and underserved areas, supported by policy guidelines.

NHI insured have access to public, faith-based, quasi-governmental and some private health facilities, as well as pharmacies and chemists accredited by and under contract with the NHIA (Kotoh et al. 2018). The benefits package of the NHI covers 95 percent of common treatments to all members and private insured, with no limits on consumption (Mensah et al. 2010; Bagnoli 2017). The benefits include outpatient and inpatient care, maternity care, oral health, eye care, diagnostic tests, generic drugs and emergency care (Teye et al. 2015; GoG 2012). There are over 4,000 public and private healthcare providers. These include community-based clinics and health centers, dental clinics, physiotherapy and diagnostic centers, eye clinics, laboratories, childbirth clinics, pharmacies, polyclinics, as well as primary, secondary and tertiary hospitals (NHIA 2018). Healthcare providers must obtain NHIA accreditation and licensing in order to provide a specified set of services and get reimbursement from the NHI.

Current provider payment mechanisms include itemized fee-for-service (FFS) for medicine for both insured and non-insured patients and case-based (diagnosis-related groupings, diagnostic-related group [DRG]) payment. Providers send their list of activities to the NHIA with a request for reimbursement (Agyepong and Nagai 2011; Agyei-Baffour et al. 2013). The DRG payments apply to all levels, from primary care up to the tertiary (teaching) hospitals (NHIS 2018). With support from the World Bank, capitation payment was piloted in Kumasi in 2013 as the payment method for first-line outpatient care. The capitation payment covers a standardized base package of services, reasonably accessible to every Ghanaian, in both urban and rural areas across the country (NHIS 2018). The defined package will be subject to regular review and if necessary, modification. Presently, the standard per capita amount translates to GH¢21 (about $5) per annum for all subscribers enrolled with a preferred primary provider (NHIS 2018).

Healthcare and Health Insurance Administration

A 13-member board oversees the operations of the NHI and NHIF. The NHIA functions as the central insurer. It provides NHI cards, accredits healthcare providers, negotiates benefit packages, sets fees, ensures quality service and reimburses providers (Kotoh et al. 2018). The NHIS Board regulates the health insurance market and monitors service providers (Fusheini et al. 2017b). The NHIA is the implementing agency of the NHIS board and provides administrative support.

The NHIA also supervises the district health insurance schemes (DHISs), but their day-to-day administration is decentralized to district offices. The NHIA established regional offices in each of the 10 regions of the country to oversee the district offices. This central control over the district offices implied a move away from the decentralized system. It enabled tighter central fiscal control over lower-level purchasing of staff and services, and to some extent it also distanced the services from the District Assemblies or local government (Agyepong et al. 2016).

Furthermore, the NHIA regulates contributions and registration fees. Health facilities have to submit quarterly reports to the NHIA, and DHISs submit annual reports to the NHIA for auditing (Kotoh et al. 2018). In collaboration with service providers, the NHIA also developed essential medicine lists to guide service provision; lastly, it sets the healthcare tariffs and reviews these with providers from time to time.

The NHIA set up health complaint committees or units in every district office to monitor the quality of services and proper handling of conflicts and complaints. This is to provide members with a voice in NHIS operations. Accountability and reporting lines are hierarchical, with district managers reporting to regions, which in turn report to the national level, but there is some overlap and blurred lines of responsibility in this reporting and communication matrix, as districts sometimes bypass regions.

Historical Developments of Ghana's Healthcare— From Independence to 1985

The Post-Independence Socialist Experiment

Following independence in 1957, the Nkrumah government sought to extend health services to the majority of the population. It abolished fees for curative services (which dated back to the 1880s; see e.g., GoG 2015) to ensure free healthcare for all, funded through general taxes and donor support (Nyonator and Kutzin 1999; Adisah-Atta 2017). It expanded healthcare and social services substantially (Carbone 2011) and shifted the focus from hospital-based curative care to preventive and community-based healthcare. Socialist, Marxists-Leninist, leftist, nationalist and Pan-Africanist ideologies all heavily influenced the Nkrumah government. The financing of free healthcare out of general taxation funding, along with similar initiatives in education and social development took its toll on the economy, however (Aikins and Koram 2017). Ghana soon found herself struggling to sustain the newly created national health system (Carbone 2011). Shortfalls in revenues weakened public services. The country's economic conditions gradually worsened in tandem with the functioning and quality of public healthcare (Van den Boom et al. 2008). By the mid-1960s, it was clear that the free healthcare approach was not sustainable.

From Full Government Financing to "Cash and Carry"

It did not take long before the post-Nkrumah governments initiated spending cuts and reintroduced co-payments for hospital care with the Hospitals

Fees Decrees of 1969, 1970 and 1971. At first, governments tried to keep the user fees low, mostly aimed to discourage unnecessary use. Meanwhile, the country plunged deeper into economic crisis, which also affected healthcare (Carbone 2011). Import restrictions, for instance, led to restrictions in the procurement of medical equipment (Aikins and Koram 2017; Arhinful 2003). By the early 1980s, there was a dramatic dearth of prescription drugs and other healthcare resources. The public health system was hardly capable of delivering any efficient services (Carbone 2011). Restoring the healthcare system became a priority for policy advocates and other civil society organizations. Successive governments appointed commissions to review possible interventions and policies between 1969 and the early 1980s (Aikins and Koram 2017).

Finally, the Provisional National Defense Council (PNDC) government of Jerry John Rawlings accepted the adjustment policies and programs urged by the World Bank and the IMF. The international agencies pressed the government to cut public spending on social services and healthcare even further. The Hospital Fees Regulation of 1985 aimed to recover 15 percent of recurrent health costs by substantially increasing the level of user fees (Agyepong and Adjei 2008; Carbone 2011). The measure infamously became known as "cash and carry," forcing patients to pay upfront for treatment at public health facilities.

The cash and carry system embodied some exemptions, for example, immunizations and infectious diseases like leprosy and tuberculosis. Pregnant women and people older than 70 years did not have to pay. The MoH extended the exemptions to indigent and poor patients. However, a major challenge was assessing who the indigents were (Atim et al. 2001; Carbone 2011). The difficulty in identifying indigents exposed the state's weak capacity to target social services (an issue not unique to Ghana). In fact, this resulted in virtually every user paying for public health services at the point of use (Carbone 2011; Aryeetey and Goldstein 2000; Atim et al. 2001; Sulzbach et al. 2005).

The consequences of the cash and carry were manifold, including low levels of health services utilization, particularly in rural communities (Waddington and Enyimayew 1989; 1990) and delays in sick patients seeking healthcare, often with grave consequences (Shaw and Griffin 1995; Oppong 2001; Mensah et al. 2010). Some patients were sharing prescription drugs among household members (Asenso-Okyere et al. 1997) and others resorted to alternative treatment from traditional medicine, healing and prayers. Access to formal healthcare was severely limited, ultimately resulting in dramatic increases in mortality rates for infectious and parasitic diseases (Quaye 1991). There was glaring evidence that the poorest population groups suffered more under the cash and carry system than richer ones. Between the late 1980s and early 1990s, the country's poorest quintile received about 11 percent of government health spending, whereas the top quintile received over 30 percent (Aryeetey and Goldstein 2000; Carbone 2011). Middle-class families were far from happy with the existing system either, as they struggled to provide for the health of their extended families (Carbone 2011).

Historical Developments from 1985 to the Adoption of the NHI in 2003

While the cash and carry policy led to improved supply of essential medicines and some other goods, other issues remained unsolved. Ineffective regulation, inconsistent implementation and widening inequities in access to essential clinical services were among the major problems (Waddington and Enyimayew 1989; 1990; Nyonator and Kutzin 1999; Blanchet et al. 2012; Agyepong and Adjei 2008). The widening inequities in access to health services and low utilization elicited two responses: non-governmental and governmental. The core challenge was to provide equitable and affordable healthcare access to all of Ghana's residents. Health financing and governance were closely interlinked in the reform efforts (Aikins and Koram 2017).

Response by Non-Government Actors

The widespread dissatisfaction with cash and carry, coupled with the lack of access to health services for the poor and other vulnerable groups prompted social organizations to find solutions. The neo-liberal economic policies adopted in the mid-1980s had opened up the idea of new players taking an active role in health financing and delivery. The response from civil society organizations came in the form of community-based mutual health organizations (MHOs) and insurance schemes.

Christian missionary organizations, in particular the Christian Health Association of Ghana (CHAG), championed the establishment of community-based insurance schemes in poor, underserved and disadvantaged areas in the late 1980s and early 1990s (Saleh 2013). St. Theresa's Catholic Mission Hospital established Ghana's first community-based health insurance scheme (CHIS) in Nkoranza in the Brong Ahafo region in 1992. The popularity of this scheme led to the emergence of several other CHISs under the label of MHOs, with a variety of target populations based on criteria such as occupation, religion and gender (IMANI 2017; Ramachandra and Hsiao 2007; Atim et al. 2001). With financial support from the US Agency for International Development (USAID) and Danish International Development Agency (DANIDA), and under MoH leadership, MHOs saw a rapid and exponential growth: from an initial 4 to 168 between 1999 and 2003 (Atim et al. 2001; Carbone 2011; Sulzbach et al. 2005). USAID and DANIDA were also instrumental in developing training manuals for MHO administrators and governing bodies (Atim 2000; Agyepong and Adjei 2008).

Other donor organizations showed interest as well, and several other sub-Saharan African nations experimented with similar schemes (see, e.g., the chapter on Tanzania in this volume). Compared with other countries, membership in Ghanaian plans appeared rather high, on average over 6,000 insured per MHO. The range of their services remained limited, however, and MHOs only covered about 2 percent of the population by 2003 (Sulzbach et al. 2005). The experience with MHOs became an important element in the agenda-setting process for Ghana's NHI a decade later.

NHI Policy Development

The second response to low utilization and access challenges was from the state. The MoH contracted national and international experts to frame recommendations for a NHI, including the International Labor Organization (ILO), the World Health Organization (WHO), the European Union (EU) and the London School of Hygiene and Tropical Medicine (LSHTM); (Atim et al. 2001). The report of a private consulting group advocated for one mandatory NHI under a central administration for contributors to SSNIT and all registered cocoa farmers (Atim et al. 2001). In parallel, for informal sector workers in rural areas, the report proposed pilot projects with community-financed schemes. The proposal thus entailed a hybrid of classical SHI and tax-financed healthcare. This would ultimately form the basis for the NHI. Key design features were (1) inclusion of non-profit and for-profit healthcare providers; (2) reimbursement of healthcare providers by capitation; (3) contribution rates equivalent to 5 percent of salary for formal sector employees and a fixed levy per ton of cocoa produced for farmers (equivalent to 7.2 percent of the producer price); and (4) registration of all insured with a single preferred provider (Atim et al. 2001).

The MoH created a special unit to administer the implementation of the NHI and to replace the cash and carry system (Agyepong and Adjei 2008). It launched a pilot project for the NHI in the Eastern region in 1997, covering four districts. The pilot had earlier roots in MoH discussions from the mid-1980s when the issue had first been tabled after user fees became more substantial (Agyepong and Adjei 2008; Carbone 2011; Atim et al. 2001; Asenso-Okyere 1995). Lack of consensus within the Ministry on the best financing strategy and particularly over the question of whether government itself should directly run an insurance scheme, stalled the project (Carbone 2011). Other factors contributing to the failure were lack of leadership and underestimation of the difficulties of implementing a centralized SHI in a low-income developing country (Agyepong and Adjei 2008; Atim et al. 2001; Arhinful 2003).

Despite earlier setbacks, the MoH once more examined insurance schemes in 1999. This time it opted for a multi-scheme approach. The Ministry itself would retain a role as "a promoter and facilitator, not an implementer" (Atim et al. 2001; Carbone 2011). This time other actors, in addition to the government, recognized the need to reform healthcare financing and organization in order to address the crisis in access, financing and utilization of services. The SSNIT, the national pension and social security agency, started planning for a centralized insurance scheme to be run by a company called the Ghana Health Care Company (Agyepong and Adjei 2008). This attempt, however, like the earlier pilot experiment, failed to materialize.

Notwithstanding the failure to establish a national insurance scheme, there were some positive outcomes. In the first place, the pilot projects had increased general awareness about alternative health financing options. Secondly, it led to greater appreciation of the issues related to establishing a national scheme, and the need to tap into native wisdom and creativity in the search for sustainable healthcare financing mechanisms. Thirdly, it underlined the need to develop policies that genuinely reflected the communities' needs and aspirations (Atim et al. 2001). In fact, the 2003 reforms incorporated both the experience of MHOs and the public sector attempts to establish population-wide insurance.

Political Developments of the NHI

Ghana's radical health reforms in 2003 occurred on the tail end of the country's transition (back) to democracy after 11 years of military rule (Handley and Mills 2001; Carbone 2011). The political reform in the early 1990s also fueled popular demands for change in the health system. Civil society organizations and other organized interests openly voiced their concerns (Carbone 2011). The pluralist system increasingly opened up the realm of health policy to new actors. Free and vigorous media became a critical tool for open debates on health issues. Interest groups mobilized to influence public discussions and had their voices heard in the health policy process. Political parties articulated their demands and presented health policy alternatives in their bid for power. All these actors gained access to the health policy-making arenas where previously the executive, ministerial and donor agencies played dominant and essentially unaccountable roles (Carbone 2011). These pressures also affected the electoral and post-election competition between the two main political parties, the National Democratic Congress (NDC) and the New Patriotic Party (NPP).

Health policy became a key opportunity for the opposition party (NPP) to challenge the ruling party (NDC). Thus, health policies contributed to shaping politics and vice versa (Carbone 2011). Ghana's 2003 health reforms represented an interesting example of the social impact of open electoral politics, and the impact of regime change on health policy. The new dynamics of electoral competition played a crucial role in prompting health policy change (Carbone 2011). Ghanaians deeply despised the existing health financing arrangements, especially the cash and carry payments. This became a core issue for the opposition party, the NPP (Carbone 2011).

During the 2000 general elections, the NPP campaigned on the promise to replace user fees with a NHI. It promised access to basic healthcare for all Ghanaians, regardless of ability to pay (Agyepong and Adjei 2008). This election promise resonated with the populace. It is usually the poorest who suffer most from regressive taxation, but middle-income groups also felt the pinch of out-of-pocket fees (Agyepong and Adjei 2008). The NPP called the fees "notoriously callous, inhumane and inequitable." It promised that "nobody in Ghana will be denied medical attention because of his or her inability to pay and that payment of fees, if any, will be discussed when the patient is out of danger" (Kofi Ayisi et al. 2018; NPP 1996; Carbone 2011). The election dynamics thus became a driving force in reshaping health policy (Fusheini 2013). Interestingly, the NPP proposal seemed quite uncharacteristic. After all, the NPP was known to favor neo-liberal policies, promoting business interests and private sector initiatives in support of the middle and upper classes, elites and the bourgeoisie of Ghanaian society. Ideologically, the liberal orientation of the NPP made it an unlikely contender for adopting such socially oriented initiatives (Carbone 2011). NPP's health policy stance was populist at best (Fusheini 2013).

The Adoption of the NHI in 2003

NPP's victory in the 2000 general elections was the first step towards actualizing the promised NHI (Osei-Akoto and Adamba 2017). With lessons from earlier failed attempts, the MoH set up a seven-member ministerial health financing task force under the chairmanship of the Director for Policy, Planning, Monitoring and Evaluation (PPME) in March 2001. The task force was to develop a framework for the NHI (Agyepong and Adjei 2008; Osei-Akoto and Adamba 2017). Over time, however, government actors felt frustrated with the slow progress due to what they saw as unnecessary technical details. The MoH changed the composition of the task force to better reflect political priorities and hasten progress (one political concern was the next elections around the corner in 2004). This time, the task force wasted no time on technical details (Carbone 2011). However, there were conflicts between the technical experts and the political nominees over issues like the incorporation of MHOs. Several of the group's technical experts, including the chair, insisted on giving the large non-formal sector access to public financing (Agyepong and Adjei 2008). Another dispute arose from the interpretation of the failed Eastern region pilot, especially the difficulty of implementing a single-payer health insurance, as favored by the then Health Minister. Internal conflicts prompted the chair of the task force to step down less than a year into the process (Agyepong and Adjei 2008; Carbone 2011). The Health Minister replaced the chair with a trusted associate who also acted as director of the PPME division. The new PPME director brought his own trusted associates on board the task force as well.

The change in leadership had far-reaching implications. With the new appointments, the process became more politicized (Carbone 2011). The political affiliations of those associates were sometimes more clear than their technical qualifications for implementing a universal health insurance. Meanwhile, task force members decided to continue the preparations, given its significance. They ultimately reached consensus by proposing a hybrid system, which incorporated a classical single-payer scheme for the formal sector and multiple-payer, semi-autonomous MHOs for the informal sector (Agyepong and Adjei 2008). Added to that model was the option of a voluntary private commercial health insurance for those who could afford it (Agyepong and Adjei 2008).

It is worth mentioning that the political leadership of the NPP did not express preference for any particular technical design. It did, however, frame four major criteria as terms of reference for the policy:

(i) The national system had to enable a quick scale-up to cover the majority of the population, by including both the formal and informal sectors.

(ii) The new proposal had to be publicly viewed as an NPP initiative, not as a continuation of the previous government's efforts like the then-existing pilot projects.

(iii) The plan had to be formulated and passed through Parliament before the next elections in 2004.

(iv) It had to result in the abolition of all user fees at the point of service (Rajkotia 2009; Fusheini 2013).

After only four months the task force succeeded in drafting a legislative proposal ready for stakeholder consultation in June 2001 (Agyepong and Adjei 2008; Osei-Akoto and Adamba 2017; Carbone 2011). Just before that date, however, a cabinet reshuffle resulted in the replacement of the then health minister who favored the single-payer centralized system. His successor continued with the process. The MoH held the first round of stakeholder forums on national and sub-national levels (Agyepong and Adjei 2008). By this time, political associates had gained a dominant position in the discussion and drafting of technical proposals. The technocrats of the MoH—some of whom were cautious, if not skeptical, about the reforms—saw their role downsized (Agyepong and Adjei 2008; Carbone 2011; Rajkotia 2007). By the end of 2002, only one original member of the task force remained involved in the policy elite group, which made the final decisions on the NHI (Agyepong and Adjei 2008).

Notwithstanding those hurdles, Parliament received the final draft of the NHI under a certificate of urgency. This allowed only one week of deliberation before the bill passed into law (Agyepong and Adjei 2008). This rushed procedure led to protests by organized labor and the Trades Union Congress, especially against the 2.5 percent surcharge on employee pension contributions channeled to the NHIF. Various interest groups requested deferment of passage of the NHI to ensure wider consultations and amendments. The minority party (the NDC) also raised objections. Responding to these concerns, the government postponed the debate and Parliament went on recess (Agyepong and Adjei 2008). However, the government took a more adversarial approach towards the extra-parliamentary union protests and NDC actions (Carbone 2011). It recalled Parliament in August and passed the bill in its original form without any changes, ignoring all protests of organized labor groups and the NDC (Agyepong and Adjei 2008). The NDC refused to be part of the passage of the bill and walked out of Parliament in protest. Organized labor groups mounted street demonstration in protest. Nonetheless, the majority NPP went ahead and passed the bill since they had the numbers to do so and the bill received presidential assent in September 2003.

Implementation of the NHI—Challenges and Further Developments

The NHI created a mixed pot of prospects and challenges for healthcare providers (Osei-Akoto and Adamba 2017). Overall, the NHI recorded some impressive results. It provides fairly equitable and affordable access to healthcare to over one-third of the population and social protection for vulnerable groups in society (Teye et al. 2015). The NHI led to a sharp increase in utilization. Fewer people had to wait to seek medical care due to financial barriers (Fusheini 2013). Outpatient visits increased from 16.9 to 27.4 million and inpatient admissions from 0.72 to 1.61 million between 2010 and 2013 (NHIA 2013; Osei-Akoto and Adamba 2017).

The NHIA accreditation also led to improved quality of services (Osei-Akoto and Adamba 2017), even if there were concerns about some private facilities skimping on the accreditation requirements. The quality assessment criteria regarded the appropriate number of qualified personnel, and led to improved amenities (e.g., clean water, electricity, beds, TV sets, comfortable seating; Osei-Akoto and Adamba 2017). Health providers in Ghana have become largely dependent on the NHI as it now constitutes the dominant revenue source, accounting for 80–90 percent of their income (Osei-Akoto and Adamba 2017; Osei-Akoto et al. 2011). Providers therefore have to live up to the new quality requirements.

Furthermore, the NHI resulted in the mobilization of additional healthcare resources (Teye et al. 2015; Hsiao and Shaw 2007). About 85–90 percent of the internally generated revenues of providers now come from the health insurance (Fusheini 2013). Consequently, providers are in a better position to purchase medicine and supplies, rather than before when they had to wait for the release of government funds, often with long delays. The additional revenues allowed for the renovation and expansion of health facilities and the hiring of additional, better-qualified professionals. Examples include the construction of a new accident and trauma center at the Komfo Anokye Teaching Hospital in Kumasi for patients from the northern and middle belt of the country, and the new children's ward at the Korle Bu teaching hospital in Accra (Fusheini 2013). The financial impact also showed in the refurbishment of outpatient departments across the country, with new, more comfortable benches for patients, and plastic chairs and televisions sets in waiting rooms (Fusheini 2013).

On the other hand, delays in reimbursement continued to frustrate administrators. Reports of unofficial and informal fees charged to subscribers due to delays undermined the ideals and implementation of the NHI (Teye et al. 2015). Providers commonly refused to provide care to NHIS insured because of outstanding deficiencies in reimbursement. Issues of underfunding, cost escalation and consistent deficits threatened the sustainability of the scheme (Parliament of Ghana 2015; Osei-Akoto and Adamba 2017). Those problems were aggravated by the low insurance premiums and contribution rates and the exemptions that extended to over 70 percent of insured; the weak gatekeeper system, whereby clients easily bypass lower-level (and lower-cost) facilities to go directly to secondary and tertiary ones; and the dominant culture of hospital-centered care (Fusheini 2016; Fusheini et al. 2017a).

Scaling up the coverage to the majority of the population remained a challenge, too. The NHI has two categories of membership: members who pay the annual premium and the (large) exempt group. The first have to register and renew their membership each year, and pay contributions ranging between GH¢7.2 and GH¢48 per year (about $8 to $52 in 2003). There is a waiting period of one month before a subscriber can access health services with the NHI card after registration. The exemptions apply to children under 18, pregnant women, mentally ill, indigents, the disabled (as determined by the Minister responsible for Social Welfare), pensioners and persons over 70 years, in addition to other categories prescribed by the MoH (GoG 2012). The coverage varies across socio-economic and age groups. For example, in 2013, the shares of insured under 18, above 70 and indigents, were 46.5, 3.8 and 12.1 percent, respectively (even while these groups were exempt from paying premiums). The average coverage in the informal sector was around 33.6 percent.

Meanwhile, active membership in the NHI varies substantially from year to year due to non-renewal of membership (in the years 2014, 2015, 2016 and 2017, the shares of the population covered were 38.0, 40.0, 38.0 and 35.3 percent, respectively). Many formal sector workers who contribute to SSNIT seemed unaware that they needed to register to enjoy the benefits of the NHI (MoH 2018; Nsiah-Boateng and Aikins 2018). There were regional differences in actual access to healthcare services due to uneven distribution of infrastructural and health workforce across the country, especially between the North and the South.

All residents have to sign up with the NHI, unless they have proof of private health insurance (which is generally quite expensive for the average Ghanaian). By 2013, the NHIA had registered 14 private mutual health insurance schemes and three private commercial health insurance plans. Together they covered 144,625 registered members, or less than one-half percent of the population (NHIA 2013).

The NHI faces further challenges of politicization and political interference. Appointments of NHIA top leaders, regional and district managers are regularly viewed as a vehicle for rewarding party members (Fusheini 2016). There is evidence that membership of the ruling political party is now a prerequisite for employment at the NHI. According to critical media reports, the NHI regularly provides "jobs for the boys" of the government of the day (Kofi Ayisi et al. 2018). Following the change of government from the NDC to NPP in 2017, NPP party followers took over local NHI offices to secure jobs (Ghanaweb.com 2017). The NHI is now seen as a political institution for rewarding party loyalists (Osei-Akoto and Adamba 2017). This does not ensure continuity and stability as every change of government means a change to the CEO and other top managers.

Access barriers due to poor infrastructural facilities and skewed distribution of health professionals and facilities between southern and northern Ghana created other critical challenges. Long travel distances and lack of facilities, or hospitals without physicians are demotivating factors to subscribe. Hard-to-reach communities in the northern part of the country and poor road conditions, exacerbated by the rainy season, make it hard to implement the health insurance (Fusheini et al. 2017a, b).

In fact, although a crucial goal of the NHI, universal coverage has remained elusive. Poor and other vulnerable groups hardly gained access to the NHI (Ramachandra and Hsiao 2007; Carbone 2011). For those groups, even the subsidized premiums created high financial barriers (Asante and Aikins 2008; Carbone 2011). The MoH and NHIA realized that they needed new strategies to reach those groups. The NHIA developed pro-poor interventions; it adopted the countrywide common targeting mechanism (CTM) for identifying, targeting and enrolling the poor. It targeted specific groups like children in orphanages; blind, deaf and mute children; children receiving free school uniforms and those in school feeding programs; as well as patients in mental health facilities; and poor people living with HIV/AIDS (NHIA 2013).

The NHIA District Offices have been responsible for implementing the new approach, in collaboration with other stakeholders like the Ghana Education Service and the Department of Social Welfare (NHIA 2013). This led to noticeable increases in enrollment, especially of indigent insured, from 23,238 to 1.2 million between 2005 and December 2013 (NHIA 2013). Yet, over 15 million people in the country are still not enrolled in the NHI, and there is no way to enforce enrollment. Many households are still lacking financial protection against catastrophic health expenditure, despite the adoption of the NHI. They depend on private insurance or out-of-pocket payment.

In addition, there is a general perception that public facilities provide poor-quality healthcare. There are anecdotes of NHI-card holders spending long hours and they often feel they receive low-quality medications (Osei-Akoto and Adamba 2017; Adamba 2011). Other complaints concern poor treatment from physicians or nurses, and bad or smelly toilet facilities (Fusheini 2013). Insured consistently mentioned negative provider attitudes and other practices that make accessing healthcare problematic (Teye et al. 2015). This in turn affected the renewal rate and retention of NHI members.

As intimated earlier, various studies identified financial sustainability as a major challenge for the NHI. A number of factors, including the rate of premiums (that presently are not actuarially based) play a role, in particular the broad exemption policy that leaves only about 30 percent of members paying premiums (Fusheini et al. 2017a). In addition, there are problems of abuse and fraud by providers, clients and district plan managers (Fusheini 2013). Initial implementation was characterized by providers engaging in over-servicing and over-prescribing of drugs, submission of fraudulent claims such as alleged cesarean sections—on men or in facilities with no capacity to perform cesareans. Clients were involved in facility shopping by moving from facility to facility, where they collected drugs for family members and for selling to roadside drug dealers, while district plan managers embezzled collected premiums, as they were not accountable at the national level but to district-level boards only (Fusheini et al. 2017a; Fusheini 2013; 2016).

One major concern about the NHI financing is its over-reliance on the VAT levy as its main source of revenue (NHIA 2010, 2011, 2012, 2013). This levy contributes about 70 percent of all NHIF revenues, more than twice the total revenue from all the other sources combined (Osei-Akoto and Adamba 2017). SSNIT contributions, the second major financing source, underwrites about 20 percent; the premiums from informal sector contributors and those who do not contribute to SSNIT only about 3.4 percent in 2013 (NHIA 2013; Osei-Akoto and Adamba 2017).

The NHI has substantial operating deficits. The net operating deficit of the NHIF amounted to GH¢96.8 million ($20 million) or 78.5 percent of total expenditure in 2013 (NHIA 2013). In April 2017, the NHIF owed service providers about GH¢1.2 billion ($247 million) in payment arrears of at least 12 months (IMANI 2017). Thus, after almost 15 years of implementation, the system is confronted with daunting financial challenges exacerbated by growing income inequality, population changes and the rise of non-communicable diseases.

Conclusion

Many commentators consider Ghana as an UHC leader in sub-Saharan Africa (Agyepong 2018) due to the radical reforms embarked upon in 2003 by the NPP government. The choice of a NHI model, principled on SHI and fashioned around the traditional welfare system of reciprocity was informed by the crises of the cash and carry system and its effects on health services utilization, and the performance of the health system in general. Employing a historical narrative perspective helps shed light on the health financing challenges Ghana has faced and the journey to the 2003 reforms. Several actors, both national and international, have been involved in the reform process, albeit in various ways ranging from commissioned studies to community-level initiatives that provided the evidence needed for the reforms.

The passage of Ghana's NHI in 2003 is a clear illustration of nimble policy entrepreneurs who successfully moved through a window of opportunity (Kingdon 1984). The cash and carry crises provided the impetus for setting the agenda. The political competition through elections brought a new political party to power, eager to implement the health reform agenda and earlier experiments with local health insurance schemes helped frame the new national insurance model.

Ghana's NHI has made significant progress with population coverage. It has facilitated access to healthcare services for over one-third of the population and led to increased utilization and reduction in out-of-pocket payments. The NHI mobilized additional resources for the health sector and led to greater income certainty for many healthcare providers.

However, major challenges remain. Reimbursement delays, low coverage, particularly of the poor and elderly, politicization and political interference in administration, poor infrastructural facilities and uneven distribution of facilities and personnel, financial sustainability and poor perceived quality of services received by subscribers threaten the operation of the NHI.

More efforts are required, and additional sources of funding need to be explored if Ghana is to achieve UHC through the NHI. The role of politics in driving this process needs to be recognized, especially in ensuring resources are made available on time to reimburse providers so as to ensure card holders are not turned away. The depoliticization of the system to ensure stability and continuity during transition from one government to the other will also go a long way to engendering trust and certainty about the sustainability and direction of the NHI.

References

Adamba, C. 2011. *The Thrills and Tears of National Health Insurance Scheme Cardholders in Ghana*. Ghana, Legon: University of Ghana, Institute of Statistical, Social and Economic Research: 1–24.

Adisah-Atta, I. 2017. "Financing health care in Ghana: are Ghanaians willing to pay higher taxes for better health care? Findings from Afrobarometer." *Social Sciences*, 6: 90.

Aikins, Ad.-G., and K. Koram. 2017. "Health and Healthcare in Ghana, 1957–2017." *The Economy of Ghana Sixty Years After Independence*. E. Aryeetey and R. Kanbur (eds.). Oxford: Oxford University Press: 365.

Agyei-Baffour, P., R. Oppong, and D. Boateng. 2013. "Knowledge, perceptions and expectations of capitation payment system in a health insurance setting: a repeated survey of clients and health providers in Kumasi, Ghana." *BMC Public Health*, 13: 1220.

Agyepong, I.A., D.N.Y. Abankwah, A. Abroso, et al. 2016. "The "Universal" in UHC and Ghana's National Health Insurance Scheme: policy and implementation challenges and dilemmas of a lower middle income country." *BMC Health Services Research*, 16(1): 504.

Agyepong, I.A., and S. Adjei. 2008. "Public social policy development and implementation: a case study of the Ghana National Health Insurance scheme." *Health Policy and Planning*, 23(2): 150–160.

Agyepong, I.A., and R.A. Nagai. 2011. "'We charge them; otherwise we cannot run the hospital' front line workers, clients and health financing policy implementation gaps in Ghana." *Health Policy*, 99(3): 226–233.

Arhinful, D.K. 2003. *The Solidarity of Self-Interest: social and Cultural Feasibility of Rural Health Insurance in Ghana.* Leiden: African Studies Centre.

Aryeetey, E., and M. Goldstein. 2000. "Ghana: social-policy reform in Africa." *Reforming Social Policy: Changing Perspectives on Sustainable Human Development.* Ottawa, ON, Canada: IDRC.

Asante, F., and M. Aikins. 2008. *Does the NHIS Cover the Poor?* Danida Health Sector Support Office Paper. Accra: DANIDA.

Asenso-Okyere, W.K. 1995. "Health Financing: Financing health care in Ghana." *World Health Forum*, 86–94.

Asenso-Okyere, W.K., I. Osei-Akoto, A. Anum, and E.N. Appiah. 1997. "Willingness to pay for health insurance in a developing economy. a pilot study of the informal sector of Ghana using contingent valuation." *Health Policy*, 42(3): 223–237.

Atim, C. 2000. *Training of Trainers Manual for Mutual Health Organisations in Ghana.* Sponsored by DANIDA Health Sector Support Office Ghana, United States Agency for International Development (USAID) and Partnerships for Health Reform (PHR).

Atim, C., S. Grey, P. Apoya, et al. 2001. *A Survey of Health Financing Schemes in Ghana. 2001.* Bethesda, MD: Abt Associates for USAID Google Scholar.

Bagnoli, L. 2017. *Does National Health Insurance Improve Children's Health? National and Regional Evidence from Ghana.* ECARES Working Papers.

Blanchet, N., G. Fink, and I. Osei-Akoto. 2012. "The effect of Ghana's National Health Insurance Scheme on health care utilisation." *Ghana Medical Journal*, 46(2): 76–84.

Carbone, G. 2011. "Democratic demands and social policies: the politics of health reform in Ghana." *J Mod Afr Stud*, 49(3): 381–408.

Cartoko. 2010. *A Map Database.* http://www.cartoko.com/2010/08/ghana-administrative-divisions/. Accessed February 2, 2018.

Fusheini, A. 2013. *The Implementation of the National Health Insurance in Ghana (2003–2013).* PhD Thesis, University of Ulster. Jordanstown: Unpublished.

Fusheini, A. 2016. "The Politico-Economic Challenges of Ghana's National Health Insurance Scheme Implementation." *Int J Health Policy Manag*, 5(9): 543–552.

Fusheini, A., G. Marnoch, and A.M. Gray. 2017a. "Implementation Challenges of the National Health Insurance Scheme in Selected Districts in Ghana: Evidence from the Field." *Int J Publ Admin*, 40(5): 416–426.

Fusheini, A., G. Marnoch, and A.M. Gray. 2017b. "Stakeholders perspectives on the success drivers in Ghana's National Health Insurance Scheme–identifying policy translation issues." *Int J Health Policy Manag*, 6(5): 273–283.

Ghanaweb.com. 2017. *Asunafo South NPP youth invade and lock up NHIS office.* Ghanaweb.com: Ghanaweb. Accessed February 2, 2018.

GoG. 2012. *National Health Insurance Act* (Act 852). Accra: Ministry of Health.

GoG. 2013. *Ghana National Health Accounts 2005 and 2010.* Accra: Ministry of Health.

GoG. 2015. *Ghana Health Financing Strategy.* Accra: Ministry of Health.

GSS. 2014. *Ghana Living Standards Survey Round 6 (GLSS 6): Poverty Profile in Ghana (2005–2013).* Accra: Ghana Statistical Service.

Handley, A., and G. Mills. 2001. *"From Military Coups to Multiparty Elections: The Ghanian Military-Civil Transition."* Den Haag: The Netherlands Institute of International Relations Clingendael.

Hsiao, W., and R.P. Shaw. 2007. *Social Health Insurance for Developing Nations*: The World Bank.

IMANI. 2017. *Reforming the National Health Insurance; Pathways to Sustainable Healthcare Financing.* IMANI: Centre for Policy and Education.

Katuu, S. 2018. "Healthcare systems: typologies, framework models, and South Africa's health sector." *Int Health Governance*, 23(2): 134–148.

Kingdon, J.W. 1984. *Agendas, Alternatives, and Public Policies.* New York, NY: Longman.

Kofi Ayisi, E., E. Yeboah-Assiamah, and J. Bawole. 2018. "Politics of Public Policy Implementation: Case of Ghana National Health Insurance Scheme." *Global Encyclopedia of Public Administration, Public Policy, and Governance.* A. Farazmand (ed.). Switzerland: Springer.

Kotoh, A.M., G.C. Aryeetey, and S. Van der Geest. 2018. "Factors that influence enrolment and retention in Ghana's National Health Insurance Scheme." *Int J Health Policy Man*, 7: 443.

Kuganab-Lem, R.B. 2007. *An Empirical Analysis of the National Health Insurance Policy Process in Ghana*. Keele University.

Mayes, R. 2004. *Universal Coverage: The Elusive Quest for National Health Insurance*: University of Michigan Press.

Mensah, J., J.R. Oppong, and C.M. Schmidt. 2010. "Ghana's National Health Insurance Scheme in the context of the health MDGs: An empirical evaluation using propensity score matching." *Health Econ*, 19: 95–106.

MoH. 2018. *Holistic Assessment of 2017 Health Sector Programme of Work*. Accra: Ministry of Health.

Myjoyonline. 2018. *Ghana's Economy Expands by 24.6%; Now Worth GH₵256bn After Rebasing*.

NHIA. 2009. *National Health Insurance Authority Annual Report 2009*. Accra: National Health Insurance Authority.

NHIA. 2010. *National Health Insurance Authority Annual Report 2010. Growing Healthier and Stronger*. Accra: National Health Insurance Authority.

NHIA. 2011. *National Health Insurance Authority Annual Report*. Accra: National Health Insurance Authority.

NHIA. 2012. *National Health Insurance Authority, 2012 Annual Report*. Accra: National Health Insurance Authority.

NHIA. 2013. *National Health Insurance Authority, 2013 Annual Report*. Accra: National Health Insurance Authority.

NHIA. 2018. *National Health Insurance Scheme Benefits package* Accra: National Health Insurance Authority. http://www.nhis.gov.gh/benefits.aspx. Accessed February 2, 2018.

NHIS. 2018. *Capitation: Provider Payment Mechanisms*. http://www.nhis.gov.gh/capitation.aspx. Accessed February 2, 2018.

NPP. 1996. *Manifesto 1996: Development in Freedom, Agenda for Change*, Accra: New Patriotic Party.

Nsiah-Boateng, E., and M. Aikins. 2018. "Trends and characteristics of enrolment in the National Health Insurance Scheme in Ghana: a quantitative analysis of longitudinal data." *Glob Health Res Policy*, 3: 32. doi:10.1186/s41256-018-0087-6.

Nyonator, F., and J. Kutzin. 1999. "Health for some? The effects of user fees in the Volta Region of Ghana." *Health Policy Plan*, 14(4): 329–341.

Oppong, J.R. 2001. "Structural Adjustment and the Health Care System." *IMF and World Bank Sponsored Structural Adjustment Programs in Africa: Ghana's Experience, 1983–1999.* K. Konadu-Agyemang (ed.). Ashgate: Aldershot: 357–370.

Osei-Akoto, I., and C. Adamba. 2017. Social Health Insurance in Ghana. *The Economy of Ghana Sixty Years After Independence*: 385.

Osei-Akoto, I., R. Atta-Ankomah, C. Adamba, et al. 2011. *Resource flow in Ghana's Health Sector: Challenges and Effects on Service Delivery.* Report prepared for Center on Budget and Policy Priorities, Washington, DC.

Parliament of Ghana. 2015. "Parliamentary Debates Official Report: Fourth Series." 90(30), March 26. Accra.

Quaye, R. 1991. "Planning the health care system in a decade of economic decline: The Ghanaian experience." *Crime, Law and Social Change*, 16(3): 303–311.

Rajkotia, Y. 2007. The political development of the Ghanaian National Health Insurance System: lessons in health governance.

Rajkotia, Y. 2009. *National Health Insurance in Ghana: Politics, Adverse Selection, and the Use of Child Health Services*: The Johns Hopkins University.

Ramachandra, S., and W.C. Hsiao. 2007. "Ghana: initiating social health insurance." *Social Health Insurance for Developing Nations*, 434: 61. doi:10.1596/978-0-8213-6949-4

RVO.nl. 2015. *Sector Report Health and Life Sciences Ghana.* Den Haag: Embassy of the Kingdom of the Netherlands in Ghana. Accessed February 2, 2018.

Sakyi, E.K., R. Atinga, and F.A. Adzei. 2012. "Managerial problems of hospitals under Ghana's National Health Insurance Scheme." *Clin Gov*, 17: 178–190.

Saleh, K. 2013. "Ghana's Universal Health Coverage." [Workshop paper] *Frontiers in Development Policy: Workshop on Innovative Development Case Studies.* Hotel Shilla Seoul, Republic of Korea (http://www.shilla.net/Seoul); Washington, DC: World Bank Institute.

Schieber, G., C. Cashin, K. Saleh, and R. Lavado. 2012. *Health Financing in Ghana*: World Bank Publications.

Shaw, R.P., and C.C. Griffin. 1995. *Financing Health Care in Sub-Saharan Africa through User Fees and Insurance.* Washington, DC: World Bank.

Sulzbach, S., B. Garshong, and G. Owusu-Banahene. 2005. *Evaluating the Effects of the National Health Insurance Act in Ghana: Baseline Report.* Partners for Health Reformplus.

Teye, J.K., A.A. Arhin, and A.S. Anamzoya. 2015. "Achievements and Challenges of the National Health Insurance Scheme in Ghana." *Curr Polit Ec of Africa*, 8(8): 487.

Van den Boom, G., N.N. Nsowah-Nuamah, G.B. Overbosch, et al. 2008. "Health-Care Provision & Self-Medication in Ghana." *The Economy of Ghana*: 392–416.

Vecchione, E., and J. Parkhurst. 2016. *Evidence Advisory System.* Briefing Notes: Ghana.

Waddington, C., and K.A. Enyimayew. 1989. "A price to pay, Part 1. The impact of user charges in the Ashanti Akim District, Ghana." *Int J Health Plann Manag*, 4(10): 17–47.

Waddington, C., and K.A. Enyimayew. 1990. "A price to pay, the impact of user charges in the Volta Region of Ghana." *Int J Health Plann Manag*, 5(4): 287–312.

Wang, H., N. Otoo, and L. Dsane-Selby. 2017. *Ghana National Health Insurance Scheme: improving Financial Sustainability Based on Expenditure Review.* Washington DC: The World Bank.

WHO/AFRO. 2018. *Comprehensive Analytical Profile, Factsheet Health Statistics 2018: Ghana.* http://www.aho.afro.who.int/profiles_information/index.php/Ghana:Index. Accessed February 2, 2018.

Witter, S., and B. Garshong. 2009. "Something old or something new? Social health insurance in Ghana." *BMC Int Health Hum Rights*, 9: 20.

WorldBank. 2018a. *GDP Per Capita (Current US$)-Selected Countries and Economies.* https://data.worldbank.org/indicator/NY.GDP.PCAP.CD?end=1960&locations=KR-GH-JP&start=1960&view=bar. Accessed February 2, 2018.

WorldBank. 2018b. *Ghana: Overview.* http://www.worldbank.org/en/country/ghana/overview. Accessed February 2, 2018.

WorldBank. 2018c. *The World Bank in Ghana: Data* (GDP-Current US$). World Bank national accounts data, and OECD National Accounts data files. Accessed February 2, 2018.

Chapter 2

Health Reforms in Tanzania: From Self-Reliance to Donor Dependency and Efforts to Return to Self-Reliance

Igor Francetic

Introduction

The United Republic of Tanzania is a mid-sized East African country, located on the Indian Ocean coast, south of the Equator. The population was about 55 million in 2016. With a land territory of about 341,700 square miles, Tanzania had the largest population and lowest population density in East Africa. Over two-thirds lived in rural areas.

Since its independence from Great Britain in 1961 and until the first democratic elections in 1995, Tanzania had been a one-party state. Ever since, the country experienced a remarkable degree of social and political stability. The fifth president elected in 2015, John P. Magufuli, pushed an agenda of socio-political change and anti-corruption policies.

The vision of post-colonial self-reliance proposed by the first President Julius Nyerere—known as the Father of the Nation—was distilled in the Arusha Declaration of 1967. Tanzania has been one of the pioneering nations in health policy development among sub-Saharan countries. Shortly after independence, President Nyerere's ruling socialist administration announced universal and free access to primary healthcare as a tool to improve the population's health and well-being, well before the 1978 Alma Ata Declaration of the World Health Organization (WHO).

It coupled specific health policies with broader social and economic development and education. The government announced a universal public health system, with budget allocations based on equity and population needs. It centralized human resources planning and training, as well as expanded investments in health infrastructure (Gilson 1995; Semali et al. 2007). Moreover, it initially discouraged private initiative in healthcare and later banned it by law in 1977 (Kumaranayake et al. 2000).

The economic hardship of the 1970s and 1980s undermined the government's ability to sustain free universal healthcare, however. The country increasingly relied on development partners and external financing for the health sector. This resulted in large vertical programs focused on specific diseases, such as HIV/AIDS, tuberculosis, malaria and vaccination programs, but also other specific financing, often driven by donor programs rather than by national priorities (Semali et al. 2007). Over time, external donors gained more significance in healthcare financing, and between 2006 and 2012, up to 50 percent of total health expenditure came from external sources. That share declined to about one-third by 2017.

Tanzania experienced robust economic growth in the early 21st century, on average 7 percent gross domestic product (GDP) growth between 2007 and 2017. Despite the increase in income and a decline in the poverty rate (from 86 to 49.1 percent between 2000 and 2010), the absolute number of people living in poverty remained among the highest in sub-Saharan Africa (World Bank 2017). Notably, high out-of-pocket healthcare costs pushed one out of 40 Tanzanian families below the poverty line (set at $1.9 PPP in 2012; World Bank 2017).

The heavy dependence on external donors caused friction. Tanzania's government felt at times overwhelmed by foreign donors who were gaining a greater say in health policy-making. For example, for many years, the World Bank and other donor agencies sponsored the community-based health insurance schemes, Community Health Fund (CHF) and TIKA, for workers in the informal sector. Those schemes aimed to increase local fundraising and improve access. The CFH and TIKA schemes were rolled out in the country despite mixed evidence about their effectiveness. It turned out to be especially hard to increase coverage in rural settings.

Similarly, international donors enthusiastically supported pay-for-performance (P4P) schemes to improve maternal and child health, but in the end, these arrangements showed only modest results and no financial sustainability. Besides lack of ownership in the policy process, the activities of multiple uncoordinated partners contributed to increased complexity, fragmentation and inequality in healthcare across the country.

The latest health policy documents (e.g., its 2015 Health Financing Strategy [HFS]) reflect the government's efforts to reach a better balance between its own priorities and donors' requests or receipts.

Healthcare and Health Financing in Tanzania, 2018

The current healthcare system and the public administration of Tanzania essentially date back to the Nyerere administration (Conyers 1981; Frumence et al. 2013). The underlying idea was to rely on primary healthcare at the village level to provide essential services for all, targeted to local needs (especially basic curative and maternal and child healthcare), with active involvement of local communities. District and regional hospitals were to oversee the lower level structures, serving as gatekeepers for referral to secondary, tertiary and specialized care (Ministry of Health 1990). The country's administration has 30 regions and 196 districts (National Bureau of Statistics 2017). After focusing on improving and expanding infrastructure, the priorities shifted in the 1980s to widening the scope of services, for example, with programs for immunization and availability of essential prescription drugs. Those programs received heavy support from external development partners and donors (Gilson 1995; Semali et al. 2004, 2007).

The Ministry of Health (MoH) presented the first comprehensive National Health Policy in 1990. That policy document incorporated principles from the 1967 Arusha Declaration by President Nyerere. The MoH presented the next update of the National Health Policy in 2007 and a third version in 2017 (Ministry of Health, Community Development, Gender, Elderly and Children 2017). In parallel, the MoH developed several specific programs and strategic plans for the health sector (Ministry of Health and Social Welfare 2015).

The earlier health policies resulted in expanded coverage and improved health outcomes in rural areas, but the economic downturns of the 1970s and 1980s created considerable pressure on the health system. Tax revenues stagnated and external development aid did not fill the gap in resources to finance free healthcare for the whole population. Severe budget cuts led to deterioration of the system (Ministry of Health 2003). The government's answer to the economic hardship was a wave of economic liberalization in the 1990s. It lifted the ban on private health practices and recognized faith-based and private hospitals, and other health facilities as proper partners in providing healthcare services (Kumaranayake et al. 2000). It allowed faith-based hospitals to serve as district hospitals in areas where no public structures were present. The government also opened a debate about new health financing options that involved patient cost sharing, prepayment and insurance plans (Ministry of Health 1990, 2003). The new economic directions and health policy options were clearly influenced by the Washington Consensus promoted by the International Monetary Fund (IMF) and the World Bank (Chimhutu et al. 2015). Other stakeholders, including non-governmental organizations (NGOs) and faith-based organizations, supported that direction.

Tanzania spent about 6 percent of its GDP on health expenditures in 2015 (35% from government expenditures, 28% from private sources and 37% from external sources). External sources served to finance disease-specific vertical programs, off-budget contributions and a Health Basket Fund (HBF) administered by the government (Ministry of Health and Social Welfare 2015; World Health Organization 2017). The share of the public budget spending for health (7.4% of the general government expenditure in 2015) remained well below the 15 percent target set in 2001 by the African Union's Abuja Declaration (Ministry of Health and Social Welfare 2015; World Health Organization 2011).

The allocation of the public basket, in line with the Arusha Declaration, takes into account the geographical distribution of income levels, population, burden of disease and density of health facilities across the country (Ministry of Health 2003). Patients paid for most private healthcare directly, contributing 26.1 percent of total health expenditure or about 93 percent of private health spending in 2015 (World Bank 2017).

To increase the availability of funds for healthcare and improve financial health protection, Tanzania decided to pursue a health insurance–based strategy in the early 1990s. With support from the World Bank, it set up the CHF to implement pilot projects in 1995 and 1996. It rolled out this scheme to about 60 districts nationwide in 2001. CHFs are district-based voluntary insurance schemes—with yearly enrollment contributions—that ultimately aimed to reach 85 percent of the (rural) population working in the informal sector.

Local government authorities (LGAs) are responsible for managing and supervising the CHFs and pooling funds to co-finance primary healthcare (Joseph and Maluka 2016). In 2009, the CHF concept expanded—with higher contribution rates reflecting higher incomes—to voluntary schemes for informal workers in both urban and suburban settings, the so-called TIKAs (acronym for the Kiswahili term *Tiba kwa Kadi*; Mtei and Mulligan 2007; Kapologwe et al. 2017).

Shortly after the first CHF pilot implementations, Tanzania's government introduced its national insurance scheme, targeting the formal sector under the National Health Insurance Fund (NHIF) act of 1999. The plan started with civil servants only, later opening enrollment to employees in the private sector. NHIF contributions are linked to salary, with a 3 percent worker contribution matched by the employer. Despite substantial support from development partners, the insurance coverage remained poor (about 16% of the population had enrolled in the CHF by 2014, and about 8% in expanded CHF and TIKA schemes; Kamuzora and Gilson 2007; Kapologwe et al. 2017; West-Slevin and Dutta 2015). Besides failing to provide financial health protection to a large share of the population, the low enrollment rates undermined the capacity of insurance schemes to effectively pool risks. Furthermore, the voluntary community-based schemes suffered from a high degree of adverse selection[1] (Wang and

---

[1]Adverse selection means that people wait to pay for insurance until they know they will face costs (because they are ill). This free-rider behavior obviously drives up the contributions for all insured and creates problems for insurance plans that accept everyone without screening.

Rosemberg 2018). There were several reasons for the low enrollment in the CHF and TIKA schemes: the regressive nature of the lump-sum annual contribution for poor households, the limited scope of services covered by CHFs (benefit package) and the low quality of healthcare services (ibidem).

The large segment of the population not covered by insurance was in principle exposed to out-of-pocket payments (OOPs). To reduce the risk of impoverishment related to healthcare costs, the MoH put targeted waivers and exemptions in place for vulnerable groups seeking care in public health facilities. Payment exemptions for fees at point of service applied to sick children, pregnant mothers, the elderly, people with chronic conditions and the disabled. Waivers for patient fees applied to poor households based on the advice of health workers and social welfare officers in consultation with local community leaders. Despite good intentions, however, the waivers and exemptions led to major problems. There was a lack of clear and consistent criteria and procedures for implementation (Mubyazi 2004; Mtei and Mulligan 2007; Mujinja and Kida 2014). The exemptions imposed a huge financial burden on the—already low—public health budget (Lee et al. 2018) and on health facilities that were not compensated for the forgone revenues of the patients exempted from payment (Wang and Rosemberg 2018).

The majority of all health facilities in the country (about 73%) are public. Non-profit faith-based organizations and other NGOs own and manage about 12 percent of health facilities, and for-profits the remaining 15 percent. Overall, 82 percent are primary care healthcare facilities (dispensaries or health posts), 10 percent secondary level health centers, and less than 4 percent are tertiary hospitals (Ministry of Health, Community Development, Gender, Elderly and Children 2017). Health facilities owned and managed by private companies, faith-based organizations or other NGOs do not benefit from direct government funding. However, some have obtained accreditation with the National Health Insurance Fund and with different CHFs and thus gained access to public financing (National Health Insurance Fund 2018; Wang and Rosemberg 2018).

Tanzania's healthcare faces serious challenges—shortages of financial and other resources and weak administrative and management capacity. The main problems can be summarized as follows: (1) inadequate quality of health services, lack of accountability and supervision; (2) severe shortages (up to 70%) of skilled human resources; (3) inadequate public financing and low patient contributions; (4) inefficient drug management and delivery, insufficient physical and technical infrastructures and poor health information systems; (5) ineffective targeting mechanisms of social protection schemes and insufficient coverage of health insurance schemes (Musau et al. 2011; Kwesigabo et al. 2012; Mujinja and Kida 2014; West-Slevin et al. 2015; World Health Organization 2016).

Despite those problems, there has been progress in the overall health of the population in the last three decades. The immunization rate of infants under 2 for measles increased from 80 to 99 percent between 1990 and 2017. The percentage of births attended by skilled health staff increased from 44 to 64 percent in that same period (Afnan-Holmes et al. 2015; Masanja et al. 2008; World Bank 2017). The infant mortality rate steadily decreased, from roughly 100 to 41 per 1,000 live births between 1990 and 2015 (see the statistical Appendix to this volume). The prevalence of underweight children decreased from 25.1 to 13.7 percent over the same period. Total HIV prevalence was kept under control, decreasing from 4.9 to 4.5 percent of the adult population between 1990 and 2017. Along with those improvements, average life expectancy at birth went up from 50 to about 63 years. Those figures suggest that the focus on primary care and the availability of healthcare services have indeed contributed to better health.

Tanzania's Health Policy-Making in the Millennium Development Goals Era

The MoH used its 2007 update of the National Health Policy to develop strategic health sector plans (HSSPs). These plans overlapped with earlier efforts to decentralize decision-making power and reform LGAs. They entailed the restructuring of regional and district administration. LGAs became responsible for the planning, budgeting and managing of public services like education and healthcare (Ministry of Health and Social Welfare 2008). The MoH further launched the Primary Healthcare Service Development Programme (PHCSDP, or *Mpango wa Maendeleo ya Afya ya Msingi* (MMAM) in Kiswahili), aimed to accelerate the provision of primary healthcare for all Tanzanians (Mujinja and Kida 2014; Ministry of Health and Social Welfare 2007, 2008).

Box 1 lists the range of specific strategies towards universal health coverage under HSSP III and HSSP IV planned for the period 2009–2020. LGAs expanded their role in administering local health services. HSSP III announced additional investments to strengthen management capacity and infrastructure of District Health Services (Strategy 1). The measures included the training, specific management and monitoring guidelines for local and district staff. It also introduced performance-based incentives, such as "P4P" or results-based financing (RBF) projects sponsored by external donors, and typically focused on service delivery targets in reproductive, maternal and child care (Binyaruka and Borghi 2017, 2018).

The government next decided to centralize the medicine supply for all public health facilities, and took steps to reduce corruption and leakages. It established a central unit, the Medical Stores Department (MSD). Strategy 3 included measures to enhance cooperation and coordination between central entities like the MoH, MSD and LGAs (Ministry of Health and Social Welfare 2008). Since its inception, however, the MSD has faced many challenges, above all shortages of essential medicines and delays in deliveries. In reaction, the MoH allowed a growing role for the private sector as an alternative supply chain for medicine (Binyaruka and Borghi 2017).

HSSP III focused on the health workforce and other resources. It noted that total staffing was substantially below standard in 2008. To address understaffing, Strategy 4 aimed to develop policies and regulation to improve human resources planning, utilization of available resources and training (initial pre-, in-service and continuous education; Ministry of Health and Social Welfare 2008). The government approved a Human

Resource for Health (HRH) Strategic Plan for the period 2008–2013. The plan included detailed multi-sector measures to address personnel shortages, as well as specific human resources management, retention and incentive policies.

With strategy 5, HSSP III addressed the crucial aspect of health financing. The main issues at the time were (and still are) the low public health budget, high OOPs, the failure of existing arrangements to protect families against the major financial risks of illness, and high dependence on external sources and vertical health programs.

As mentioned earlier, external development partners have played a major role in framing Tanzania's health policy since the early 2000s. They supported projects and programs with financial resources and technical assistance. The World Bank remained a major sponsor of CHF and pilot schemes with P4P and other RBF (Binyaruka and Borghi 2017; Chimhutu et al. 2015; Mayumana et al. 2017). These policy options are part of HSSP III, the updated National Health Policy and later strategic documents described later.

Another indication of the importance of development partners is the 1999 decision of the Tanzanian government to pursue a so-called sector-wide approach (SWAP) for health. The SWAP coordinates health reforms through sector-level committees involving all relevant stakeholders. It allows development partners to participate directly in the policy-making process. Two essential components of the SWAP are (1) the HBF and (2) the technical working groups (TWGs). The HBF is a financing mechanism supported by a set of development partners. It pools financial resources into a general fund aimed to support the implementation of strategic health sector plans and reforms. Notably, the rollout of voluntary CHF schemes across the country benefitted from a matching contribution for enrollment fees by the HBF (Wang and Rosemberg 2018). The partners contributing to the HBF participate in the SWAP committee to periodically assess the use of funds (Development Partners Group Tanzania 2005). The SWAP approach further includes TWGs and sub-committees working on specific components of the health sector reform. TWGs allow development partners, academics and other stakeholders to participate in the shaping of health policies down to detail (Hutton and Tanner 2004; Ministry of Health and Social Welfare 2015). The MoH continued to involve a wide range of stakeholders in the development of the fourth health sector plan—HSSP IV (2015–2020)—through the SWAPs and TWGs. Stakeholders included government agencies, WHO, NGOs, the private sector, the Prime Minister's Office for Regional Administration and, notably, foreign development partners.

Health Policy in the Sustainable Development Goals Era

One major inspirational source for HSSP IV was the idea of Sustainable Development Goals (SDGs). Another influence was Tanzania's large multi-sector development program launched in 2013, known as Big Results Now (BRN), inspired by the principle of results-based aid.[2] BRN focused on four main principles: prioritization, coordination of implementation, methodical approaches and inter-ministerial cooperation and management systems. It aimed to accelerate the realization of the core ambition of Tanzania's Development Vision 2025 (namely becoming a middle-income nation by 2025). It sought to attract external development support in different key areas (national key results areas; NKRAs), linking financing to clear and measurable results. The cabinet designated healthcare as a specific NKRA in 2014. HSSP IV, therefore, incorporated many BRN principles (Janus and Keijzer 2015). While the overall strategies and goals of HSSP IV (listed in Box 1) are in line with HSSP III, there is more emphasis on implementation, management and multi-sector coordination (Ministry of Health and Social Welfare 2015).

The government again took up health financing as a major issue in its 2015 HFS, a crucial component of HSSP IV. The 2015 HFS included five main elements: (1) a mandatory Single National Health Insurance (SNHI); (2) a minimum benefits package; (3) financing of public health activities; (4) mobilization of resources for health and social welfare; and

---

[2]We have not come across anyone supporting the principle of non-results-based aid.

Box 1. Health Sector Strategies in HSSP III and HSSP IV

HSSP III (July 2009 to June 2015)	HSSP IV (July 2015 to June 2020)
Strategy 1: District Health Services Strategy 2: Referral Hospital Services Strategy 3: Central Support Strategy 4: Human Resources for Health Strategy 5: Healthcare Financing Strategy 6: Public Private Partnerships Strategy 7: Maternal, Newborn and Child Health Strategy 8: Disease Prevention and Control Strategy 9: Emergency Preparedness Strategy 10: Social Welfare and Social Protection Strategy 11: Monitoring and Evaluation <u>Cross-cutting issues</u>: quality, equity, gender sensitivity, community ownership and coherence in governance.	• Quality assurance • Package of Intervention by levels of care • Health service provision by type of service • Inter-sector collaboration for health • Emergency preparedness and response • Social welfare service delivery • Human resources for health and social welfare • Essential medicines and health products • Infrastructure, transport and equipment • Monitoring and evaluation system • ICT and e-health • Health financing • Financial management system • Management of implementation and governance • Gender in health • Stepwise approach coordination and management

Source: Ministry of Health and Social Welfare (2008, 2015).

(5) allocation of resources to the health sector. HSSP IV went a step further than HSSP III in presenting reliable cost estimates and framing explicit policy priorities and goals for the health sector (Ministry of Health and Social Welfare 2015).

The proposed SNHI aimed to integrate Tanzania's fragmented health insurance schemes (NHIF, CHF and TIKA) into a single financial risk pool by 2020. This would create economies of scale and allow for effective cross-subsidization across the different systems. The implementation of the SNHI faced big challenges, however: low health insurance enrollment rates, low contribution compliance, the difficulty of targeting the informal sector and the problematic task of enforcing mandatory coverage (Prabhakaran and Dutta 2017).

One important political barrier to the reforms remained the need for substantial cross-subsidization between the formal and informal sectors. The proposed financing model discriminates between the salary-based contributions for the formal sector employees and the annual CFH and TIKA contributions for unemployed, informal sector workers and the poor. The SNHI would also need to harmonize different benefit packages into one standard, minimum package. The current contributions collected by the plans targeting the informal sector are generally too low to ensure financial sustainability. To operate, they receive heavy subsidy from development partners in the form of matching funds for the yearly contributions. At present, NHIF-insured pay a 3 percent contribution, matched by identical contributions from their employers. The merger into a unique risk pool requires the richer enrollees of the formal sector to cover part of the gap in contributions generated by the informal sector enrollees. Higher contributions, however, will likely decrease the enrollment rate—especially among informal workers—and thus further shrink the financial resources available (Prabhakaran and Dutta 2017).

The proposed SNHI portion of the HFS marked a move away from the current waivers and exemptions for OOPs (user fees and contributions) towards an insurance-based model with wider risk pooling. Under this new model, poor and vulnerable groups would be required to enroll in the health insurance. Instead of exempting them from payments at the point of service, the government would subsidize the enrollment of targeted groups, defined as people living below the national poverty line. The latest budget analysis estimated that about 28 percent of the population (in the informal sector) is eligible for subsidized insurance (Lee et al. 2018).

The HFS also sought to tackle the big issue of provider payment. As mentioned earlier, the HFS would separate the functions of providing and purchasing healthcare services. The insurance fund would mediate all payments to health providers for treatment included in the benefit package (Health Sector Technical Working Group 2017). The second main component of the proposal was the introduction of capitation-based payments by the CHFs, as well as improvement of the allocation formula for the public HBF (Lee et al. 2018).

Finally, the 2015 HFS aimed to diversify and increase the financial resources through new sources such as earmarked taxes. This would help decrease the high dependency on external development partners and donors (Ministry of Health and Social Welfare 2015), especially for insurance schemes targeting the informal sector and rural populations (Lee et al. 2018).

The HFS proposal underwent several rounds of reviews in the Inter-Ministerial Technical Committee (IMTC). The IMTC accepted the idea of mandatory insurance, the new public financing (except earmarked taxes) and a standardized, minimum benefits package. The cabinet rejected the SNHI in favor of reforming and harmonizing all CHF and TIKA schemes, however. The current way forward for the HFS in Tanzania—while waiting for future approval of the SNHI proposal—appears to be twofold. First, they include mandatory enrollment in the NHIF for workers in the formal sector. Second, they include efforts to improve and harmonize the CHFs and TIKAs, with effective targeting of vulnerable groups in the informal sector (Health Sector Technical Working Group 2017). Capacity building and training of LGAs for effective management of the system started in early 2018. The underwriting of the matching fund (financed primarily by development partners through the HBF) that currently supports the CHFs remains unclear, however (Lee et al. 2018).

Summary

Tanzania's experience shows, first, that it is possible to improve the health of a country's population even with very modest levels of public health spending.

Second, as one of the poorest nations in sub-Saharan Africa, Tanzania has been a major recipient of foreign aid for its healthcare. While external contributions helped expand investments in health services that contributed to the improvement of the population's health, they also created problems. They added to the fragmentation by setting up disease-specific programs ("silos"), and commonly appeared to follow the priorities of the donor rather than the recipient. This fragmentation added to administrative costs and duplication of services.

Third, Tanzania's experience in the framing of national health policy illustrates a high degree of path dependency. Its popular first President Nyerere established the tradition of central planning and control over public services. That tradition is still visible today. It assumes a central role of government in the financing and provision of healthcare service—at least, on paper—while sometimes ignoring the importance of the non-profit and for-profit sectors of modern western and traditional medicine.

Fourth, the experience illustrates the importance of distinguishing policy-making, the formal statements in government documents, such as in health sector plans or legislation passed by Parliament, and the ultimate policy outcome (Palmer and Short 1968). As seen in other countries in this volume, the policy rhetoric as presented in formal government plans and proposals often deviates from reality.

The reality, then, of Tanzania's health, healthcare and health policy-making by the end of the second decade of the 20th century shows a complicated picture. There has been progress in the health of the population, as noted earlier. Moreover, even with modest amounts of public investment, the public health infrastructure has benefitted from the expanded investments. Nonetheless, efforts to develop voluntary pre-paid insurance plans for low-income populations in rural and urban areas have not been very successful. These schemes were often plagued by chronic underfunding due to low contributions and low subscription rates, and developed a high dependency on long-term government support and external donor financing. They also faced inefficient management, fraud and abuse (Wang and Rosemberg 2018). The insurance for the formal sector reached less than 10 percent of the population by 2018. The proposal for a universal health insurance died in the Cabinet in 2015.

The abovementioned problems are not unique to Tanzania, as we will show in this volume. In that regard, the lessons from Germany's health insurance history are important to all nations eager to implement population-wide social insurance. It took decades, if not more than a century, for Germany's local, regional and craft-based mutual health insurances to become viable and sustainable income protection schemes for their members. Many of those plans struggled to survive as their small membership and unstable revenues did not provide a solid base for long-term insurance. That only changed with mandatory membership after the passage of the social health insurance by Chancellor Bismarck in 1883. That step codified social insurance and mandated industrial workers (and later, other groups) to become member of a sick fund at the end of the 19th century. It also allowed for a larger scale of operations of the funds. Their long experience with the running of local and regional mutual insurance schemes also contributed to build up of administrative capacity, active membership control and trust.

References

Afnan-Holmes, H., M. Magoma, T. John, et al. 2015. "Tanzania's Countdown to 2015: an analysis of two decades of progress and gaps for reproductive, maternal, newborn, and child health, to inform priorities for post-2015." *Lancet Glob Health*, 3(7): e396–e409.

Binyaruka, P. and J. Borghi. 2017. "Improving quality of care through payment for performance: examining effects on the availability and stock-out of essential medical commodities in Tanzania." *Trop Med Int Health*, 22(1): 92–102. doi:10.1111/tmi.12809

Binyaruka, P. and J. Borghi. 2018. "Does payment for performance increase performance inequalities across health providers? A case study of Tanzania." *Health Policy Plan*, 33, 1026–1036. doi:10.1093/heapol/czy084

Buse, K., D. Booth, and A. Harmer. 2008. *Donors and the Political Dimensions of Health Sector Reform: The Cases of Tanzania and Uganda.* London: Overseas Development Institute.

Chimhutu, V., M. Tjomsland, N.G. Songstad, et al. 2015. "Introducing payment for performance in the health sector of Tanzania–the policy process." *Global Health*, 11: 38. doi:10.1186/s12992-015-0125-9.

Conyers, D. 1981. "Decentralization for regional development: a comparative study of Tanzania, Zambia and Papua New Guinea." *Public Adm Dev*, 1(2): 107–120.

Development Partners Group Tanzania. 2005. *Terms of Reference for Development Partners Group on Health (DPG Health)*. Dar es Salaam: DPG.

Frumence, G., T. Nyamhanga, M. Mwangu, and A.-K. Hurtig. 2013. "Challenges to the implementation of health sector decentralization in Tanzania: experiences from Kongwa district council." *Global Health Action*, 6(1): 20983. doi:10.3402/gha.v6i0.20983

Gilson, L. 1995. "Management and healthcare reform in sub-Saharan Africa." *Soc Sci Med*, 40(5), 695–710.

Health Sector Technical Working Group. 2017. *Update on HFS. Feedback from IMTC*. Presented at the Presentation at the Joint HF & PFM TWGs, November 9, 2017. Unpublished.

Hirschman, A.O. 1970. *Exit, Voice and Loyalty. Responses to Decline in Firms, Organizations, and States*. Cambridge: Harvard University Press.

Hutton, G. and M. Tanner. 2004. "The sector-wide approach: a blessing for public health?" *Bull of the World Health Organization*, 82: 893–893.

Janus, H. and N. Keijzer. 2015. *Big Results Now? Emerging Lessons from Results-Based Aid in Tanzania* (SSRN Scholarly Paper No. ID 2673227). Rochester, NY: Social Science Research Network.

Joseph, C. and S.O. Maluka. 2016. "Do management and leadership practices in the context of decentralisation influence performance of community health fund? Evidence from Iramba and Iringa districts in Tanzania." *Int J Health Policy Manag*, 6(5): 257–265.

Kamuzora, P. and L. Gilson. 2007. "Factors influencing implementation of the Community Health Fund in Tanzania." *Health Policy Plan*, 22(2): 95–102.

Kapologwe, N.A., G.B. Kagaruki, A. Kalolo, et al. 2017. "Barriers and facilitators to enrollment and re-enrollment into the community health funds/Tiba Kwa Kadi (CHF/TIKA) in Tanzania: a cross-sectional inquiry on the effects of socio-demographic factors and social marketing strategies." *BMC Health Serv Res*, 17(308). doi:10.1186/s12913-017-2250-z

Kumaranayake, L., S. Lake, P. Mujinja, et al. 2000. "How do countries regulate the health sector? Evidence from Tanzania and Zimbabwe." *Health Policy Plan*, 15(4): 357–367.

Kwesigabo, G., M.A. Mwangu, D.C. Kakoko, et al. 2012. "Tanzania's health system and workforce crisis." *J Public Health Policy*, 33: 35–44.

Lambo, E. and L.G. Sambo. 2003. "Health Sector Reform in sub-Saharan Africa: a synthesis of country experiences." *East Afr Med J*, 80(6), S1–S20.

Lee, B., K. Tarimo, and A. Dutta. 2018. *Tanzania's Improved Community Health Fund. An Analysis of Scale-Up Plans and Design*. Health Policy Plus Policy Brief, October 2018, Washington, DC: Health Policy Plus.

Maluka, S. and D. Chitama. 2017. *Primary Health Care Systems (PRIMASYS): Comprehensive Case Study from United Republic of Tanzania*. http://hdl. handle.net/20.500.11810/4738.

Masanja, H., D. de Savigny, P. Smithson, et al. 2008. "Child survival gains in Tanzania: analysis of data from demographic and health surveys." *The Lancet*, 371(9620): 1276–1283.

Mayumana, I., J. Borghi, L. Anselmi, et al. 2017. "Effects of Payment for performance on accountability mechanisms: evidence from Pwani, Tanzania." *Soc Sci Med*, 179: 61–73. doi:10.1016/j.socscimed.2017.02.022

Ministry of Health. 1990. *National Health Policy*. Dodoma: The United Republic of Tanzania.

Ministry of Health. 2003. *National Health Policy*. Dodoma: The United Republic of Tanzania.

Ministry of Health. 2007. *National Health Policy*. Dodoma: The United Republic of Tanzania.

Ministry of Health, Community Development, Gender, Elderly and Children. 2017a. *HFR Web Portal-Facilities*. http://hfrportal.ehealth.go.tz/index. php?r=facilities/facilitiesList. Accessed December 29, 2017.

Ministry of Health, Community Development, Gender, Elderly and Children. 2017b. *The National Health Policy 2017. Sixth Draft Version for External Consultation with Ministries, Departments and Agencies*. Dodoma: The United Republic of Tanzania.

Mtei, G. and J. Mulligan. 2007. *Community Health Funds in Tanzania: A Literature Review*. Ifakara: Ifakara Health Research and Development Centre.

Mubyazi, G.M. 2004. "The Tanzanian policy on health-care fee waivers and exemptions in practice as compared with other developing countries: evidence from recent local studies and international literature." *East Afr J Publ Health*, 1(1).

Mujinja, P.G. and T.M. Kida. 2014. *Implications of health sector reforms in Tanzania: Policies, indicators and accessibility to health services*. ESRF Discussion Paper 62. Dar es Salaam: Economic and Social Research Foundation.

Musau, S., G. Chee, R. Patsika, et al. 2011. *Tanzania Health System Assessment 2010 Report* (HFG Project). Bethesda, MD: Health Systems 20/20 project, Abt Associates Inc. https://www.hfgproject.org/tanzania-health-system-assessment-2010-report/. Accessed December 29, 2017.

National Bureau of Statistics (NBS). 2017. *Tanzania Total Population by District–Regions*, 2016–2017. http://www.nbs.go.tz/nbstz/index.php/english/statistics-by-subject/population-and-housing-census/844-tanzania-total-population-by-district-regions-2016. Accessed January 9, 2018.

National Health Insurance Fund (NHIF). 2018. *Accredited Vituo*. http://www.nhif.or.tz/facilities. Accessed November 9, 2018.

Prabhakaran, S. and A. Dutta. 2017. *Actuarial study of the proposed single national health insurance scheme in Tanzania*. Health Policy Project Policy Brief, Palladium Group, 11/17.

Semali, I.A.J., D. de Savigny, M. Tanner, and C. Akim. 2004. "Health sector reforms and decentralization in Tanzania: the case of expanded program on immunization at national level." *East Afr J Publ Health*, 1(1): 33–40.

Semali, I.A.J., M. Tanner, and D. de Savigny. 2007. "Health reform cycles in Tanzania: 1924–1994." *Tanzania J Dev Stud*, 7(2): 89–102.

Wang, H. and N. Rosemberg. 2018. "Universal health coverage in low-income countries: Tanzania's efforts to overcome barriers to equitable health service access." *Universal Health Coverage Study Series*. Washington DC: World Bank Group: 39.

West-Slevin, K., C. Barker, and M. Hickman. 2015. "Snapshot: Tanzania's health system." *Health Policy Project Policy Brief*. Futures Group.

West-Slevin, K. and A. Dutta. 2015. "Prospects for sustainable health financing in Tanzania." *Health Policy Project Policy Brief*. Futures Group.

World Bank. 2017. *World Development Indicators*. http://databank.worldbank.org/ data/reports.aspx?source=2&country=TZA. Accessed December 29, 2017.

WHO. 2011. *The Abuja Declaration: Ten Years On.* Geneva: World Health Organization.

WHO. 2016. *United Republic of Tanzania WHO Country Cooperation Strategy 2016–2020*. Brazzaville: WHO Regional Office for Africa. World Health Organization.

WHO. 2017. *Global Health Expenditure Database*. World Health Organization. http://apps.who.int/nha/database/ViewData/Indicators/en. Accessed December 29, 2017.

Section II

Health Reforms in Latin America: Chile and Ecuador

Some of the world's most dramatic political transformations in the late 20th century took place with the 'bloodless revolutions' of Latin American nations shedding their military dictatorships. None of those bloodless revolutions were simple or without conflict, but they ultimately resulted in relatively stable democracies across the continent. Periods of high economic growth, well-educated elites strongly in favor of establishing democratic governance and earlier traditions of civic society organizations (e.g., labor unions supporting social health insurance) were factors that contributed to relative stability. While periods of high economic growth alternated with stagnation (and populist, if democratically elected, leaders often turned more autocratic over time), Latin American countries generally succeeded in improving incomes, education levels and the health of their populations.

Still, they also faced the legacies of economic inequalities, weak or absent democratic institutions, the exclusion and abuse of minorities, environmental damage and one-sided economies dependent on primary resources (e.g., mining, wine, meat or other agriculture) with relatively low levels of manufactured exports. After the economic downturn in the 1980s, some nations were pressured by the International Monetary Fund (IMF) and World Bank to follow the policy recommendations of the

Washington Consensus.[1] In healthcare, that translated into measures to replace state-financed healthcare with private health insurance and for-profit services. Not all nations embraced that route, however, and the nations analyzed in this regional section took diverging pathways in their efforts to expand access to healthcare.

Their experience illustrates how exclusionary regimes can implement major change in a relatively short period of time. The military dictatorship of Chile, for example, restricted access to policy-making, crushed protests and banished actors and public opinion from discussions. While the regime encouraged private health insurance and cut down public spending, it did not do away with public health services or public insurance. Likewise, there was strong support for public healthcare as a human right after the restoration of democracy in 1990, but that did not lead to the abolishment or even substantial reform of private health insurance. The changes in political regime thus created windows of opportunity for change, but the Chilean experience also illustrates how dominant values as well as institutional legacies impose limits on what government can do.

While Ecuador had a more stable history than many other Latin American nations, it also had weaker institutions. Democratically elected administrations alternated with military juntas and authoritarian rulers for much of the 20th century. President Rafael Correa stepped into office with very high approval rates in 2007, and was reelected in 2009 (he became one of the longest serving presidents of Ecuador). Rejecting the Washington Consensus, he presented a new constitution in 2008 and the national 'Good Living Plan' of 2010 that reaffirmed a strong role of the state,

---

[1] The Washington Consensus, the (informal) agreement between the IMF, World Bank and US Department of the Treasury, became popular during the 1980s. It entailed a set of economic policy recommendations for developing countries. The Consensus reflected the neoliberal view favoring free markets and a reduced role of the state, with reforms that included debt management, control of inflation, reduction of government deficits, open trade policies and privatization. Over time, the term became associated with the dogmatic "trickle-down" (or voodoo) economics, and more and more critics and civic society organizations pointed out by the late 1990s that the recommendations of the Consensus had failed to deliver their promises.

participatory public policy-making and programs to eradicate inequity, exclusion and discrimination. Health regained its status as a human right, supported by the goal of universal coverage. Other elements of the reforms included additional financing (helped by a boom in oil revenues). They targeted specific populations (e.g., mothers, rural and indigenous groups) and sought administrative decentralization and improved coordination of services.

The reform initially seemed successful in reestablishing the state as a central actor, but there was growing concern over the slow pace of implementation and lack of resources. The system remained fragmented and the private sector gained ground as the health ministry increasingly contracted out services. At first, Correa's successor, Moreno, promised to continue the social policies of his predecessor. Moreno did increase the freedom of the press and undid some measures of his predecessor, which were widely seen as improper interference in the judiciary system. Under growing fiscal and budgetary pressure, however, he shifted to a more conservative course and after a referendum in early 2018, there were concerns that Moreno was heading in the same direction as prior regimes with a more authoritarian course.

Map 3. Population, Income Level and Health Expenditure in Ghana and Tanzania, 1960–2015

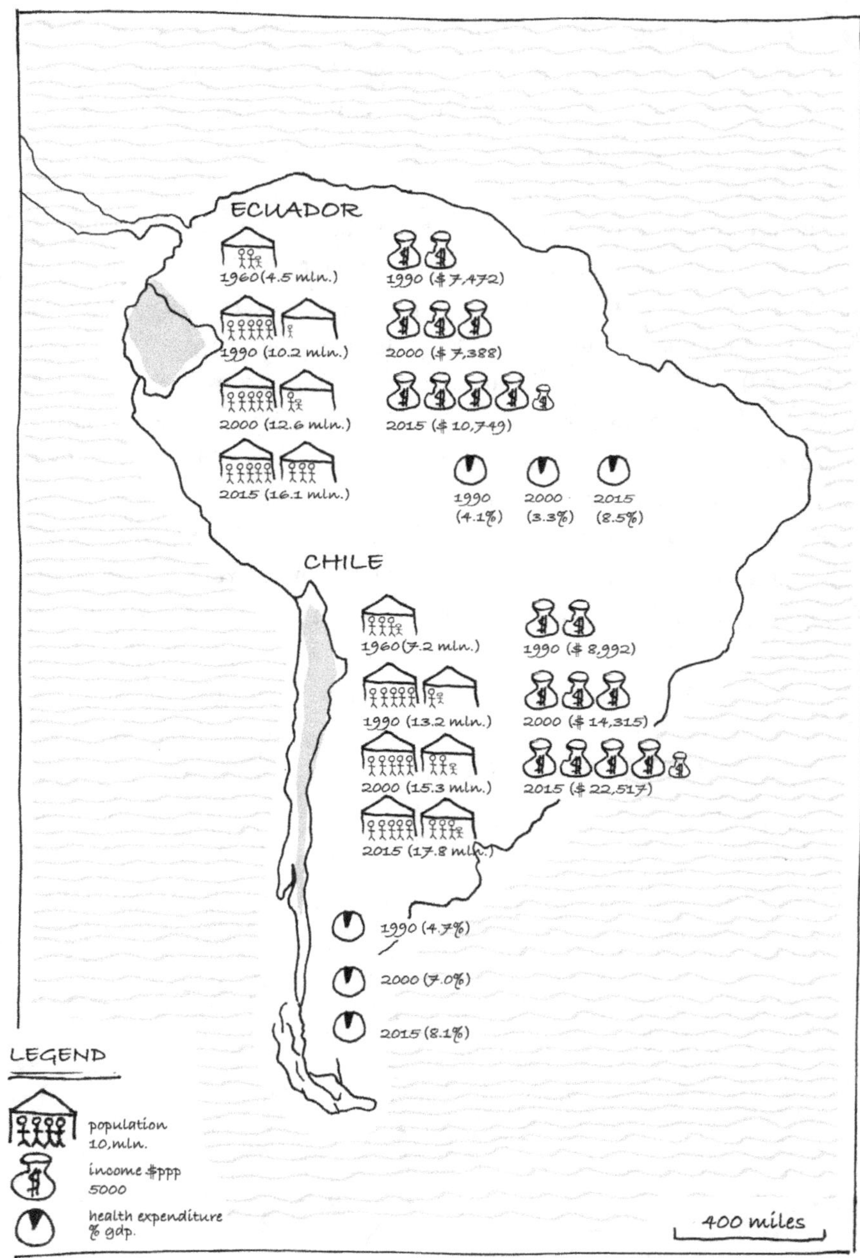

Map 4. Number of Physicians, Infant Mortality and Life Expectancy in Ghana and Tanzania, 1960–2015

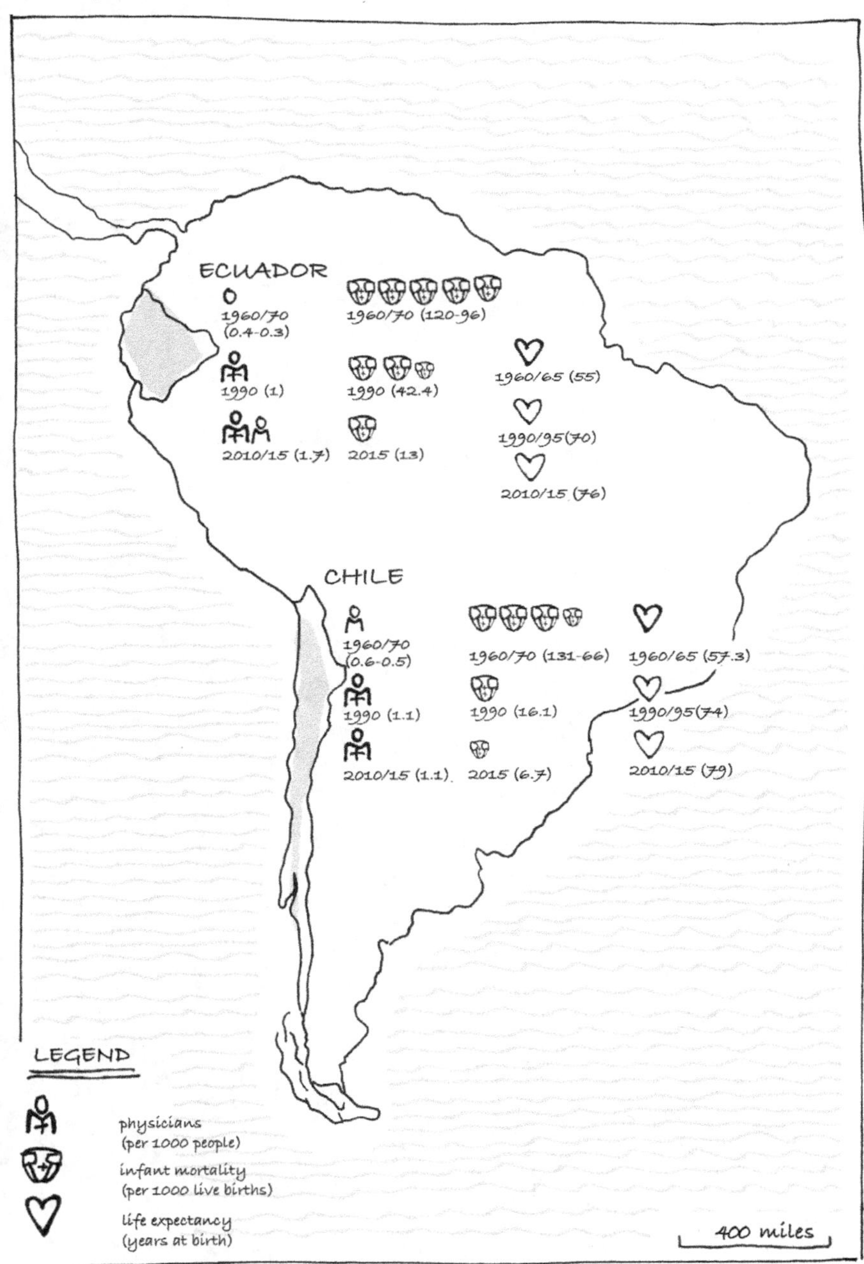

Chapter 3

Health Reforms in Chile

Guillermo Paraje

Introduction

Chile is a mid-sized country in southwestern Latin America with a population of about 17.6 million in 2018. The Andes mountain range provides much of the natural border with Argentina in the east, the Pacific Ocean in the west. In the north, Chile borders Peru and in the northeast, Bolivia. Easter Island also falls under Chile's jurisdiction. The country emerged as a unitary democratic republic in 1833. A modern liberal charter replaced the conservative constitution in 1925. The charter was in effect until September 1973 when general Pinochet's military coup ended the democratic rein of Salvador Allende. In fact, until then, Chile had been one of the Americas' most stable democracies. Pinochet imposed a new constitution in 1980. His dictatorship ended in 1990 with general elections, which restored democratic authorities. The sharp political reversals during the 20th century created windows of opportunity for major shifts in policy directions, but did not result in the abandonment of every institution created by previous regimes.

Major Changes in Chile's Health Financing in the 20th Century

Chile was one of the first countries in Latin America with social insurance systems for public sector workers and urban, manual workers in the early 20th century. Modeled after the Bismarckian social insurance of 1883, the

Caja del Seguro Obrero (SO) covered blue-collar urban workers from 1924. The SO entitlements included sick leave and medical benefits, maternity and child healthcare and benefits in case of old age, disability and death. The SO ran its own health facilities and reimbursed charity care for the poor in hospitals of the colonial institution *Beneficencia Pública*. It faced internal problems: shortages of funds, internal disputes over its administrative structure and opposition from physicians wary of external control over their liberal practices. While the insured had free choice of doctor, many physicians simply did not accept SO patients.

The SO merged with the *Caja de Previsión de Empleados Particulares*, the scheme for white-collar workers, to create the *Servicio Médico Nacional de Empleados*, the National Health Service for Employees (SERMENA) in 1942 (De Viado and Flores 1944). The armed forces have had their own health service since 1915. The development of the social insurance systems prompted physicians to establish their own association in 1958, the *Colegio Médico de Chile*. Over time, the Colegio became one of the strongest stakeholders in the healthcare arena. That institutional legacy is still visible today.

The three major political parties took widely divergent positions regarding future policy directions. The left preferred a centrally planned state-run National Health Service (NHS), which would include all health services—a plan heavily opposed by white-collar workers and the medical association in favor of liberal medicine. The center-left *Partido Radical* favored the Western European model of social insurance as administered by the SO, complemented by extensive public health programs. The conservative right favored voluntary private insurance with prevention programs for the working population, modeled after the *Ley de Medicina Preventiva*, the Preventive Medicine Law of 1938, with compulsory medical examinations for syphilis, tuberculosis and heart disease. In the early 1950s, the new Social Christian party (later renamed Christian Democratic Party, PDC) joined the left-center coalition government. This unlocked a window of opportunity (Kingdon 1984) for the proponents of a NHS modeled after the British NHS. Two leading health experts, Dr. Benjamin Viel and the lawyer Francisco Pinto, visited the United Kingdom to study the new NHS (Pinto Santa Cruz and Viel 1950). In 1952, the government begun the implementation of the universal *Sistema Nacional de Salud* (SNS) based on the citizens' right to healthcare. The SNS was the first of its type in Latin America and several other nations followed.

Implementation was slow, however. The SNS faced several problems: lack of finances and manpower, fragmentation and unequal access to healthcare, as some groups were left out (e.g., white-collar workers, rural workers and the unemployed). The system mostly covered formal blue-collar workers. The SNS thus did not lead to genuine universal or equal access.

The first PDC government under President Eduardo Frei (1964–1970) represented the new entrepreneurial spirit of the modern middle class. It decided to address the unequal access to the SNS. The center-left parties advocated for a transformation of the SNS into a NHS, entirely financed out of general taxation. The medical association, *Colegio Médico*, opposed the proposal; however, together with the (white-collar) employees who did not want to be equated with (blue-collar) workers. It instead proposed to extend SERMENA's free-choice model. Chile's Parliament finally passed a law in 1968 offering a free-choice scheme for public and private employees and a separate insurance for blue-collar workers. SERMENA would administer the latter, to be reimbursed by SNS. President Frei, Senator Salvador Allende and others realized that this would lead to further fragmentation and a stronger class bias of the SNS, but considered the law a transitory agreement. When Allende became president in November 1970, he announced the creation of the *Sistema Unico de Salud*, the universal health system, evoking strong political opposition from most physicians.

Almost two years later, the military coup directed by general Pinochet led to Allende's death in September 1973. The dictatorship engaged in a radical neoliberal experiment. It sought to reduce the role of the state, privatize pensions and social security, and introduce markets and consumer choice in healthcare (Foxley 1988; Jost 1999). It drastically reduced public spending and cut public health services. It also banned all political parties and corporations, including the medical association.

The regime opened the private healthcare market in 1982. Under the new public scheme (created from SERMENA), *Fondo Nacional de Salud* (FONASA, National Health Fund), insured were allowed to opt out and seek private coverage, with heavy subsidies for the private health insurers, the *Instituciones de Salud Previsional* (ISAPREs; Jost 1999; Unger et al. 2008; Barrientos and Loyd-Sherlock 2000). As in other countries, the option to exit from the public system without restrictions, expressive of the neoliberal consumer's right to choose, led to a spiraling process of risk selection as private insurers did not have to accept everyone seeking coverage. The young and healthy went mostly private, but a disproportionally high number of sick and elderly (as well as females of reproductive age) had to remain in (or return to) the public scheme, as they faced serious access barriers to the private market (Barrientos 2002; Höfter 2006). The contribution rates for FONASA (and later the rates for ISAPREs as well) went up from 2 to 7 percent of income (with a monthly income ceiling that today would be about $2,700). Those who chose (and were accepted for enrollment by) one of the private ISAPREs, insurers were exempt from paying contributions to FONASA (unlike the National Insurance schemes of Canada, Israel or Taiwan, where there is no opting out). The ISAPREs initially grew rapidly. By 1995, they covered about 30 percent of the population, but lost ground again after the return to democracy (see below).

The Pinochet dictatorship next created the National System of Health Services, the *Sistema Nacional de Servicios de Salud* (SNSS). It decentralized the SNSS into 26 semi-autonomous regional boards, financed out of the national FONASA health fund. The responsibility for providing primary care shifted to the municipalities.

With those steps, access to healthcare became even more fragmented and stratified. FONASA beneficiaries fell into four categories, depending on taxable household income. Categories A and B included the unemployed, indigents with no income and very low-income households, while categories C and D covered higher income groups. Beneficiaries could choose to use two different modalities for healthcare. The first, the *Modalidad de Atentión Institucional* (MAI, or Public Institutions

Modality), was mandatory for those in the FONASA A and B categories, with no co-payment. Those in groups B, C and D could voluntarily use this modality, but with co-payments (10 percent for group C and 20 percent for group D). The *Modalidad Libre Elección* (MLE, the free-choice modality) reimbursed the cost of care by independent professionals and private facilities. For this care, FONASA gave providers vouchers according to the set fee schedule, while patients had to cover the difference between those vouchers and the actual price (Superintendencia de Salud 2009). MLE charged three levels of co-payments, ranging from 25 to 60 percent, depending on the category of healthcare. Most physicians billed for services with the highest co-payments (Labra 2007). A small proportion of uninsured (those who were working informally and were not contributing 7 percent of their incomes) paid for their care out-of-pocket. FONASA and ISAPREs agencies received employees' contributions directly from employers. At no point did workers have to pay themselves, since employers automatically deducted contributions from their gross wages.

The proportion of uninsured has been decreasing over time. A recent reform mandated that the self-employed contribute either to FONASA or to ISAPREs. This reform was scheduled for full implementation in 2018.

After the return to democracy in 1990, President Patricio Aylwin announced massive new investments to improve the quality of public health services and reduce waitlists. While embracing the principles of equity, solidarity and universal access, the new regime did not abolish the dual insurance system. It did impose more regulation on private insurance. For example, insurers had to offer a minimum coverage with uniform community-rated premiums within each health plan (though there were thousands of plans offered in the market, creating the possibility for insurers to 'cream-skim') and accept dependents. Spouses were no longer permitted to split membership between public and private insurance, with one partner under public, the other under private coverage. The government phased out subsidies for the privately insured, causing a drop in ISAPRE membership from about 25 to 19 percent between 1997 and 2016 (ISAPRES 2016).

The ISAPREs continued to function as traditional for-profit insurers offering sick leave and healthcare coverage. Some ISAPREs owned health facilities, and some had preferred provider arrangements (Jost 1999). Predictably, they attracted mostly affluent, young, urban males. Since they charged risk-rated premiums for each group of insured (until regulation banned that practice), women paid more than men (and got lower financial coverage), and people over 60 sometimes faced premiums up to eight times more than young adults (Unger et al. 2008). Most ISAPREs charged user fees, subject to legal caps aimed to mitigate the financial burden for low-income families. The ISAPREs faced increased competition by American-style HMOs (Barrientos and Lloyd-Sherlock 2000), though the number of such plans remained low.

Health of Chile's Population

Aggregate health indicators are relatively good in Chile, though there are important socio-economic disparities. Life expectancy at birth is currently 80 years, higher than some developed countries including the US Infant mortality (under the age of one) saw a rapid decline, from 66.5 to 6.3 per 1,000 live births between 1970 and 2017 (World Bank 2017). Maternal mortality went down from 55 to 22 per 100,000 live births between 1990 and 2013 (WHO 2018). There were over 17,000 physicians in 2010 or just over 1 per 1,000 people in the population; and barely 0.15 nurses and midwives per 1,000 people in that year (WHO 2018). The general level of health, as shown by numerous studies since the famous Lalonde Report of 1974, is narrowly associated with non-medical determinants of health like genetic disposition, income, work environment and living conditions. Nonetheless, healthcare plays a role, too, especially in reducing child and maternal mortality, and Chile has obviously made good progress with those indicators by investing in child vaccination and maternal and pediatric healthcare. Child vaccination rates are now similar to those in high-income industrialized nations.

Total fertility rates dropped to 1.8 percent, below the replacement rate, and the country's population is rapidly aging. The elderly dependency ratio (the ratio between the population over 60 and the population age 15–59) went up from 14.7 to 20.1 between 1970 and 2010 and is expected to reach 38.7 in 2030 (Fajnzylber and Paraje 2014).

Apart from this demographic transition, the country experienced an epidemiological transition from contagious to non-communicable diseases (NCDs). The prevalence of risk factors like alcohol and tobacco use, obesity, and sedentary lifestyle are among the highest in the Americas (WHO 2018). This casts a shadow over future health gains. NCDs pose new challenges to the health system, and will require more money and long-term care.

Healthcare and Health Financing in Chile, 2018

The current mix of financing sources for Chile's healthcare reflects the 20th century development as pictured earlier: it combines social insurance plans for employees, civil servants and other groups with voluntary private insurance for the self-employed and some higher income groups and tax-funded subsidies for public healthcare.

Facing opposition against the market-oriented policies of the former military dictatorship, the democratic government reaffirmed its strong commitment to the public health system in the late 1990s. Most hospitals, clinics and municipal primary care centers remained under public ownership and control. Physicians working at public hospitals are public employees but they can work as private physicians when they are not working for the hospitals. Some public hospitals have been allowed, for a certain number of years, to function as semi-private autonomous operators. FONASA settled long-term contracts with hospitals for the payment of inpatient care. These payments funded the largest share of the hospitals' revenues; only about 15 percent came from private-insured patients.

The government announced a shift towards capitation payment for primary care (a fixed amount per patient registered with a physician's practice) and case-based (diagnosis-related-group based, [DRG-based]) payment for hospital care in the late 1990s, paid through FONASA. Implementation of those changes was slow, however. The DRG-based payments initially covered a limited number of conditions, expanding slowly over time. By the mid-2000s, DRGs only covered about 10 percent of hospital revenues—an experience similar to that in other nations (see e.g., the chapters on Taiwan or the Netherlands in this volume).

The Health Reform Commission of 2000, with representatives from physician associations, health worker unions and private providers, identified four sector objectives: improving health indicators, addressing changing demand due to aging and other factors, reducing health inequalities across socio-economic groups and improving the accessibility and quality of healthcare services (Labra and Tapia 2005). These recommendations led to several legislative proposals to improve administration and management, further regulations to ISAPREs and improvement of access to high-cost treatment. The latter step became known as the *Plan AUGE* of 2005.

AUGE started with only 25 conditions but rapidly expanded. It covered 80 conditions by 2018, representing close to 60 percent of the country's disease burden. It includes several types of cancer (both pediatric and adult), cardiovascular disease, HIV/AIDS, chronic conditions (like diabetes, hypertension or depression) and life-improving interventions (e.g., hip replacement, cataract surgery and hearing devices). The program has universal coverage (ISAPREs also have to cover their beneficiaries, though they can charge an extra premium), but there is some restriction on the choice of providers, as insurance agencies define a closed provider network.

AUGE conditions have well-defined medical protocols, which have helped keep costs under control, for both ISAPREs and FONASA insured. ISAPREs insurers receive reimbursement for the cost of treating AUGE conditions though a risk equalization fund. It uses age and sex as criteria for the reallocation of funds. The ISAPREs cannot discriminate and have to charge their insured populations community-rated premiums for AUGE coverage (Paraje and Infante 2014).

The AUGE scheme emphasizes prevention, early detection and primary care. It set maximum wait times and annual limits on the amounts that families spend on healthcare (Bossert and Leisewitz 2016). Generally, the plan has been considered an important starting point in ensuring universal access to (high-cost) healthcare, but it also raised issues regarding the definition of entitlements, persistent gender inequalities in health and the exclusion of certain population groups (e.g., the indigenous, women and unpaid caregivers) in decision-making (Dannreuther and Gideon 2008).

Initially, health professionals resisted the plan, especially members of the *Colegio Médico*, who resisted the idea of intervention in their medical practices, the imposition of clinical protocols and limited freedom of patients to choose among providers. The general public, on the other hand, expressed support for the plan, especially for the financial protection it offered, even though after more than 12 years a significant portion of the population is not yet familiar with the details (Paraje and Infante 2014).

Administration of Healthcare in Chile, 2018

The overall stewardship of the health system is, exclusively, in the hands of the Ministry of Health (MoH). Apart from providing public health guidelines and general supervision, the MoH is in charge of supervising the activities of five autonomous organizations: (1) the *Sistema de Servicios Nacional de Salud* (SSNS, the NHSs System), with 29 regional branches, provides health promotion and healthcare through a network of public primary health centers, hospitals and other public providers; (2) FONASA; (3) the *Instituto Nacional de Salud Pública* (INSP, the National Public Health Institute), in charge of authorizing and supervising pharmaceutical production and sales; (4) the *Central Nacional de Abastecimiento* (CENABAST, the National Supply Center), which centralizes purchases of prescription drugs and public hospital inputs; and (5) the *Superintendencia de Salud* (SoS, Superintendence of Health), in charge of supervising and regulating health insurance agencies, both FONASA and ISAPREs (Becerril-Montekio et al. 2011).

The regional branches of the SSNS are responsible for the implementation of national health policies and the allocation of available health resources. The SNSS budget is part of the MoH budget, approved by Congress as part of the general state budget.

Though FONASA falls, in theory, under the supervision of the SoS, in practice it is relatively autonomous. FONASA is technically an insurance agent, but it is also in charge of allocating resources to local health authorities and even for certain investments in health facilities.

Since 1920, the municipalities have been the backbone of the Chilean health system, responsible for primary healthcare. The MoH determines the available budgets for these services based on population numbers. As most resources for health at the municipality level come from this budget, the primary health services have an incentive to refer complex (and expensive) cases to secondary level hospitals. This weakens their role as gatekeeper, which aims to reduce excess use of hospital care by FONASA beneficiaries. In contrast, the ISAPRE beneficiaries are not covered for services in municipal health centers, and this too has an effect of increasing health expenditures.

Conclusions

Chile's current healthcare system reflects the numerous shifts in political direction during the 20th century. It combines contributory social and private health insurance, separate schemes for specific populations like the police and army, with tax-financed public health services. The social insurance systems started in the early 20th century and followed the Bismarckian model, which offered healthcare coverage for industrial workers. Over time the populations covered and range of benefits expanded, but effective opposition from physicians and other interested parties led to the development of parallel structures for higher income groups, such as white-collar workers and the self-employed. Mounting access problems in the private insurance market for the elderly, women in reproductive age, chronically ill or disabled, and increased risk selection prompted more and more government intervention. That experience is not unique to Chile. All countries with parallel public and private systems have faced this problem (see e.g., the chapter on the Netherlands in this volume).

The Chilean experience illustrates how exclusionary regimes can implement major change in a relatively short period of time (Labra 2007). The Pinochet dictatorship restricted access to policy-making, crushed protests and banished public opinion from discussions. It cut down on public spending and encouraged private health insurance, but it did not do away with public health services or public insurance. Likewise, strong support for public healthcare as a human right after the restoration of democracy in 1990 led to more inclusionary policy-making, but did not result in the elimination or even substantial reform of private health insurance.

This chapter illustrates how the changes in Chile's political regimes created windows of opportunity for change. Yet, the dominant values, as well as institutional legacies restricted what government could actually amend. Even while the military regime encouraged private health insurance and cut public spending, it did not abolish the social insurance structures or public health services. Likewise, while there was strong support for public healthcare as a universal right after the restoration of democracy in 1990, that did not lead to the abolishment of private insurance. As Paul Pierson (1994) argued: institutions, once in place, tend to create their own constituencies (e.g., beneficiaries, administrators and political supporters) that will resist their demise.

References

Barrientos, A. 2002. "Health policy in Chile: the return of the public sector." *Bull Latin Am Res*, 21(3): 442–459.

Barrientos, A. and P. Lloyd-Sherlock. 2000. "Reforming health insurance in Argentina and Chile." *Health Policy Plan*, 15(4): 417–423.

Becerril-Montekio, V., J.D. Dios Reyes, and A. Manuel. 2011. "Sistema de salud de Chile." *Salud Pública de México*, 53(Suplemento 2). Atlas de los sistemas de salud de América Latina y el Caribe.

Bossert, T.J. and T. Leisewitz. January 7, 2016. "Innovation and change in the Chilean Health System." *N Engl J Med*, 374(1): 1–5.

Dannreuther, C. and J. Gideon. 2008. "Entitled to health? Social protection in Chile's Plan AUGE." *Dev Change*, 39(5): 845–864.

De Viado, M., and A. Flores. 1944. "Health insurance in Chile." *CMAJ*, 51(6): 564–570.

Fajnzylber, E. and G. Paraje. 2014. "Chile." *Beyond Contributory Pensions: Fourteen Experiences with Coverage Expansion in Latin America.* Washington, DC: The World Bank.

Foxley, A. 1988. *Experimentos Neoliberales en América Latina.* Mexico City: Fondo de Cultura Económic.

Höfter, R.H. 2006. "Private health insurance and utilization of health services in Chile." *Appl Econ*, 38(4): 423–439.

ISAPRES. 2016. *ISAPRES 1981–2016: 35 Years Developing Chile's Private Health System.* Santiago de Chile: ISAPRES

Jost, T.S. 1999. "Managed care regulation: can we learn from others? The Chilean experience." *Mich J Law Reform*, 32(4): 863–98.

Kingdon, J.W. 1984. *Agendas, Alternatives, and Public Policies.* New York, NY: Longman.

Labra, M.E. 2007. "Modes of health policy making and medical interests in Chile in the 20th century." (Updated English version). M.E. "Padrões de Formulação de Políticas de Saúde no Chile no Século XX". *DADOS-Revista de Ciências Sociais*, 2000, 43(1):153–182.

Labra, M.E. and A. Tapia. 2005. *Reformas del Sector Salud y Salud Sexual y Reproductiva en América Latina y el Caribe: Tendencias e interrelaciones– una revisión. El caso de Chile.* Mexico City: UNFPA: 69–80.

Paraje, G. and A. Infante. 2014. "La Reforma AUGE 10 años después." *Las Nuevas Políticas de Protección Social en Chile* (2nd ed.). O. Larrañaga and D. Contreras (eds). Santiago de Chile, Chile: Uqbar Editores: 73–111.

Pierson, P. 1994. *Dismantling the Welfare State? Reagan, Thatcher and the Politics of Retrenchment.* Cambridge: Cambridge University Press.

Pinto Santa Cruz, F. and B. Viel. 1950. *Seguridad Social chilena: puntos para una reforma.* Santiago: Editora del Pacífico.

Reichard, S. 1996. "Ideology drives health care reforms in Chile." *J Public Health Policy*, 17(1): 80–98.

Superintendencia de Salud. 2009. *Estadísticas.* http://www.supersalud.gob.cl. Accessed August 3, 2011.

Unger, J.P., P. De Paepe, G.S. Cantuarias, and O.A. Herrera. 2008. "Chile's neoliberal health reform: an assessment and a critique." *PLOS Med*, 5(4): e79.

WHO. 2018. *WHO Health Data.* The World Health Organization. http://www. who.int/gho/maternal_health/countries/en/. Accessed January 30, 2018.

World Bank. 2008. *Realizing Rights through Social Guarantees. Analysis of New Approaches to Social Policy in Latin America and South Africa.* Social Development Department, Report No 40047-GLB. http://go.worldbank.org/ P2LXPQU1Z0. Accessed August 2, 2011.

World Bank. 2017. *The World Bank Database.* http://data.worldbank.org. Accessed May 21, 2017.

Chapter 4

Public Health Policy in Ecuador

Santiago Illescas Correa

Introduction

Ecuador is a small nation in northwest Latin America, with 16.8 million inhabitants in 2018. It is divided into four regions: the Pacific coast, the Andes, the Amazon and the insular region, which includes the Galapagos Islands. Ecuador is home to some of the highest volcanoes of Latin America: the Chimborazo, the Cotopaxi and the Tungurahua. Due to its geographical position, it has a huge variety of flora and fauna, with some of the greatest biodiversity in the world. The country has been independent since 1809. Almost 50 percent of the population was economically active, with less than 20 percent working in the formal sector. Almost one quarter lived below the poverty line. These characteristics of the country's economy obviously affect the structure of (potential) health financing.

Most nations in Latin America and the Caribbean share the political commitment to provide a basic level of social protection for the health of all their citizens. They face challenges of uneven economic growth, inequality and the legacies of military dictatorships that all but excluded civic society from social policy-making. Despite great efforts to improve that situation, and nearly two decades of health reform efforts, about 20 percent of the populations remain excluded from existing protection mechanisms, and reform results do not always match the lofty ambitions and expectations (Atun et al. 2015).

Ecuador presents an interesting case of how regime change can create windows of opportunity for social change. In this case, the Correa administration brought about a radical shift in social and health policies, based on its new Constitution and explicit reform ambitions framed in the "Good Living Plan." These reforms showed that determined leadership, along with strong popular support for explicit values of solidarity and citizenship, can develop its own course and not follow the commonly adopted neoliberal economics embraced by many other Latin American nations.

Ecuador's experience also illustrates how formally stated policies are not always the same as the policies actually implemented or the ultimate outcomes of reforms. Lack of capital, disappointment with results and opposition from the private sector and other entrenched interests led to delays in reform implementation. As Pierson (1994) argued, institutions, once in place, tend to create their own constituencies and will resist major change. Indeed, "ideas, interests and institutions" (Klein and Marmor 2006) were major factors affecting the health reform process in Ecuador.

Pressures for Change: Economic and Social Factors and Health Reform Directions

Ecuador has had a more stable history than many other nations in Latin America, but frailer democratic institutions. Weak, if democratically elected administrations alternated with military juntas and authoritarian rulers for much of the 20th century. During periods of relative calm and growing prosperity (at least for the elites) in the 1950s and 1960s, there were some efforts to modernize the economy and restore democracy. Still, the basic features of a strong, inclusive democracy were lacking: large groups of the population were restricted or excluded from access to political decision-making, as well as a lack of civic organizations and divided labor unions (Coffey 2016). In general, administrations remained more representative of elite business interests than that of the population at large.

The economic downturn of the 1980s, combined with low oil prices and skyrocketing external debt added to the political instability, in addition to a succession of ineffective and unpopular presidents (WHO 2006). The regimes of populist leaders regularly turned autocratic, marked by poor governance, corruption, abuse of power and the suppression of civil liberties and freedom of press; however, next they often found themselves ousted by the disaffected middle class who had elected them in the first place. For decades, Ecuador struggled between the utopian policies of economic efficiency and the actual deterioration in health, social, economic and political conditions and quality of life.

President Rafael Correa stepped into office with high approval rates in 2007 (he became one of Ecuador's longest serving presidents). Correa presented a new Constitution in 2008 and the *Plan National del Buen Vivir 2013–2017* ("National Good Living Plan") in 2010, which emphasized a strong role of the state, participatory public policy-making and programs to eradicate inequity, exclusion and discrimination. The government considered social policy a crucial part in the recovery of the State's role, based on principles of solidarity, universal coverage and free delivery of education, health, social protection and security. It viewed those key services as public goods rather than merchandise (Villacrés 2003).

The Correa regime explicitly rejected the Washington Consensus, the neoliberal reform recommendations of the International Monetary Fund, World Bank and European Union, which had become popular in other Latin American countries since the 1980s (Weisbrot 2017). In its health policies it opted instead for a more universal, tax-based National Health System (NHS)-model of de-commodified healthcare and health financing, with a public safety net for those excluded from the formal labor market.

The new direction included community-based programs aimed to secure universal access to healthcare and infrastructure. Health regained its status as a human right, supported by universal coverage.[1] Additional financing, improved coordination, targeted policies for specific populations (e.g., mothers and infants, rural populations and indigenous groups), integrated primary services and public networks of independent providers

---

[1]This was an interesting example of policy-making by framing certain rights in the Constitution. The problem with that approach is that governments often make sweeping promises (with statements like "healthcare for all," or "seamless care") without operationalization of those terms. The constitutional "right to health" faces the realities of shortages in public health budgets, uneven distribution of resources, feeble administration and the outright fraud and abuse that many countries struggle with.

were other elements of the reforms. The government realized that this required improved coordination and measures to reduce fragmentation of the health system, duplication of activities and waste.

The Correa administration (the "Government of the Citizens' Revolution") substantially increased agricultural subsidies and spending on social programs, most notably for healthcare and education. The government seized companies owned by a handful of powerful families who had been implicated in a 1990s banking scandal. While antagonizing some business and media groups, his reformist agenda received strong popular support from voters. In September 2008, the electorate approved a new constitutional referendum that increased presidential powers over economic and monetary policy.

The reform agenda included the establishment of a NHS. It presented basic principles for other sectorial reforms—social development and labor relations, for example—that aimed to transform the welfare matrix. That is to say, it aimed to transform the conservative corporate regime (with a Bismarckian employment-based health insurance) into a universal tax-based model. This transformation had obvious implications for the positions of certain stakeholder coalitions supporting or opposing the changes, the coverage of services, the form of financing and the degree and type of state intervention.

Ecuador's Healthcare Services, 2018

Ecuador has a mixed public–private health system. The public sector includes the providers financed by the Ministry of Public Health (MSP) and the national System of Social Security: the Ecuadorian Institute of Social Security (IESS), including the Rural Social Insurance (SSC), the Armed Forces Social Security Institute (ISSFA) and the National Police Social Security Institute (ISSPOL). The MSP system (services paid for by the *Ministerio de Salud Publica*) covers a wide range of healthcare, but with variability in access and availability. Despite efforts to enforce legal mandates and improvements in the access to prescription drugs and medical devices, the system does not guarantee a constant supply.

Table 1. MSP Coverage and Health Insurance Membership in Ecuador, 2017

	Beneficiaries	Share of Population (%)
MSP	16,503,120	100
IESS	4,316,057	26.2
SSC	820,008	5.0
ISSFA	231,507	1.4
ISSPOL	215,501	1.3
Private insurance	4,614,210	28.0

Source: INEC 2017.

As shown in Table 1, slightly more than 50 percent of the population is covered by public or private insurance. Most patients still rely on the private sector and out-of-pocket payments. The government sought to improve access to services and, above all, strengthen financial protection for certain conditions and catastrophic illnesses. It developed a separate financing system for free maternity care (SENPLADES 2010).

In principle, MSP-financed facilities are accessible to all. In practice, however, they are mostly used by the uninsured, thus people without private or public health insurance. Other ministries play a role in the health system too, for example, the Ministries of Defense, Transportation and Public Works, Education, Economic and Social Inclusion and the Coordinating Ministry of Social Development.

While IESS' role is primarily to provide insurance (it is the largest social insurance fund), it also offers healthcare services through general hospitals in large urban centers and dozens of clinics in smaller communities. Services are available to those who have made their mandatory contributions into the IESS system (through payroll deductions). IESS has been open to voluntary members since the early 2010s. Benefits include emergency care, inpatient preventive and curative care and outpatient consultation. It also covers home care as well as compensation for medical care in private clinics that have contracts with IESS. Patients generally feel that affiliation to the public social security subsystem offers the greatest coverage of medical, dental and pharmaceutical services.

Private healthcare includes both for-profit providers (health maintenance organizations [HMOs], private insurers, independent physicians, private clinics and hospitals) and non-profits like NGOs, civil society organizations or social associations. Certified private entities can act as service providers in the public system and receive reimbursement from the Social Security System. Both private insurers and HMOs are under the surveillance of the Superintendence of Companies.

Non-profits play a key role in Ecuadorian healthcare. The most important ones are the Guayaquil Welfare Board, a charity serving medium- and low-income individuals, the Guayaquil Children's Protection Society, the Cancer Society (providing specialized diagnostic and cancer treatment services in the country's main cities) and the Ecuadorian Red Cross. The Guayaquil Welfare Board and the Cancer Society are under the regulatory control of the MSP, with whom they also maintain service provision contracts. These private institutions thus act as public sector service providers.

Healthcare Financing in Ecuador, 2018

Total health expenditure in Ecuador went up from 8.6 to 9.3 percent of gross domestic product (GDP) between 2010 and 2017. Of this, 4.5 percent was public expenditure (out of the social security and MSP budgets) and 4.1 percent was private (insurance premiums and out-of-pocket payments).

The four main financing sources for Ecuador's healthcare were (1) general taxation for government-offered healthcare services, mainly through the MSP; (2) social health insurance contributions from workers in the formal sector, with general (IESS) or specific schemes (ISSFA, ISSPOL, SSC); (3) premiums for the mandatory Traffic Accident Insurance Fund (FONSAT) established in 2009, responsible for compensating victims of traffic accidents and (4) private insurance premiums and out-of-pocket payments.

Each agency of the social security system collects the contributions to finance services for specific diseases and maternity care, as covered by its insurance institutions (IESS, ISSFA and ISSPOL). The same applies to private insurers. There is a parallel system for the MSP. The financing and organization of healthcare is thus quite fragmented.

The 2008 Constitution states that health financing must "come from permanent sources of the General Government budget" to be distributed according to demographic and epidemiological criteria (population and health needs). Likewise, it defines which institutions can receive public financing. It set budget allocations for healthcare to guarantee the availability of resources, as well as annual increases in public health spending until it reaches 4 percent of GDP. The MSP budget increased from \$669 million to \$2.4 billion between 2007 and 2014.

There are no co-payments in the public system, with the exception of some health services in the ISSFA and ISSPOL subsystems. The Correa administration proposed earmarked taxes on alcohol, tobacco, and some other activities as additional health financing. There are no financial contributions from subnational governments (provinces, municipalities) for public health, as they do not have that competency (Figure 1).

Public health financing thus consisted of general taxation, specific taxes and social insurance contributions. The private sector received its resources from insurance premiums, co-payments and other direct patient payments, as well as supplemental payments and premiums for the traffic accident insurance. There were modest amounts of charitable donations and foreign development aid for specific activities (Kliksberg 2000).

Table 1 shows the relative shares of the insurance subsystems. In 2017, about 28 percent of the population had private insurance. This share was expected to go down as the Labor Ministry announced a new workers' insurance.

Resource allocation is based on national priorities. That is to say, institutional planning must correspond with the National Development Plan and MSP's social and health policy agendas. Most of the provinces' budgets (for hospitals and regional health facilities) are determined by regular activities. They can barely spend 15–20 percent of their revenue

Figure 1. Financing Ecuador's Healthcare, 2014.

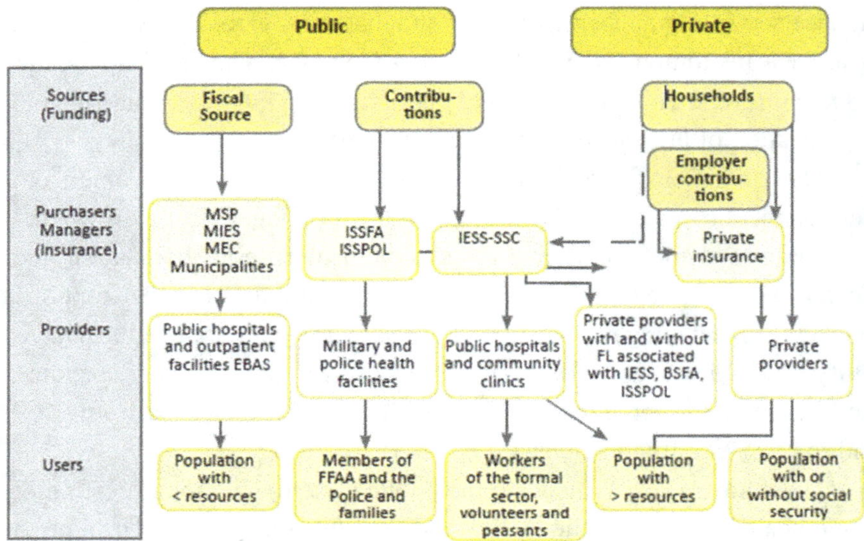

Source: MCDS 2013.

for reprogramming and adaptation to policy priorities. The situation for the Health Ministry is hardly better, as more than 85 percent of its regular budget consists of personnel salaries. The health units thus have limited capacity to obtain supplies. There is no resource allocation for autonomous subnational governments.

Two policy initiatives sought to separate the purchase and provision functions of benefits in 2006: the Law of the Provision of Free Maternity Care and a new tariff schedule. Both introduced elements of demand subsidy. The mandatory tariff schedule aims to improve universal access to the system and applies to all public and private providers. The schedule facilitates payments similar to earlier agreements with private clinics, which aimed to guarantee access to surgeries for poor patients. It also introduced rules for licensing and qualifications of all providers in the NHS, the Public Health Network and the Supplementary Network (both for-profit and non-profit organizations).

Likewise, the Law for the Provision of Free Maternity Care incorporated new elements in financing and resource management. It separated financing from provision and transferred resources to the municipalities. The law allowed for greater diversification of providers outside of services traditionally provided by the units of the Ministry itself, by including non-profit organizations and traditional providers like midwives. The Maternity and Child Care law now covers non-governmental organizations, the IESS and even traditional medicine. The MSP created an execution unit to supervise payments and increase accountability.

The MSP announced the implementation of a standardized system of accounts across healthcare institutions to allow for more transparency and easier transfer of patients. It expected that this would result in better use of (unused) capacity and a progressive leveling of the per capita expenditure across the country.

Stewardship of Ecuador's Healthcare

The MSP performs the role of national health authority. It "must create, comply with and enforce public policies of the State, developed and executed according to the Constitution" (Art. 363). The MSP is responsible for the framing and implementation of national health policies. One major plan, the Comprehensive Healthcare Model (MAIS), aimed at a new territorial organization of health services networks with an expansion of public health services and Basic Health Teams (EBAs).

The National Health Authority (thus the MSP) has overall responsibility for the NHS. That includes defining national health policy, regulation and control and setting standards for health-related activities. MSP responsibilities further include (1) expanding coverage to ensure universal healthcare coverage, and improving the quality of healthcare; (2) improving government-provided services; (3) safeguarding respect for ancestral practices; (4) special attention to priority groups; (5) implementing sexual and reproductive health-related actions, and guaranteeing women's integral health, particularly during pregnancy, delivery and postpartum; (6) ensuring the availability of safe and effective medication; and (7) improving health-care for the workforce (López-Cevallos and Chunhuei 2010).

The National Health Council (CONASA), a semi-independent legal entity with administrative and financial autonomy is responsible for inter-sector coordination, consensus-building and inter-sector health policies. It shares the stewardship function with the MSP.

Decentralization and De-concentration of Health Administration

The policy directions guided by the "Good Living" principles entailed the decentralization and deconcentration[2] of budgetary responsibilities and decision-making powers. This aimed to improve policy coordination and functional consistency in the administrations of the Ministry of Health and Social Security.

The MSP can be labeled a Type 2 organization, characterized by a high degree of deconcentration but low decentralization in the framing of its policies and articulating of processes, products and services. It has strong control over its stewardship and regulation at the central level. The regional or intermediate level is responsible for regional planning, while the local level is in charge of actually coordinating and managing services. Administrative districts (territorial entities common to the Ministries of Health, Education, Economic and Social Inclusion, and Labor) enable streamlining of public service provision at the local level. There have been shifts in political power since 2007, with greater authority, resources and decision-making powers granted to regional and local governments. Figure 2 shows the country's political and administrative territorial structure: autonomous governments and territorial structures created to perform the national executive function at the zonal and districts levels.

These changes redefined the roles of national, regional, provincial and municipal authorities. They sought to pave the way for greater social

---

[2]Decentralization means the shift in financing and decision-making power from central government to regional and local authorities; de-concentrating entails the shift of certain administrative functions from the central (Health) Ministry to regional offices.

Figure 2. Territorial Structure of Ecuador's (Health) Administration, 2018.

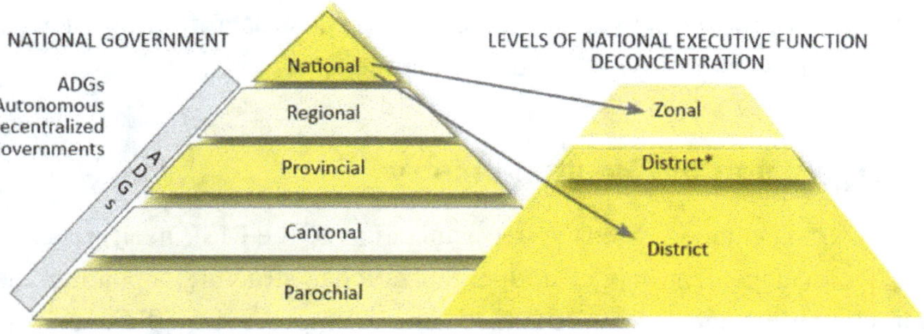

Source: MSP 2010.

participation in public administration. The government next proposed redrawing the country's administrative districts to enhance the local provision of public services, and announced it would adjust the existing scheme of provincial offices (MSP 2010).

Strengthening the National Health Authority

The MSP announced the creation of three specialized entities: the General Coordination of Strategic Development in Health, the Health Governance Undersecretariat and the semi-independent Control Agency for Health Facilities. The General Coordination of Strategic Development in Health is responsible for setting priorities and policy guidelines based on an analysis of the population's health. It takes into account health trends and determinants such as costs and medical practices. This unit's recommendations enable the National Health Authority's informed decision-making. It provides a space for reflection, vision and analysis to support the strategic orientation of the NHS, aimed to improve the population's health.

The Health Governance Undersecretariat stewards the NHS. It will enact and enforce legal instruments, give direction to NHS actors, support contract negotiations and coordination of policies.

The Control Agency for Health Facilities would be in charge of controlling the provision of healthcare as financed by the NHS. It is tasked with monitoring compliance with current standards for infrastructure, equipment, human resources and licensing regulations.

Reorganizing the Health Ministry

The reforms entailed extensive reorganization of the MSP itself, redefining its management model and organizational structure, updating the administration and internal management to improve its efficiency and transparency. The reorganization sought to strengthen the capacity of the MSP in performing its role of health authority and implementing its mission, institutional objectives and mandates.

The new management model also involved the decentralization of financial and administrative responsibilities to newly created territorial structures, defined as zones and districts. This intended to separate the policy-making and stewardship functions at the central level. At the local level, it would allow for the administration of healthcare services to be intrinsically linked to the epidemiological, social and demographic needs of the territories. The shift also aimed to create faster, more efficient resource management and improvements in management, productivity and service provision.

The main focus of the Undersecretariat of Health Prevention and Promotion is to support the primary care model focused on health promotion, prevention and the restructuring of inter-sector networks. The Undersecretariat is tasked with developing and promoting specific actions regarding health determinants. In addition, the reforms included the creation of two new ministries, the Ministry of Economic and Social Inclusion and the Ministry of Education, as well as common districts to enable the development of integrated services.

Outcome of the Correa Reforms

The Correa reforms re-established a central role of government in the framing of health policy. The reforms led to marked improvements in the healthcare system and in some health indicators, like reduced child mortality and longer life expectancy. It strengthened government control over healthcare and health insurance and included efforts to decentralize governance. Additional government investment expanded hospital capacity and increased the number of smaller clinics (OIT 2001).

Healthcare and social security in Ecuador made substantial improvements. The Correa administration doubled the healthcare budget, built new public hospitals and clinics and upgraded existing facilities. It purchased high-tech diagnostic and treatment equipment (that were previously not even available in private hospitals) and hired a large number of doctors, including medical specialists from Spain and Cuba (PAHO-WHO 2006).

Various surveys indicate that the country's ranking advanced to one of the top five Latin American countries in terms of healthcare quality. A 2014 Bloomberg survey of overall healthcare efficiency, factoring in both cost and quality, listed Ecuador 20th in the world (Bloomberg 2014). By contrast, the same survey ranked the United States 46th.

The reforms gained support from unions of physicians and other health workers, who saw a rise in salaries and improvements in training, professional career planning and a new code for their professional work. Ecuador became a benchmark country in the region with a nutrition policy aimed to promote healthy behavior by implementing new food labeling rules (Bolis 2001).

The reforms also evoked criticism, however. The pace of the implementation of the reform program was extremely slow, and healthcare remained fragmented. A large share of the population hardly saw any improvement in its health status or access to healthcare services. The expansion of hospital capacity was mostly concentrated in urban areas, and the number of smaller clinics remained trivial. In fact, the expansion actually caused a certain concentration (Coppedge 1996). Critics argued that there was less of a paradigm shift than a gradual adjustment of some institutions and management practices.

The government announced further increases in public health budgets for healthcare in the national 21st-Century Revolution health plan, but these promises faced the reality of severe reductions in public budgets caused by economic downturns. Increasingly, the government had to contract out health services to private providers. Some commentators concluded that Ecuador's health sector suffered a "silent" neoliberal reform (De Paepe et al. 2012).

Despite some of the abovementioned successes, many problems remained: the fragmented system, lack of coordination between services, underfunded public hospitals and very high out-of-pocket payments. In sum, there were clear gaps between government ambitions and current realities.

Conclusion

Ecuador's recent health reforms illustrate how the newly elected populist regime, under President Correa, took its mandate to gain support for a new constitution and new directions in social and fiscal policy. Indeed, the victory of the Government of the Citizens' Revolution in the 2007 election (also enabled by the boom in oil prices) constituted a major window of opportunity (Kingdon 1984), for sweeping and ambitious social reforms. The health reforms sought to transform the traditional social insurance that only covered workers in the formal sector into a universal NHS. That broadened the eligibility base from employment to citizenship. The health reforms included the decentralization of decision-making power and budgetary responsibilities in line with other sectors. This decentralization aspired to bring decision-making power closer to the people and improve coordination with other public services like housing and education.

Both the Social Security System and the NHS are responsible for universal access to healthcare as well as for actually providing health services. That sometimes leads to confusion. The Social Security System is not intended to provide healthcare services itself (but as seen earlier, IESS actually does provide healthcare to its members). Its main duty is to provide insurance coverage so that its beneficiaries have access to healthcare when needed. The actual service delivery is within the purview of the NHS.

It is at the central level of the definition and regulation of the NHS's functioning where the greatest inconsistencies are found, between the new constitutional framework and the current operational reality. There is a clear need to reform the secondary legislation of the NHS with updated standards in a new health code and new organizational proposals (PAHO-WHO 2010).

At first sight, the Correa government seemed successful in re-establishing the state as a central actor in social policy-making. It increased the public healthcare budget to reduce access barriers and protect family incomes from high medical costs. It established the principle of free healthcare for all, and sought to expand the provision of medical care, medicine and diagnostics, as well as a range of medical specialties in the public hospitals. It improved the physical infrastructure and increased human resources.

Despite the strong directive and popular support for the Correa administration, however, the results of the health reforms did not match expectations. Institutional legacies, opposition from powerful stake-holders with veto powers, and mounting dissatisfaction with the lack of positive results—aggravated by growing deficits and public spending cuts prompted by the economic downturn—all added to the faltering of the reforms.

Critics noted the slow implementation of reforms. Ecuador's health-care remains fragmented, the population's health lagging and the private sector gains ground as the government increasingly contracts out services it cannot deliver itself. In short, as noted earlier, the country is suffering a silent neoliberal reform (De Paepe et al. 2012).

Agenda for the Future: Remaining Challenges

The new constitution of 2008 provided the legal framework to strengthen the active participation of civil society in the development of the new NHS. For example, it contemplated the creation of the Citizens' Participation and Social Control Council. Thus far, this effort has not made much progress.

Another issue concerns the growing role of the private sector. Under the economic duress of fiscal pressure and public budget shortages, the government extended contracts with private healthcare providers. The last decades have seen a substantial growth in supplemental health services through private networks, especially for IESS insured. Some estimates suggest that such private payments cover about 8 percent of total health spending. That development raises questions about both the role of the private sector and the total level of health spending. While shifting towards a more public system, Ecuador did not eliminate private organizations and it does not seem likely that their role will end anytime soon. Is the current level of health funding enough? No country in the world has publicly financed universal health coverage with lower (public) spending than about nine percent of GDP. This suggests that Ecuador will have to escalate its total health spending (Figueras et al. 2002).

Another element of the reform proposals concerned the integration of primary services to the first level of care, to be financed out of the national Basic Healthcare Fund. The second aim of this program is to develop second- and third-level public networks that improve the functional integration of services offered by independent health providers. Thus far there had been limited progress in the development of such networks, and it is unclear whether Correa's successor, Moreno, will continue in this direction. Related to this issue are the more detailed questions regarding the stakeholders at the different levels of health policy-making: Who are the main stakeholders, who are the winners and losers of further changes in the system of governance, who will likely support those policies?

The experience of Correa's health reforms show the gap between ambitions of major structural transformation and the reality of more gradual adjustments of existing institutions. Evaluating the final outcome of the reforms is not easy, as it involves a complex interlinkage of institutional and programmatic changes and shifts in decision-making power and budgetary authority.

The Correa administration presented the health reforms as part of a wider program of administrative decentralization to enable better coordination of services across different social policy fields like housing, education and health. This entailed administrative reforms across different governmental agencies in a relatively short period of time. That administrative reform coincided with the proposed shift towards an integrated NHS (estimated to take six years to implement). On top of those two complex campaigns, the administration also proposed major reforms within the Health Ministry itself, by establishing three new agencies. The multifaceted interaction between all those reforms prompts the question of administrative capacity. Is it reasonable to expect that those three processes can be successfully implemented within a short period of time?

References

Atun, R., L.O. de Andrade, G. Almeida, et al. March 28, 2015. "Health-system reform and universal coverage in Latin America." *Lancet*, 385(9974): 1230–1247.

Bloomberg. 2014. "Where do you get the most for your healthcare dollar?" *Bloomberg Business*, September 18, 2015.

Bolis, M. 2001. "Marco jurídico para la regulación del financiamiento y aseguramiento del sector de la salud." *Taller Regulación del Sector Salud*. Santiago: OPS—World Health Organization.

Coffey, G. 2016. *The State of Health in Ecuador*. OpenDemocracy.

Coppedge, M. 1996. "El concepto de gobernabilidad. Modelos positivos y negativos." *En Ecuador: un problema de gobernabilidad*. Quito: CORDES-PNUD.

De Paepe, P., R. Echeverría Tapia, E. Aguilar Santacruz, and J.P. Unger. 2012. "Ecuador's silent health reform." *Int J Health Serv*, 42(2): 219–233.

Figueras, J., P. Musgrove, G. Carrin, and A. Durán. 2002. "Retos para los sistemas sanitarios de Latinoamérica: ¿qué puede aprenderse de la experiencia europea?" Barcelona: *Gac Sani*, 16(1): 5–17.

INEC. 2017. *Ecuador en cifras*. National Institute of Statistics and Censuses. www.inec.gob.ec.

Kingdon, J.W. 1984. *Agendas, Alternatives, and Public Policies*. New York: Longman.

Klein, R., and T.R. Marmor. 2006. "Reflections on Policy Analysis: Putting it Together Again." *The Oxford Handbook of Political Science*. R. Goodin (ed). Oxford: Oxford University Press: 982–912.

Kliksberg, B. 2000. "¿Cómo reformar el Estado para enfrentar los desafíos sociales del 2000?" *Revista de la Facultad de Ciencias Económicas. UNMSM,* 16: 235–269.

López-Cevallos, D., and C. Chunhuei. 2010. "Assessing the context of healthcare utilization in Ecuador: a spatial and multilevel analysis." *BMC Health Serv Res,* 10: 64. Published online March 12, 2010. doi:10.1186/1472-6963-10-64

MSP. 2010. *Nuevo Modelo de gestión del MSP.* Quito, Ecuador: Ministry of Health.

OIT. 2001. *"Hacia un trabajo decente: Una protección social en salud para todos los trabajadores y sus familias".* Programa Estrategias y Técnicas contra la Exclusión Social y la Pobreza, Sector de la Protección Social. PAHO-WHO. World Health Organization.

PAHO-WHO. 2006. *Situación de salud del Ecuador 2006.* Quito, Ecuador: Organización Panamericana de la Salud.

PAHO-WHO. 2010. *Sistemas de Salud: Mejorar el Desempeño.* Ginebra: World Health Organization.

Pierson, P. 1994. *Dismantling the Welfare State? Reagan, Thatcher and the Politics of Retrenchment.* Cambridge: Cambridge University Press.

SENPLADES. 2010. *Plan de Desarrollo del Ecuador: 2009–2013.* Quito, Ecuador: SENPLADES.

Villacrés, A.N. 2003. *Sistemas de salud: diseño, organización y evaluación* (Syllabus). Módulo Organización de los Sistemas de Salud. Maestría de Políticas Públicas y Gestión. Quito, Ecuador: FLACSO.

Villacrés, A.N. 2008. "Buen gobierno en salud: un desafio de todos." *Trasformaciones sociales y sistemas de salud en America Latina* (Primera ed.). B. Espinoza and W. Waters (eds). Quito, Pichincha, Ecuador: Rispergraf: 27. http://www.flacsoandes.edu.ec. Accessed June 21, 2015.

Weisbrot, M. 2017. "Ecuadors decade of reform." *Huffpost,* February 15, 2017.

WHO. 2006. *Informe Mundial de la Salud 2000.* Geneva: World Health Organization.

Section III

Healthcare Reforms in Western Europe: The Netherlands and Switzerland

Responding to fiscal and budgetary pressures and rising demand for healthcare services since the mid-1970s, governments across Western Europe sought to rein in public spending with a mix of old mechanisms (e.g., general budgets, price and volume controls) and new techniques (financial incentives for patients, insured and healthcare providers, in addition to the delisting of entitlements). The reality of retrenchment turned out to be far less substantial than the rhetoric that accompanied reform efforts, however. In most cases, public health spending expanded to cover new population groups, treatment for new diseases, such as HIV/AIDS, and expensive new medical technology and drugs.

The Netherlands and Switzerland—two nations that already had universal or near-universal coverage in the mid-20th century—replaced their public and private health insurance schemes with "consumer-driven healthcare." Switzerland took the lead in 1996 with a population-wide health insurance offered by competing (but non-profit) private insurers under extensive public regulation. Ten years later, the Netherlands replaced its mix of public and private health insurance with a quasi-private insurance. Both nations require that all (legal) residents retain basic health coverage with an insurer of their choice. Insured can opt for supplemental coverage and alternative plans with conditions different from the standard coverage.

The Swiss and Dutch schemes became, for some international commentators, leading examples of consumer-driven healthcare and a potential model for the United States and other countries. However, much of the commentary focused on the theoretical promises of the model rather than on actual results. For example, rather than relying on market competition to control health expenditure, both countries combined private insurance with a heavy dose of cross-subsidization and government regulation. In both cases, within a few years of the introduction of the new insurance, there was a sharp decline in the numbers of people switching plans (in Switzerland the rate of changing policies increased again after insurers offered major rebates for high deductible plans). An unexpected consequence in both countries—at least, in the eyes of policy-makers—was the administrative complexity and costliness of the cross-subsidization, and the monitoring and supervision of the insurance mandate. Both nations saw an accelerated process of market concentration for health insurances and a substantial rise in overall health expenditure, from well below to well above the OECD average. Other issues were the increasing numbers of uninsured and delinquent payers, and declining consumer trust in health insurers.

Holland and Switzerland remain the only two nations to have embraced consumer-driven health reforms, but two decades later, there does not seem to be much popular support or political enthusiasm to continue that course in either nation.

Map 5. Population, Income Level and Health Expenditure in The Netherlands and Switzerland, 1960–2015

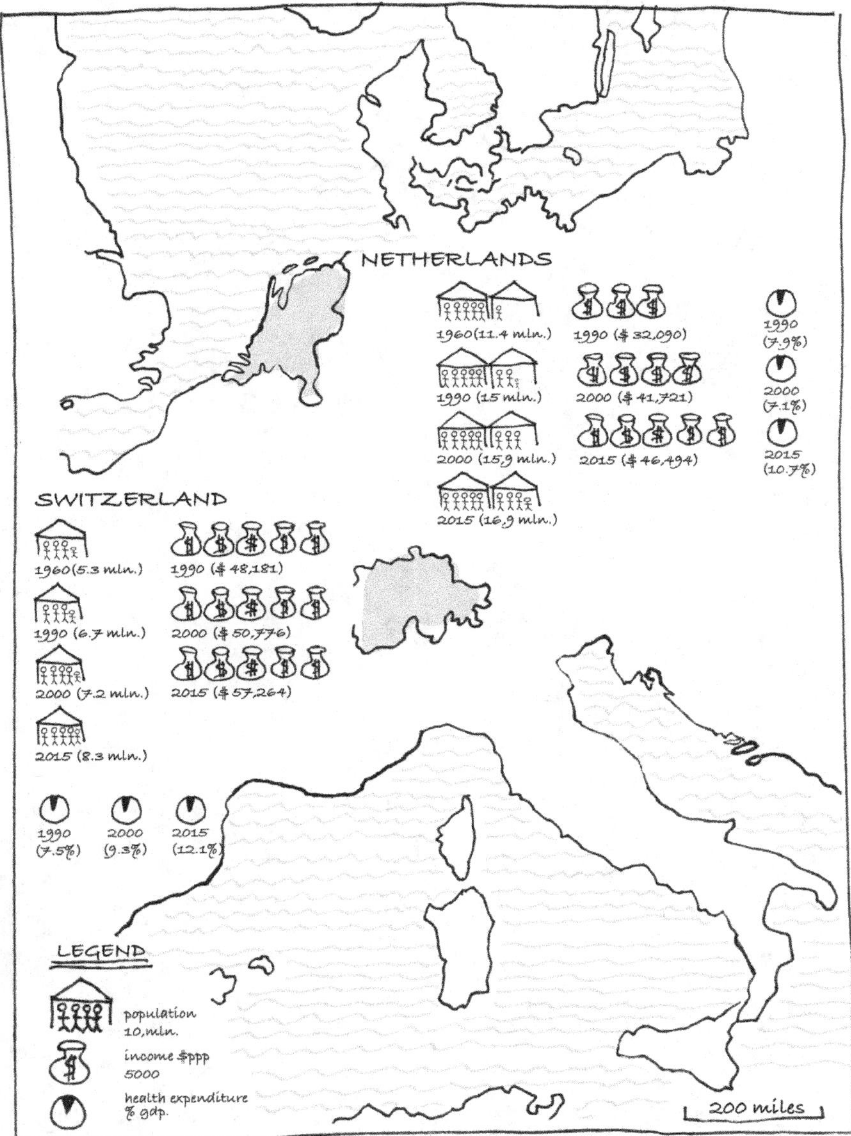

Map 6. Number of Physicians, Infant Mortality and Life Expectancy in The Netherlands and Switzerland, 1960–2015

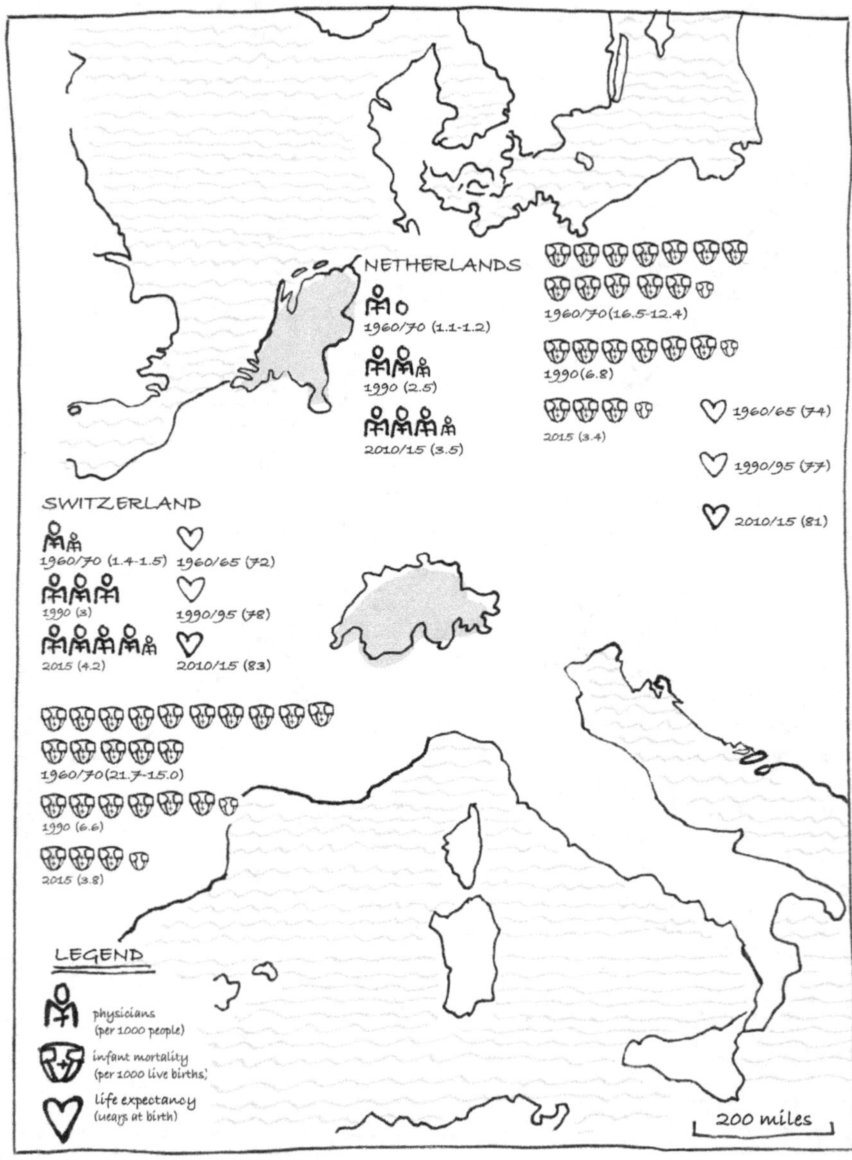

Change and Continuity in Dutch Healthcare: Origins and Consequences of the 2006 Health Insurance Reforms

Kieke G.H. Okma, Aad de Roo and Hans Maarse

Introduction

The Dutch government introduced a population-wide mandate to obtain health insurance in 2006, replacing the existing public and private health insurance. What led to this new insurance? Did it represent a dramatic break with the past, heralding consumer-driven healthcare under the new regime of managed competition? What happened after its introduction, and what do we expect to happen to Dutch healthcare in the future?

To answer these questions, this chapter starts with a brief sketch of Dutch health insurance and healthcare in the early 21st century. It analyzes the core characteristics of social policy-making in much of the 20th century (including the tradition of neo-corporatism and non-state healthcare provision) and the pressures for health reform since the late 1970s. It shows how the main stakeholders in Dutch healthcare, especially insurers and providers, adjusted their attitudes and behaviors in anticipation of reforms—even while some of those reforms were never implemented. Finally, we look at the new role of patients as consumers.

In principle, the 2006 policy expanded options for insured to choose insurers and health plans. Interest in shopping around for health plans dropped sharply after the first year, however. Initially, the new law did not affect providers' and insurers' behavior much either. While no longer legally obligated to contract with every provider, insurers rarely broke off long-standing contractual relations, anxious to avoid angry reactions in their insured or physicians. A decade later, there was still little evidence of selective contracting (some insurers did not renew contracts based on quality considerations), but the accelerated concentration of the health insurance market caused a sharp drop in the number of independent insurers. Since the early 2000s, four main insurance conglomerates have covered over 90 percent of the market.

Likewise, hospitals and other providers fortified their regional market positions by engaging in processes of horizontal and vertical integration. They sought to improve their services, and there was a flurry of organizational changes in healthcare. New providers offered substitutes for traditional services but the scale of their operations remained modest.

Importantly, the 2006 scheme did not replace previous governance models. Nor did the market replace the government in healthcare and insurance. Rather than a sudden transformation or dramatic break with the past, there was a gradual change. As Carolyn Tuohy argued (2018), the Dutch reforms were originally designed as a blueprint. Over time, however, the reforms stagnated and the process of change had become much more incremental—in fact, by the early 21st century, Lindblom's *The Science of Muddling Through* (1959) had become a more appropriate term. The reforms did result in a complicated and inconsistent overlay of governance models.

Health Insurance in the Netherlands, 2017

The Health Insurance Law (*Zorgverzekeringswet* or ZVW) of 2006 mandates that all adult legal residents in the Netherlands acquire basic coverage for medical care with an insurer of their own choice.[1,2] Coverage is on an individual basis, excluding dependents.[3] The government determines the entitlements, essentially: medical care in hospitals and physicians' offices, prescription drugs, dental care for under age 18 and some other health services. While insurers can act as for-profit companies, most remained non-profits. They have to accept any applicant for basic coverage, and charge community-rated premiums (thus, similar to the rules of America's Obamacare of 2010). The revenue of insurers consists of income-related contributions and flat-rate premiums (on average about €100 per month) paid directly by insured. Low-income insured are eligible for fiscal subsidies. About five million persons or 31 percent of the

---

[1] One unsolved question regard the legal status of the Health Insurance Act ZVW (Okma 2002). The Dutch government initially presented the insurance, mandated by law, as private, but changed its mind realizing such privatization might run afoul of international treaties. Treaties of the International Labor Organization, the Council of Europe and the EU, for example, require member states to cover a minimum share of the population with social insurance. Some experts have argued that the ZVW cannot be labeled social insurance as the mandate requires residents to take out insurance but does not automatically register everyone. The only authority to determine the nature of the system is the European Court of Justice (ECJ). The ECJ will only give a formal ruling, however, if and when someone brings a case to the Court. That has not (yet) happened. This is not just a semantic question. Regulatory regimes of social and private insurance differ substantially. Under the EU Treaty, national governments can freely determine the nature of national social policies (e.g., a National Health Service model or social health insurance). Once providers and insurers are free to negotiate over the volume and prices of their services, however, they clearly engage in economic activity and, the ECJ has ruled, are thus subject to EU competition law. EU rules for (private) insurance and banking restrict government intervention in setting prices, allowing collective bargaining, or favoring national providers or insurers over international actors.

[2] The term "basic" is somewhat misleading. The ZVW covers a broad range of entitlements, including medical care in hospitals and family practices, prescription drugs, dental care for insured under 18 and other services, with modest amounts of co-payments.

[3] Introduced in an era with dominance of the one-income family, the Bismarckian social insurance covered both wage earners and their dependents. It protected families against the financial risks of illness, disability, unemployment, old age and death of the family breadwinner.

population received this subsidy in 2017 that, on average, compensated for about 40 percent of their ZWV premiums (CBS 2015; *Zorgwijzer.nl* 2017).

Employers collect the income-related contributions for the ZVW as earmarked taxation, 6.7 percent for employers and 5.4 percent of gross incomes for employees (up to a ceiling of €53,700) in 2017. The Tax Department then allocates this money to insurers based on a risk equalization formula to compensate insurers with more high-risk (high cost) patients in their portfolio. This way, it is hoped, insurers will pay more attention to contracting efficient healthcare than on selecting healthy and wealthy—and on average, less costly—insured. Insured can chose a plan with a lower premium, which offers reimbursement (patients initially pay for their physician or hospital bills themselves) instead of benefits in-kind or other financial conditions.

All insured face a mandatory deductible, €385 per year in 2018; they can add a voluntary deductible of up to €500 in exchange for lower premiums, and take out supplemental coverage for entitlements not covered by the ZVW. As the latter is voluntary, the ZVW rules do not apply (e.g., the requirement to accept all applicants). Initially, the vast majority of insured (90 percent) had supplemental coverage, perhaps reflecting the general affinity of Dutch households for high insurance against financial risks, but that share had dropped to 85 percent in 2017.

Patients face user fees for certain services, for example, prescription drugs, mental health and long-term care. With the rise of mandatory deductibles and co-payments, the level of out-of-pocket payments (OOPs) increased from 9.45 to 12.25 percent of total health expenditure between 2000 and 2017. Still, it remained one of the lowest of all industrialized nations (World Bank 2017).

In addition, all legal residents contributed 9.65 percent of taxable income for long-term care insurance in 2018 (*Wet Langdurige Zorg*, WLZ), and all taxpayers share the burden of the fiscal subsidies that cover the premiums for the unemployed, welfare recipients and insured younger than 18, as well as for administration and some other costs.

The financing of long-term care split four ways in 2015 (Maarse and Jeurissen 2016). Stay in nursing homes and specialized facilities shifted to the WLZ, administered by the Health Ministry (Ministry of Health [MoH]). Home help and some other services became the responsibility of local authorities as part of the Welfare Support Act (*Wet Maatschappelijke Ondersteuning*, WMO). Non-institutional mental health and community nursing shifted to the ZVW. Thus, health insurers gained control over part of long-term care. Finally, some of the long-term care institutions for the handicapped remained under direct control of the MoH.

Dutch Healthcare, Health Insurance and Health Administration in the 20th Century

Dutch healthcare shares some core policy goals with other European countries: universal access, solidarity in sharing the financial burden, cost control, patient choice and professional autonomy for healthcare providers (OECD 1992). It also has some particular features: a relatively high share of private financing (at least until 2006, see below), non-government provision of care and a neo-corporatist style of social policy-making.

Holland's social policy has borrowed heavily from its eastern neighbor, including the Bismarckian model of social insurance. During the Second World War, the German occupational forces imposed the Sick Funds Degree (*Ziekenfondsbesluit*) mandating sick fund membership for certain categories of workers. This resolved the decades-long dispute within Dutch government about the governance arrangement of social health insurance, in particular the question of which groups should be represented on the board of the sick funds: employers and employees or also government? When the Sick Fund Law (*Ziekenfondswet*, ZFW) passed in 1964, private insurance already covered about 35 percent of the population. The government accepted this reality, informally labeled the "peace border," and agreed to keep ZFW membership below 65 percent of the population (when Germany introduced its own social health insurance in 1883, only about 10 percent of its population had private insurance, hence its peace border was set at a much higher income level). For over five decades, all changes in Dutch health policy respected this peace border.

The ZFW covered hospital care, dentists, general physicians, prescription drugs and some other services. The sick funds, the voluntary mutual insurances active since the 19th century, became responsible for administering the social insurance. In exchange for taking on this public role, they gained virtually unrestricted access to public finance: when health expenditures rose, their contribution rates (and often government subsidies) went up, too. Dutch social insurance expanded gradually by including more and more population groups, and by covering more and more entitlements. It added a separate population-wide plan for long-term care, the Exceptional Medical Expenses Act (*Algemene Wet Bijzondere Ziektekosten*, AWBZ) in 1968. The AWBZ covered the cost of hospitalization longer than 365 days, stays in mental institutions, nursing homes, home care and some other health-related services. The AWBZ relieved families, charities and local communities of the financial burden of long-term care. It also fueled a rapid expansion of long-term care institutions and a very high rate of institutional care. With the AWBZ, Holland was the first nation with population-wide long-term care insurance.

The second important feature of Dutch healthcare was the dominance of non-state provision of services. The tradition of providing collective goods by voluntary, non-government organizations traces back to middle ages (De Swaan 1988). The medieval guilds (associations of craftsmen) offered financial support to their members in case of illness or death. Local communities, churches and monasteries set up hospitals as shelters for the homeless, elderly, sick and mentally ill. This tradition is still visible today, even while the denominational backgrounds have faded due to recent waves of mergers.

Dutch healthcare included about 90 independent hospitals, about 22,000 medical specialists and 9,000 general practitioners (GPs), over 500,000 nurses and auxiliary nurses and tens of thousands other health professionals in 2017 (NIVEL 2017). One-third of GPs worked solo, the others in small group practices. Medical specialists are employed by academic centers, while the ones in general hospitals mostly work for group practices; but there is an increasing trend of employment contracts, especially for female doctors. Most patients are registered with a GP, and remain with their GP unless they change residencies. A GP's referral is required for specialist or hospital care.

GP incomes consisted of a mix of capitation (a fixed amount for each patient registered with the practice), fee for service, payments for special activity (e.g., preventive activities or after hours service), bundled payments for patients with specific chronic diseases, and subsidies for investment in information technology or hiring specialized staff like practice nurses or dieticians. Altogether these payments have driven up the income level of Dutch GPs (together with that of their English counterparts) to the highest in the world in the last two decades. Hospital revenues are largely based on a unique Dutch model of case-based payments or "diagnosis-treatment combinations" (see below).

Despite the dominance of private not-for-profit healthcare, the system always contained for-profit elements. GPs and many other health professionals, for example, are self-employed entrepreneurs. As in most other industrialized nations, the drug and medical device industries are almost exclusively for-profit. Several hospitals developed for-profit subsidiaries. Dutch governments traditionally played a modest role in the provision of healthcare, mostly limited to public health, family welfare services by local authorities, public regional psychiatric institutions and the financing of medical research.

The third feature of Dutch healthcare is the neo-corporatist tradition of social policy-making, with organized interest groups sharing the responsibility with governments for the shaping and outcome of social policy-making (Lijphart 1968). In healthcare, stakeholders included labor unions, employers, providers, insurers and organized patient groups. The basic assumption of this governance model was a certain hierarchy in responsibilities labeled sovereignty in one's own sphere by Protestants, or subsidiarity by Catholics—the latter term is still common in European Union (EU) politics, expressive of preference for national over EU-level decision-making. Individual families were to take care of their own members, and next, the denominational organizations to which most Dutch families belonged, like churches, schools, housing corporations, home care associations and welfare organizations. Only when those two levels failed to meet the basic needs of their members would the state step in as a residual safety net.

For much of the second half of the 20th century, Dutch healthcare combined a mix of public and private financing with mostly non-government healthcare provision, independent and decentralized administration of healthcare and insurance, with extensive involvement of organized stakeholders—but under extensive government regulation.

Origins and Shape of Market-Oriented Healthcare Reforms in Holland

The Dutch social insurance for disability, unemployment and sickness benefits, old-age pensions and social health insurance, expanded steadily in the decades after World War II. There were concerns about rising costs and disputes about administrative responsibilities, but the majority of the population welcomed the expansion as part of the modern welfare state.

As in other industrialized countries, a confluence of economic, ideological and demographic factors fueled widespread debate about the future of the welfare state (Timmins 1995). The oil crises and economic stagflation of the 1970s, changing ideological views of the role of the state and revised demographic projections that revealed a faster aging of the population than earlier predictions, all created pressures for change. After decades of consensual neo-corporatist policy-making, the attention shifted—at least rhetorically—to models of individualized and decentralized decision-making.

An expert committee headed by Wisse Dekker, the former CEO of Philips Electronics, proposed a major overhaul of Dutch healthcare in 1987 (Commissie Dekker 1987). Its problem analysis was not new; earlier reports also pointed to the fragmented funding, lack of consumer choice and financial incentives, as well as the rigid regulations and government control inhibiting flexible and coordinated services. The Committee proposed to amalgamate the existing financing streams (public and private insurance and AWBZ) into one mandatory social health insurance covering acute medical care and long-term care. It advocated a stronger role for the insurers as third-party payers in healthcare, free choice of insurer and health plan, fewer entitlements under the basic insurance and partial replacement of the income-related contributions by (community-rated) flat-rate premiums. The plan further included options for insured to take on supplemental coverage and accept deductibles or coinsurance in exchange for lower premiums. Finally, the plan implied a reduced role of government by deregulating planning and fee-setting legislation. This would not completely eliminate the role of the state in healthcare, however. The government was to determine the entitlements of the basic health insurance and the budgets of health insurers and monitor market outcomes. Yet the responsibility for negotiations over the quantity, quality and prices of health services was to shift to (competing) healthcare providers and (competing—but not-for-profit) health insurers.

The underlying idea was that consumer choice combined with selective contracting would create incentives for insurers and providers to keep premiums down and improve the quality, efficiency and patient-friendliness of healthcare services. Some commentators saw the Dutch reform as a triumph of consumerism and a shining example for other nations (Naik 2007; Harris 2007; Van de Ven and Schut 2008; Enthoven and Van de Ven 2007). Others labeled the changes market-oriented reforms instead, as the market principles were matched with extensive public regulation (Van Ginneken 2015; Maarse et al. 2015).

The proposal caused much uproar, and it took lengthy debate to pass Parliament. The Health Ministry framed an ambitious four-year implementation plan. It shifted some services (e.g., ambulatory mental healthcare and prescription drugs) from the public and private insurances to the long-term care insurance AWBZ, which was to become the new social health insurance for all.[4] The MoH relaxed rules for hospital planning and fee setting. Local authorities lost control over the establishment of new

---

[4] At the time, this approach seemed a sensible choice as the AWBZ already applied to the entire population. A gradual shift of entitlements from the public and private insurance schemes to the AWBZ would require the least legislative and administrative change.

practices of family doctors, and provincial authorities lost their role in hospital planning.[5]

After the first implementation steps in the early 1990s, however, stakeholder opposition resurfaced, public support eroded and the political backing for the reforms weakened. The Dutch Parliament shelved the next steps—but remarkably, did not reverse the measures already taken. In 1994, a left-center-conservative coalition of Labor (PvdA), Conservative (VVD), and Liberal Democrat (D66) parties replaced the coalition of Christian Democrats (CDA), VVD and D66. Its governing manifesto announced a shift from wholesale reforms to incremental adjustments (*Regeerakkoord* 1994). The coalition announced plans for a universal basic health insurance a few years later (MOH 2001). The next two decades saw regular changes in coalition governments, always including at least two of the major parties and sometimes one of the smaller ones. Their successive governing manifestos reflected some shift in emphasis, but rarely major change in policy directions.

The next center-conservative coalition government finally passed the 2006 ZVW law. The ZVW replaced the ZFW and private health insurances with a population-wide mandate to acquire insurance. Growing waitlists, especially in long-term care, played a crucial role in the rapid passage of the ZVW. In several cases during the late 1990s, patients and their families had successfully taken the government to court to enforce their rights. The Cabinet decided to reduce waitlists by substantially increasing health spending in the years 2000–2003. Many politicians agreed with this spending increase at the time, but shortly afterward seemed to have forgotten the episode, when they then supported the ZVW. Health Minister Hans Hoogervorst cited runaway costs as the main reason for privatizing health insurance, convincing Dutch Parliament to pass the ZVW in 2005.

---

[5] To compensate Dutch provinces for their loss of control over healthcare planning, they gained the responsibility over the newly created regional Patient and Consumer Platforms in the late 1990s. The platforms became meeting grounds for patient groups, but not prominent actors in the negotiations between governments, insurers and healthcare providers over covenants (that in fact, represented a return to neo-corporatist consensual decision-making—see below).

The 2006 ZVW was substantially similar to the earlier Dekker proposals. While it left out long-term care from the basic insurance coverage (increasing the role of local governments instead), it pushed the notion of market competition even further by allowing more room for for-profit healthcare and health insurance. The ZVW passed Parliament with remarkably little public debate. The Senate (the First Chamber of Parliament) passed the bill in one day—the day before summer recess—a stunningly short time for passing such far-reaching change in social health insurance.

The 2017 coalition of VVD, CDA, D66 and the small, conservative Christian Union (CU) seemed to take some distance from the market-oriented course of its predecessors, however. Its governing manifesto hardly mentioned individual choice or competition, instead emphasizing cost control (read: more out-of-pocket payment and lower collective financing), individual responsibility (read: more informal long-term care at home) and the need for (regional) collaboration. Medical ethics regained a dominant position on the policy agenda (*Regeerakkoord* 2017).

In the end, Dutch health policies of the 1980s through the early 21st century showed a remarkable degree of stability. Changing political coalitions caused shifts in emphasis from structural reform to incremental policies and vice versa, but hardly affected the core elements of the market-oriented reforms. Yet, despite this orientation, the market did not replace government as the leading force in healthcare. As none of the political parties have an absolute majority, coalition governments always included at least two or more of the four major parties: CDA, VVD, PvdA and D66. Moreover, in a small nation like the Netherlands, all the leading politicians know each other personally. These political realities explain a great deal of the continuity in policy-making.

Governance of Dutch Healthcare: From Neo-Corporatism to Market to Neo-Neo-Corporatism?

As the entitlements and eligibility criteria for the ZFW social health insurance expanded after its inception in 1964, so did government control over healthcare planning and financing. Still, GPs, dentists and physiotherapists continued to practice as self-employed health professionals, and the ownership and management of health facilities remained largely non-governmental. The market-oriented health reforms did not always sit easily with this non-profit tradition. Dutch hospitals, and other actors, suddenly faced financial risks. They had to operate like market actors, but did not always feel comfortable with that role (Rosenberg 2006, 2007).

The market-oriented policies (that brought individual choice and competition) did not replace existing governance instruments (e.g., macro budgets with price and volume controls). Dutch healthcare institutions had expanded since the 1960s with a wide array of quasi-independent administrative and advisory bodies. Many stakeholders had formal representation in those bodies. This corporatist form of governance in social policy-making, sometimes labeled the Dutch Polder model, was vilified as the Dutch disease, and further implicated as the main cause of stagnating growth and high unemployment in the late 1980s (Visser and Hemerijck 1997). The discovery of huge oil and natural gas reserves had boosted public spending, and critics argued that this windfall was blocking efforts to loosen up labor markets and increase efficiency in the economy. Ironically, the very same model of corporatist policy-making was widely heralded as the Dutch Miracle when economic growth and employment in Holland rose faster than in neighboring European countries in the early 1990s.

As part of a broader reassessment of the Dutch welfare state, a study commissioned by Parliament found that there were several hundred expert committees and agencies in the healthcare domain (Commissie De Jong 1991). Parliament decided to drastically reduce the number and size of these bodies (as well as its own standing committees) and eliminate direct stakeholder representation to create "efficient, expert-only" advisory committees (Okma 1997a). This obviously curtailed the scope for organized interests to influence health policy. The relatively easy passage of the 2006 ZVW illustrated that the erosion of neo-corporatist structures had made life easier for governments eager to implement rapid change.

The polder mentality did not completely disappear, however. Dutch interest groups remained willing to sit down with government to discuss and implement social policy. One particular policy instrument that made a remarkable comeback was the covenant (Klee and Okma 2001). Less official than law and not legally binding (but more than an informal agreement), covenants were considered by Dutch governments to be a convenient way to engage major stakeholders in fiscal and social policy-making. Covenants operate under the shadow of hierarchy as governments can ultimately revert to formal legislation (Scharpf 1997; Maarse et al. 2015).

Time and again, Dutch governments sought agreement with hospitals, insurers and other stakeholders on soft spending limits and other policy goals. When hospital expenditures exceeded budget estimates in 2004, for example, the MoH framed a covenant with the national associations of hospitals and health insurers (MoH 2006). It established similar covenants with the pharmaceutical industry and medical specialists, and a second one with hospitals and insurers in 2011 (NVZ 2011). Likewise, the Dutch Healthcare Institute (*Netherlands Zorginstituut*, formerly Healthcare Authority or *Zorgautoriteit*), the regulatory body for healthcare markets, concluded covenants with providers to encourage the proper use of healthcare (MoH 2017). Other covenants aimed to improve the efficiency of mental health services and patient safety in ambulances. The proliferation of covenants raised concerns about the unclear allocation of responsibilities. In a few cases, parties walked out; for example, the producers of generic drugs, who disagreed with the covenant between government and the pharmaceutical industry.

This "neo-neo-corporatism" brought major stakeholders to the policy table but no longer in a systematic way. The new agreements, often concluded behind closed doors, resulted in more opaque policy networks. Participants in the previous neo-corporatist policy-making deliberations were no longer commonly included, for example, the consumer and patient platforms. The informal character of the new covenants (even while the government increasingly used the agreements as a form of 'soft budget ceilings') meant that some parties only felt obliged to live up to its agreement for as long as it served their interests. The old neo-corporatist structures caused delays due to long deliberations, but they were often effective, since in the end, the outcomes were widely supported by the parties who had been at the table.

Establishing the new model with competing (private) actors, hands-off government, "managed competition as a driving force" and the "shift from supply control to the demand side"[6] (e.g., Wammes et al. 2013; ACM 2016) became more complicated and time-consuming than originally envisioned. Dutch citizens—like other Europeans—generally expect government to safeguard access to good quality healthcare. Facing public outcry over the delisting of certain entitlements, the government frequently reinstated (part of) those services and took other measures to moderate the financial consequences for particular patient groups. Expansion of coverage remained at least as common as delisting, despite efforts to reduce the basic insurance.

The government extended its role in monitoring healthcare quality, developing case-based payment models and implementing information technology. It set up several new agencies (sometimes replacing old ones with a new name), for example, the National Healthcare Institute (formerly the Health Insurance Board), the Medicine Evaluation Board, the Health Council, the Dutch Healthcare Authority, the Diagnosis Combination Maintenance Organization, the NICTIZ Institute supporting the development of information technology and electronic medical records and the Quality Institute (Wammes et al. 2013; Van Ginneken 2015).

The rules of the game had changed, but the new rules did not fully replace old ones. Providers and insurers had to compete, but at the same time, governments encouraged them to collaborate on the regional and national levels. Government announced it would step back, but it also kept tight control over health expenditure and the allocation of public funds. This resulted in complementary governance models (Helderman 2007) or perhaps more accurately, in a complicated overlay (Okma and de Roo

---

[6]Those terms are not self-explanatory. Supply regulation refers to government control of the allocation of resources, planning of health facilities, price-setting, as well as quality supervision. Demand regulation assumes that individual choice of health plans and providers will prompt (competing) health insurers to contract (competing) providers to ensure efficient and good quality care on behalf of their insured.

2009; Okma 2009) reflecting rather divergent and sometimes conflicting ideas on the role of the state, citizens and organized interests.

Changing Positions of Dutch Health Insurers

The overlay of governance models created managerial dilemmas for Dutch healthcare providers and insurers. The health reforms introduced risks to players who had traditionally enjoyed high levels of certainty and income protection. Population groups eligible for social insurance were automatically insured. Their employers withheld the insurance contributions as earmarked taxes, making them less visible than the nominal (flat-rate) premiums insured had to pay directly. Traditionally, sick fund members had virtually unrestricted access to healthcare, with modest amounts of user fees for certain services. Sick funds had enjoyed nearly unrestricted access to public funding, since higher health costs translated into higher contributions and tax subsidies. They had to contract with all healthcare providers in their region, who in turn were all but certain to receive their annual budgets.

All those financial certainties evaporated in 1991. The open-ended financing shifted to capitated budgets for insurers, gradually increasing their financial risk (Leu et al. 2008; Schut and Van de Ven 2005). Hospitals saw a shift in their payment model, which increased their financial exposure. The share of hospital finances covered by case-based payments rose from 10 to 81 percent between 2006 and 2016 (Vektis 2017).

Reacting to the market-oriented health reforms, Dutch health insurers initially appeared more concerned with expanding and consolidating their market positions than improving the quality of healthcare (Okma and de Roo 2009; ACM 2016). Insurers improved their administration, expanded (and sometimes reduced) their coverage and merged with others. Anticipating the new insurance law in 2006, several set their premiums below cost and ran up high bills on marketing and advertising to lure in new customers. To recoup those losses, some increased premiums by about 10 percent in 2007 (Smit and Mokveld 2007). In 2017, insurers announced substantial premium increases to compensate for losses, but in

Healthcare spending and financing in the Netherlands, 1972–2015

According to the Central Bureau for Statistics (CBS), total spending on healthcare and related welfare services (including long-term care) increased 13-fold, from 6.5 to 94.6 billion euros between 1972 and 2015 (CBS 2017). The growth of these categories exceeded that of the national income. Their share of GDP increased from 8.7 to 14.0 percent (although these percentages would be about 1 percent point lower excluding the related welfare services). Healthcare spending also exceeded overall population growth; expressed as index numbers (with 2010 = 100), the population increased from 80 to 102, health expenditure went from 8 to 109 and per capita spending from 9 to 106, a twelvefold increase (CBS 2017). With that level of spending, Holland had reached the top five of the OECD nations.

While those spending figures include some services that do not typically fall under the international definition of healthcare (e.g., long-term care in institutions) the overall trends still show very high growth rates.

Table 1. Healthcare Financing in the Netherlands, 1972–2015

		1972	1980	1990	1995	2000	2005	2010	2015
Health expenditure (millions of euros)	Total care and welfare	6,450	17,310	26,658	35,148	46,452	67,151	87,632	94,608
	Health and long-term care	5,638	15,237	23,123	30,047	39,070	57,452	74,691	81,783
Financing source (millions of euro)	Total	6,450	17,310	26,658	35,148	46,452	67,151	87,632	94,608
	Government	1,615	4,065	5,018	6,706	6,761	8,417	13,123	17,092
	Health insurance	2,081	5,525	7,241	7,570	12,862	17,566	34,633	40,675
	AWBZ/WLZ	1,003	3,485	6,940	12,030	13,109	20,192	22,612	17,694
	Other	1,751	4,235	7,459	8,842	13,718	20,977	17,263	19,146
Expenses as share of GDP (percent)		8.7	10.6	10.9	10.8	10.4	12.3	13.9	14.0
Indices (2010 = 100)	Healthcare and long-term care	8	20	31	40	52	77	100	109
	Population	80	85	90	93	96	98	100	102
	Spending per capita	9	23	34	43	55	78	100	106

Source: CBS 2017 (data for 2015 estimates).

(*Continued*)

> Health expenditure (excluding long-term care) amounted to, on average, €4,000 per person, or €6,700 per adult per year in 2014 (children under 18 do not pay contributions). That amount consisted of almost €900 ZVW flat-rate premium, €1,340 ZVW contribution and €1,220 AWBZ/WLZ contribution, plus co-payments of €310 and €250 for other spending. About 85 percent of the population had procured supplemental coverage, with annual premiums averaging €250 in 2017. Aside from those payments for premiums, contributions and out-of-pocket payments, taxpayers faced an average tax burden of €1,200.
>
> The annual growth rate of publicly financed health expenditure leveled off, from 5.2 percent between 2000 and 2010, to 2.9 percent after 2010 (Van Strien and Bhageloe-Datadin 2015). Opinions differ as to the causes of that decrease: sharper price negotiations by insurers, shifts to generic drugs, the delisting of entitlements from the ZVW or the decline in economic growth. At the same time, administrative costs, fiscal subsidies for low-income families, local welfare services previously under the long-term care insurance, AWBZ and other long-term care expenses continued to grow, in particular the popular vouchers (*persoonsgebonden budget*, PGB).
>
> As the individual payments for the ZVW and long-term care (flat-rate premiums, deductibles and other direct payments) rose, there was a slight drop in the share of collective financing (income related-contributions and tax subsidies), from about 73 to 70.5 percent between 2006 and 2014 (Van Strien and Bhageloe-Datadin 2015).

the end, actual increases were lower than expected (*Zorgverzekering Informatie Centrum Nl* 2017).

Some health insurers pressured hospitals to work more efficiently and contracted with for-profit clinics to manage waitlists. Others offered memberships to sports clinics or regular check-ups in their supplemental coverage. A few experimented with preferred provider arrangements, but this never became popular in Holland. Most insurers offered collective employment-based insurance contracts; in 2007, almost 70 percent of insured were members of such collective contracts (Vektis 2017). That implied a substantial role for employment-based contracting and the return of employers and their national association (VNO) to the health policy arena. There is clearly an element of risk selection in such collective contracting. In general, employment-based collective groups represent lower risks (lower costs). Such lower premiums for certain groups generally resulted in higher individual premiums.

These practices raised concerns about risk selection to lure in young, healthy (and less costly) clients (Maarse et al. 2015). To counteract this trend—as another example of public intervention in the private market—the government ruled that collective contracts could not offer more than a 10 percent discount (Smit and Mokveld 2007). Dutch health insurers traditionally faced strong social norms condemning risk discriminatory practices, and therefore refrained from applying risk ratings that fully reflected the risk of certain groups (Okma 1997a; ACM 2016). The NZA signaled some evidence of risk selection, but not enough to take action (NZA 2016).

Regional monopolies of sick funds were abolished in 1991, allowing for new entrants into the social health insurance field. In practice, however, it accelerated the ongoing process of mergers and acquisitions. There were over 1,200 independent sick funds at the beginning of the 20th century. That number dropped to 600 in 1950 and to around 60 in the early 1980s (Okma 2002). By 2006, anticipating new legislation, sick funds disappeared as independent agencies, as all had merged with private insurers. Consequently, there were 33 health insurers, both former sick funds and private insurers in 2006, and following further consolidation, that number dropped to 24 in 2018 (Vektis 2018). Most of these operated as part of broader conglomerates. Four major insurance groups (Achmea, VGZ, CZ and Menzis) covered about 90 percent of insured. Despite formally competing, their relative market shares have remained remarkably stable since 2008 (ACM 2016; Vektis 2017). The number of plans, especially supplemental policies, increased but their coverage remained very similar.

In the late 1990s, a few international insurers tried their hand in the Dutch market, for example, the French AXA and the German DKV, but they soon left the country again. The Luxemburg insurer Iptiq announced

Uninsured in the Netherlands

Traditionally, Holland had few uninsured. The 35 percent or so of the population not eligible for social insurance were not legally obligated to acquire (private) health insurance until 2006, but the vast majority had actually done so. Perhaps reflecting the general tendency of Dutch families to purchase extensive coverage for homes, cars and other property, the rate of non-insurance was less than 2 percent in the late 1990s (Ministry of Health 1996)—thus quite different from the United States—where at the time of the introduction of the 2010 Patient Protection and Affordable Care Act over 15 percent of the population did not have coverage.

That changed after the passage of the 2006 ZVW. The number of both uninsured and delinquent payers rose rapidly. At first, the Health Ministry announced that uninsured people requiring hospitalization would face the bills themselves (MoH 2007). They also had to obtain insurance retroactively and pay a fine. Enforcing such fines turned out challenging, however. Observing high rates of non-compliance, the MoH reduced the amounts in 2017. The GAK (the administrative office for welfare payments) became responsible for tracing the uninsured—illustrating another shift of policy to the national level. Based on administrative controls of central and local registries, its actions led to a sharp reduction in number of uninsured, from almost 150,000 to 30,000 between 2006 and 2016 (Vektis 2017).

The GAK was also charged with addressing payment delinquency. There were about 200,000 delinquent payers in mid-2007—who, lacking government action would become uninsured—as insurers could bar someone who had not paid monthly premiums for over three months (CBS 2007). The number grew to over 320,000 in 2015, with an over-representation of young immigrants, single-parent families and welfare recipients; groups generally unable to pay high fines or hospital bills out-of-pocket. Though still a modest share, out-of-pocket payments nonetheless became a significant political issue (as in Israel, see the chapter in this volume). After notification by insurers, the GAK was to impose a fine and enforce payment. Insurers themselves, also, became more active to prevent delinquency. The number of delinquents declined again, but the measures resulted in a sharp rise of debt settlement by local welfare offices.

The Dutch experience illustrates that insurance mandates are hard to enforce and administratively costly. They require the insured take active steps to enroll, with the probability that young and immigrant population groups and low-income families are less likely to retain insurance than others (Van Ginneken and Rice 2015).

its intention in 2017 to take over three smaller insurance plans, Promovendum, National Academic and Besured, from VGZ (*Zorgverzekering Informatie Centrum NL* 2017). Those very designations suggested another form of risk selection: obviously targeting highly educated insured, on average wealthier and healthier groups.

Changing Positions of Dutch Healthcare Providers

Managers of hospitals and other healthcare services reacted in different ways to the new challenges (De Roo 1995, 2003). To reduce costs, they contracted out maintenance and hotel functions, and initiated collective purchasing of medical goods. They built up financial reserves by improving their administration, realizing economies of scale and replacing skilled staff with less expensive labor. While remaining non-profits (by law), some hospitals created for-profit subsidiaries to provide customized luxury care and extended services. A few ventured into extended services like home care, meals-on-wheels and sports clinics or rapid access clinics for employees. Public polls and debates in Dutch Parliament revealed strong opposition to such preferential services for certain groups, however (ACM 2016).

At first, the MoH sought to restrain the independent for-profit clinics (*zelfstandige behandelcentra*, or ZBCs). A few years later, however, the government supported these clinics as a solution to long waitlists for elective surgery. ZBCs are mostly smaller facilities, with total revenues of less than 4 percent of all hospital expenditure in 2016 (Vektis 2018). Not all fared well. The number of ZBCs rose from about 200 to 350 between 2006 and 2011, but declined again to 245 in 2017 (Vektis 2017). They faced competition from hospital-related clinics, with numbers rising from 88 to 144 between 2011 and 2016 (*Volksgezondheidenzorg.nl* 2017).

Providers—like insurers—also strengthened their market position by collaborating with others. Many hospitals engaged in horizontal integration, developing informal networks and merging with others. They took over nursing homes, retirement facilities and ambulatory care in their region. The number of hospitals (including academic medical centers) declined from

91 to 79 between 2014 and 2016, though the number of locations (120) remained the same (Volksgezondheidenzorg.nl 2017). In some cases, this regional collaboration eliminated competition altogether—limiting consumer choice and defeating pro-competitive government policies. The two largest academic centers of Holland, the Free University hospital and the Academic Medical Center Amsterdam, each with over 1,000 beds and thousands of medical specialists, announced plans to merge in 2017. Despite concerns about the large scale of the new medical conglomerate, the Dutch anti-trust authority did not veto the merger, which went ahead in 2018.

In principle, hospitals negotiate each year with insurers over the price and volume of their services, based on a case-based payment model specially developed in the Netherlands. The decentralized development of this Diagnosis-Treatment Combination Model (DBC) resulted in over 30,000 different DBCs. This obviously caused heavy administrative burdens on hospitals and others. The MoH decided to reduce the number to about 4,000 in 2012, covering both inpatient and outpatient care (Wammes et al. 2013). It also relabeled the DBCs "Diagnosis-Treatment Model On Its Way To Transparency" (DOTs). Rather than resulting in extensive bargaining with insurers, however, increasing transparency and promoting competition, the bundled payment model prompted providers to collaborate in formal regional groups (Bal et al. 2017). For example, Dutch GPs created regional cooperatives to avoid individual contract negotiations. Also, increasingly, hospitals and other health facilities now seek multiyear contracts with health insurance—a return to the earlier social insurance practice.

There is obvious tension amid the contracting role of healthcare providers (based on the assumption that they negotiate with—competing—insurers over contracts), growing market concentration, renewed efforts of the Health Ministry to encourage regional collaboration and the rise of multiyear contracts between insurers and hospitals. There is also tension between the traditional non-profit status of hospitals and the way they have to deal with new financial risks, for example, in attracting commercial loans for capital extensions. Healthcare managers face the competing (and sometimes conflicting) external demands of price-based negotiations, participation in collective covenants and new forms of long-term regional collaboration, as well as traditional concerns of maintaining their regional patient base.

New Roles for Patients and Consumers in Dutch Healthcare

Dutch citizens and patient organizations have assumed new roles, too. This has hardly resulted in consumer-driven healthcare, however. Since the abolition of regional boundaries for sick funds in 1991, almost all funds expanded their activities nationwide.[7] To encourage the mobility of insured, the government sponsored websites with comparative information about healthcare and insurances. The main consumer association in the Netherlands, *Consumentenbond*, started to publish systematic assessments of the costs and quality of healthcare and health insurance in the 1990s. The weekly *Elsevier* published lists of the "best and worst" hospitals. New websites with information about healthcare and insurances spread rapidly, for example, *www.Zorgwijzer.NL* (Care Compass), *www.Kiesbeter.NL* (Better Choice), *www.ZorgverzekeringInformatieCentrum* (Care Insurance Information Center) and *www.Zorgpremie.net* (Care Premium).

The comparative information had limited effect. Dutch citizens tired of the bombardment of information, suggesting a backlash against consumerism in healthcare (Okma and Ooijens 2005). The mobility of insured remained modest (Laske-Aldershof et al. 2004) until the introduction of the ZVW in 2006, when 18 percent of insured changed insurance. Then, less than 5 percent of insured changed plans in 2007. That share has hovered between 6 and 7 percent since 2014 (Vektis 2017). In theory, Dutch consumers would all benefit from switching to cheaper policies, but they rarely voted with their feet (ACM 2016). The ACM concluded that there was perhaps not enough consumer info or transparency.

---

[7] A seemingly contradictory consequence of the option to switch sick funds was that persons with social insurance had more choice than private insured, as the latter were facing denial of coverage due to pre-existing medical conditions or other reasons. This created "job lock" when people feared losing their (supplemental) health insurance.

As in other countries, there was a marked bias in the composition of populations that switched plans versus the less discriminating ones who stayed put (see also the chapter in Chile in this volume). Young, healthy and higher income groups are (much) more inclined to switch plans than elderly, disabled or chronically ill (De Jong et al. 2008; Okma and Crivelli 2013; ACM 2016). For the more promiscuous consumers, the premium is more important than the quality of healthcare (Nivel 2009; Zorgwijzer 2011; Brabers et al. 2016). In short, the insured that need healthcare most are least likely to exert their consumer power to force insurers to contract good quality, efficient and patient-friendly care.

Interestingly, consumer action has been more effective in long-term care than in acute medical care (Okma 1997b). For example, patient representatives of the mentally handicapped and their relatives have successfully lobbied for better quality services in many cases. This consumerism found its origins in the "lunatics movement" of Dutch psychiatric patients in the 1960s, and subsequently, with relatives of people with developmental handicaps. Families of elderly and chronically ill patients took the government to court—and won—in the 1990s. This prompted the government to allocate additional financing for long-term care. Again in the early 2010s and in 2018, Dutch government rapidly agreed on additional budgets following media coverage of long waitlists and poor quality care in nursing homes. The strategy of "voice" (Hirschman 1970) worked well in these domains.

There has also been some "exit." The long-term care insurance AWBZ, and its successor the WLZ, has offered certain categories of patients the option of cash benefits or vouchers (PGB) instead of services in-kind since the mid-1990s. Those vouchers became very popular. Over 50,000 patients chose this option in 2003, receiving an average amount of about €20,000 per year, or over one billion euros. That amount doubled to over two billion euros in 2010. The budget for vouchers split over different budgets after the reorganization of the AWBZ in 2015, and it has since become hard to trace the total numbers of recipients or expenditures. There were estimates of 150,000 persons with a PGB in 2017, receiving up to €40,000 per person per year (over six billion euros; *Zorginstituut* 2016).

In contrast, (Dutch) patients expressed far less interest in exit within the domain of acute medical care. Most stayed with their GP for many years, usually following his or her advise about medical specialists and hospitals. Dutch patients traditionally showed a high degree of loyalty to hospitals (particularly the ones with a religious background) and to their former regional sick funds (Laske-Aldershof et al. 2004). The assumption of "satisficing behavior" found by March and Simon (1958) seems to apply to the Dutch situation: most people limit their choice to the first few alternatives they can clearly comprehend and feel comfortable with. The majority of patients are not willing or able to shop around extensively (with some of the abovementioned exceptions). The bombardment of information on websites, newspapers, specialized journals and other media has not done much to change that satisficing behavior in Dutch healthcare.

The role of citizens, insured and patients as collective actors in the policy arena gained some weight with the creation of regional Patient and Consumer Platforms (see footnote 7). The platforms became meeting grounds for existing patient groups, but not prominent actors in the health policy arena. For example, they were no formal parties in most covenants between governments, insurers and healthcare providers.

Summary and Conclusions: Results of the 2006 Healthcare Reforms 10 Years Later; Outlook for the Future

This chapter analyzed the origins and fate of the market-oriented health reforms in the Netherlands since the late 1980s. Both the acceptance of the original Dekker proposals of 1987 and the universal mandate to obtain health insurance (ZVW) in 2006 reflect the opening of windows of opportunity for major reforms. A few years after the partial implementation of the original legislation, however, opposition resurfaced and political support faded, ultimately leading Parliament to shelve the reforms altogether. A decade and several coalition governments later, the market-oriented plans came back as an even bigger bang reform. This time, helped by strong fiscal pressure and a more conservative coalition, Health Minister

Hoogervorst gained enough support for the rapid passage of the 2006 ZVW law by Dutch Parliament. The underlying assumption of those reforms was that the critical choice of health plans by individual citizens would prompt (competing) insurers to selectively contract with (competing) providers, thus safeguarding the best, cheapest and most patient-friendly care for their insured.

How did those expectations work out?

We noted how after the first year of the implementation of the 2006 ZVW Health Insurance Law, which introduced consumer choice and managed competition, there was a marked drop in the number of insured switching plans. Younger, higher educated and healthier groups changed more often than elderly or disabled insured. Since 2006, more than 70 percent of Dutch insured never changed plan. In short, the people who need healthcare most were the least likely to act as critical consumers of health insurance.

The chapter also indicated how health insurers generally paid more attention to consolidating their market positions than to the quality of healthcare. Healthcare providers also merged and created regional networks. This market concentration obviously reduced the scope of competition. Reflecting a lack of confidence in the cost-controlling capacity of market competition, governments regularly turned to traditional controls like macro budgets, delisting of entitlements and increased user fees—the latter two aimed more to shift costs than control them.

Some commentators concluded that the reforms were successful in bringing about universal coverage with identical benefits for all, solidarity and expanded patient choice, a competitive health insurance market and better information about healthcare (Van de Ven et al. 2011).[8] At the same time, they noted that insurers hardly developed new products or engaged in selective contracting due to public pressure and the fear of reputation

---

[8] Here is a problem of attribution: Were the low numbers of uninsured due to the new insurance, to government action, or to the former mix of public and private insurance? Likewise, can we attribute good population health to a new insurance scheme only three years after its introduction?

damage. Other problems continued: government interference, the dysfunctional payment system for hospitals (the very slow implementation of the newly developed DOTs), capacity shortages and the question of whether the regulation of private insurance is compatible with EU banking and insurance law. In a follow-up reaction, Schut and Van de Ven (2011b) argued that increased purchaser competition had already changed Dutch healthcare. They noted some price drops in hospital care (but with increases in the volume of services, no cost savings and lack of evidence of improved efficiency of the system). Other problems were "diagnosis creep," supply-induced demand, lack of reliable information about the quality of care and declining consumer trust in insurers. To address these problems, they advocated for better performance indicators, product classification and improved risk equalization (not surprising as the authors themselves were involved with those technical issues during the last four decades). Still, in a marked departure from their earlier position as warm advocates of the managed competition model, they concluded that it is unlikely that Dutch governments will expand purchaser competition any time soon with the global financial crisis and budget pressure.

Other commentators pointed to the political opposition to the reforms, the unpopularity of hospital closures, preferential patient treatment, for-profit healthcare and for-profit insurance, as well as lack of progress with the risk equalization system[9] and the new payment system for hospitals. Everywhere, price reductions led to increased volume of services, resulting in higher premiums and contributions (Maarse and Paulus 2011). Furthermore, the model had not shown success in controlling costs (Bal and Zuiderend-Jerak 2011; Lynch and Van Altenburg-Van den Broek 2010).

---

[9]All countries that use such risk equalization schemes struggle with the trade-off between costs and the degree of detail in estimating the costs of certain patient categories (see e.g., the chapters about Switzerland and Israel in this volume). Adding criteria to the schemes (apart from the "easy" ones like age or gender or postal area) greatly adds to administrative complexity and costs. Insurers will always have some opportunity to find out which patients will likely generate high future expenses, and this creates a financial incentive to "shed" those insured.

Predictably, the proponents of consumer-driven healthcare claimed that the reforms had not been implemented enough for the competition to be functioning well, whereas opponents were more skeptical about the potential benefits. For example, Van de Ven et al. (2011) argued that some necessary conditions were not yet in place, like performance indicators, transparent product classification and risk equalization. They insisted, however, that the "underlying political mainstream" supported further steps towards managed competition. In their view, there were two alternatives: (1) a return to the former social health insurance, with the general problems of government controls and long waitlists or (2) a tax-based single payer system, alien to Holland.[10]

We addressed the question of whether the 2006 system denoted a dramatic change in Dutch healthcare. Yes and No is the short answer. Yes, because the 2006 legislation effectively ended the more than 100-year-old tradition of sick funds, plunging Dutch healthcare into uncharted territory with quasi-private health insurance (the legal question of whether the current health insurance is private or public remains to be answered, see footnote 1).

No, because the new orientation towards market competition has not driven out the robust popular support for social solidarity in Dutch society. For-profit health services are tolerated on a modest scale—as long as governments safeguard access to a wide range of services without undue financial barriers. Efforts to engage in risk selection by insurers and providers are frowned upon. There is consumerism at the margin, but Dutch citizens have not embraced consumer-driven acute medical care. Insofar as they favor choice and exit, those apply much more to (long-term)

---

[10]This choice of only two alternative courses of action seems too narrow. The first, and most likely, outcome is obviously Lindblom's "muddling through" (1959). This permits political players to insist they are on the way to a better system without admitting the road may be a dead end. Another alternative is the Canadian national health insurance under de-centralized administration. Given the high concentration of the current insurance market, there is reason to question whether it will ever be truly competitive. Replacing the four main health insurers with the public administration of a population-wide health insurance does not seem incompatible with dominant values in Dutch society.

healthcare services than to the choice of plan. Citizens feel strongly about the quality of long-term care for their elderly and handicapped relatives, and are willing to take an active position, as we saw through the rapid growth of the voucher system.

We also exhibited how the new "private" health insurance greatly added to administrative complexity and costs. As Glied (2008) observed, mandates are both difficult and costly to implement, an experience not unique to the Netherlands. Ten years after the passage of the 2006 health insurance law, total health expenditure in Holland had risen from eight to over 13 percent of GDP—not quite the picture of successful cost control by private markets.

The Dutch case also illustrates how competitive markets require extensive regulation and supervision. The partially implemented health reforms did not replace the existing governance models. Despite the announced shifts from supply regulation to demand regulation, both categories of regulation remained firmly in place. Governments actually extended their presence by creating new agencies to monitor and control markets. Consequently, by the second decade of the 21st century, Dutch healthcare revealed a complex mix of public and private governance with an intricate overlay of state control and deregulation, patient choice and paternalistic government, market competition and market concentration, individual choice and collective action.

Finally, what do we expect for the future? The governing manifesto of the 2017 coalition government appeared to have taken some distance from the market-oriented reforms. It hardly mentioned competition or consumer choice but emphasized the need for individual responsibility, lower public health spending (implying the delisting of benefits, stronger government budget controls and a shift from institutional to home care), with more regional collaboration (and thus less competition). Combined with the high degree of concentration in the health insurance markets and some hospital regions, this implies, in fact, a shift in the direction of the Canadian model of universal health insurance. The four major insurance conglomerates have hardly changed their relative market shares in the last decades. In fact, they function more like public agencies than active contractors competing on behalf of their insured.

References

ACM. 2016. *Competition in the Dutch Health Insurance Market. Interim Report.* Authority for Consumers and Markets. Amsterdam: AFM.

Bal, R. and T. Zuiderend-Jerak. 2011. "The practice of markets in Dutch healthcare: are we drinking from the same glass?" *Health Econ Policy Law,* 6(1): 139–145.

Brabers, A., A. Verleun, R. Hoefman, and J. de Jong. 2016. *Percentage wisselaars blijft gelijk. Premie net als in eerdere jaren de belangrijkste reden om te wisselen.* [Share Insured Switching Plans Remains Unchanged. Premium Most Important Reason to Switch as in Previous Years.] Factsheet. Utrecht: Nivel.

CBS. 2007. *Kenmerken van Wanbetalers Zorgverzekeringswet.* [Characteristics Delinquent Payers of the Health Insurance Premiums]. Voorburg: Centraal Bureau voor de Statistiek.

CBS. 2015. *De Nederlandse Economie.* Voorburg: Centraal Bureau voor de Statistiek.

CBS. 2017. *Kerncijfers Zorguitgaven.* Den Haag/Heerlen: Centraal Bureau voor de Statistiek.

Commissie De Jong. 1991. *Raad op Maat. Rapport van de Bijzondere Commissie Vraagpunten Adviesorganen.* [Measured Advice. Report on Special Advisory Committees]. The Hague: SDU.

Commissie Dekker. 1987. *Bereidheid tot Verandering.* [Willingness to Change; Report of the Advisory Committee on Healthcare Reform]. The Hague: Distributiecentrum Overheidspublicaties.

De Jong, D.J., A. van den Brink-Muinen, and P.P. Groenewegen. 2008. "The Dutch health insurance reform: switching between insurers, a comparison between the general population and the chronically ill and disabled." *BMC Health Serv Res*, 8: 58.

De Roo, A.A. 1995. "Contracting and Solidarity: Market-Oriented Changes in Dutch Health Insurance Systems." *Implementing Planned Markets in*

Healthcare. R.B. Saltman and C. Von Otter (eds). Buckingham: Open University Press: 45–64.

De Roo, A.A. 2003. *De Zorgsector als Bedrijfstak in Wording*. [Healthcare Becoming a Grown Up Sector]. Inaugural Lecture. Tilburg: Tilburg University.

De Swaan, A. 1998. *In Care of the State: Healthcare, Education and Welfare in Europe and the USA in the Modern Era*. Oxford: Polity Press.

Enthoven, A. and W.P.M.M. Van de Ven. 2007. "Going Dutch—Managed-competition health insurance in the Netherlands." *N Engl J Med*, 357(24): 2421–2426.

Glied, S.A. 2008. "Universal coverage one head at a time—the risks and benefits of individual health insurance mandates." *N Engl J Med*, 358(15): 1540–1542.

Harris, G. 2007. "Looking at Dutch and Swiss health systems." *NYT*, October 30, 2007.

Helderman, J.-K. April 19–20, 2007. *Institutional Complementarity in Dutch Healthcare Reforms. Going Beyond the Pre-occupation with Choice*. European Health Policy Group, Berlin.

Hirschman, A.O. 1970. *Exit, Voice and Loyalty. Responses to Decline in Firms, Organizations, and States*. Cambridge: Harvard University Press.

Kingdon, J. 1984. *Agendas, Alternatives, and Public Policies*. New York: Longman.

Klee, M. and K.G.H. Okma. 2001. "Convenanten: Nieuw Instrument Van Beleid?" [Covenants: a new policy instrument?] *Zorg en Verzekering*, 8(1): 8–20.

Laske-Aldershof, T., E. Schut, K. Beck, et al. 2004. "Consumer mobility in vasocial health insurance markets. A five-country comparison." *Appl Health Econ Health Policy*, 3(4): 229–241.

Leu, R.E., F.H. Rutten, W. Brouwer, et al. 2009. "The Swiss and Dutch health insurance systems: universal coverage and regulated competitive insurance markets." *Health Policy, Health Reform, Perform Improv*, (104): 1–4.

Lijphart, A. 1968. *Verzuiling, Pacificatie en Kentering in de Nederlandse Politiek*. [Pillarization, Pacification and Turnaround in Dutch Policies]. Amsterdam: J.H. de Bussy.

Lindblom, C.E. 1959. "The science of muddling through." *Public Adm Rev*, 19(2): 79–99.

Lynch, R. and E. Altenburg-Van den Broek. 2010. *The Drawbacks of Dutch-Style Healthcare Rules: Lessons for America.* (Backgrounder). Washington: The Heritage Foundation.

Maarse, J.A.M. and P.P. Jeurissen. 2016. "The policy and politics of the 2015 long-term care reform in the Netherlands." *Health Policy*, 120: 241–245. doi:10.1016/j.healthpol.2016.01.014.

Maarse, J.A.M., P.P. Jeurissen, and D. Ruwaard. 2015. "Results of the market-oriented reform in the Netherlands: a review." *Health Econ Policy Law*, 2015: 161–178. doi:10.1017/S1744133115000353

Maarse, J.A.M. and A. Paulus. 2011. "The politics of health-care reform in the Netherlands since 2006." *Health Econ Policy Law*, 6(1): 125–134.

March, J., and H. Simons. 1958. *Organizations.* New York: John Wiley and Sons.

Marmor, T.R., R. Freeman, and K.G.H. Okma. 2003. "Comparative perspectives and policy learning in the world of healthcare." *J Comp Policy Anal*, 7(4): 331–348.

MoH. 1996. *Rijksbegroting Volksgezondheid, Welzijn en Sport 1996.* [Health Budget 1996.] Rijswijk: Ministerie van Volksgezondheid, Welzijn en Sport.

MoH. 2006. *Rijksbegroting Volksgezondheid, Welzijn en Sport 2007.* [Health Budget 2007.] The Hague: Ministerie van Volksgezondheid, Welzijn en Sport.

MoH. November 12, 2007. Oplossing Wanbetalersproblematiek (Nominale) Zorgpremie [Solution Delinquency Nominal Premiums]. *Letter to Parliament.* The Hague: SDU.

MoH. 2017. *Hoofdlijnenakkoord medisch-specialistische zorg 2018 ondertekend.* Press Release. [MoH Signs Covenant with Medical Specialists.] Nieuwsbericht, June 8. The Hague: Rijksoverheid.

Naik, G. 2007. "Dutch treatment: In Holland, some see model for U.S. Healthcare System." *Wall Street J*, September 6.

NVZ. 2011. *Bestuurlijk Hoofdlijnenakkoord 2012–2015* [Covenant MoH with Hospital Association and Health Insurers]. Zeist: NVZ.

NZA. 2016. Nederlandse Zorgautoriteit. *Kwalitatief onderzoek naar risicoselectie and risicosolidariteit op de zorgverzekeringsmarkt.* [Risk Selection and Solidarity in the Health Insurance Market.] Rapport: NZA.

OECD. 1992. *The Reform of Health Care: A Comparative Analysis of Seven OECD Countries.* Paris: Organisation for Economic Co-operation and Development.

OECD. 2017. *OECD Health Statistics 2017*. http://www.oecd.org/els/health-systems/health-data.htm. Accessed April 6, 2018.

OECD.stat. *Health Expenditure and Financing*, 2018. http://stats.oecd.org/index.aspx?DataSetCode=HEALTH_STAT. Accessed April 6, 2018.

Okma, K.G.H. 1997a. *Studies on Dutch Health Politics, Policies and Law*. PhD Diss. Amsterdam: Free University.

Okma, K.G.H. 1997b. "Concurrentie, Markten en Marktwerking in de Gezondheidszorg." [Competition and markets in healthcare]. *Tijdschrift voor Politieke Economie, Themanummer Marktwerking*, 20(2): 164–178.

Okma, K.G.H. 2002. "Health Care and the Welfare State: Two Worlds of Welfare Drifting Apart?" *Social Security in Transition*. J. Berghman, A. Nagelkerke, and K. Boos, et al. (eds). Leiden: Kluwer Law International: 229–38.

Okma, K.G.H. 2009. "Recent Changes in Dutch Health Insurance. Individual Mandate or Social Health Insurance?" *Expanding Access to Healthcare. A Management Approach*. T.F. Buss and P.N. Van de Water (eds). Armonk, NY, USA: M.E. Sharpe: 144–161.

Okma, K.G.H. and L. Crivelli. 2013. "Swiss and Dutch 'Consumer-driven health care: ideal model or reality?" *Health Pol*, 109(2): 105–112.

Okma, K.G.H. and A.A. de Roo. 2009. "The Netherlands: From Polder Model to Modern Management." *Comparative Studies & the Politics of Modern Medicine*. T.R. Marmor, R. Freeman, and K.G.H. Okma (eds). New Haven: Yale University Press: 120–152.

Okma, K.G.H. and T.R. Marmor. 2013. "Comparative studies and healthcare policy: learning and mislearning across borders." *Clin Med*, 13(5): 487–491.

Okma, K.G.H. T.R. Marmor, and J. Oberlander. July 2011. "Managed competition for medicare? Sobering lessons from the Netherlands." *N Engl J Med*, 12: 1–3.

Palmer, G.R. and S.D. Short. 1989. *Healthcare and Public Policy—An Australian Analysis*. Melbourne: The Macmillan Company of Australia.

Regeerakkoord. 1994. [Governing Manifesto 1994]. The Hague: SDU.

Regeerakkoord. 2017. [Governing Manifesto 2017]. The Hague: SDU.

Rose, R. 1993. *Lesson-Drawing in Public Policy. A Guide to Learning Across Time and Space*. Chatham, NJ: Chatham House Publishers.

Rosenberg, E. 2006. "Ziekenhuizen Moeten Hard Zijn." [Hospitals Must Be Ruthless]. *NRC Handelsblad,* January 18.

Rosenberg, E. 2007. "Concurrentie in de Zorg Blijft Uit." [Competition in Healthcare Does Not Materialize]. *NRC Handelsblad*, May 15.

Scharpf, F. 1997. *Games Real People Play. Actor-oriented Institutionalism in Policy Research.* Boulder: Westview.

Schneider, E.C., D.O. Sarnak, S. Squires, et al. 2017. *Mirror, Mirror 2017: International Comparison Reflects Flaws and Opportunities for Better U.S. Healthcare.* The Commonwealth Fund.

Schut, F.T. and W.P.M.M. van de Ven. 2005. "Rationing and competition in the Dutch health-care system." *Health Econ*, 14: S59–S74.

Schut, F.T. and W.P.M.M. van de Ven. 2011a. "Effects of purchaser competition in the Dutch health system: is the glass half full or half empty?" *Health Econ Policy Law*, 6(1): 109–123.

Schut, F.T. and W.P.M.M. van de Ven. 2011b. "Managed competition the Dutch health system: is there a realistic alternative?" *Health Econ Policy Law*, 2001 6(1): 135–137.

Smit, M. and P. Mokveld. 2007. *Verzekerdenmobiliteit en Keuzegedrag.* [Mobility and Choice in Dutch Health Insurance]. Zeist: Vektis.

Timmins, N. 1995. *The Five Giants. A Biography of the Welfare State.* London: HarperCollins.

Tuohy Hughes, C. 2018. *Remaking Policy. Scale, Pace and Policy Strategy in Healthcare Reforms.* Toronto: University of Toronto Press.

Van den Berg, M., R. Heijink, L. Zwakhals, et al. 2011. "Healthcare performance in the Netherlands: easy access, varying quality, rising costs." *Eurohealth*, 16(4): 27–29.

Van de Ven, W.P.P.M., and F.T. Schut. 2008. "Universal mandatory health insurance in the Netherlands: a model for the United States?" *Health Affairs*, 27(3): 771–781.

Van de Ven, W.P.M.M., F.T. Schut, H.E.C.M. Hermans. 2011. *Evaluatie Zorgverzekeringswet en Wet op de Zorgtoeslag.* [Evaluation ZVW and Fiscal Subsidy Act ZVW.] Den Haag: ZonNW.

Van Ginneken, E., and T. Rice. 2015. "Enforcing enrollment in health insurance exchanges: evidence from the Netherlands, Switzerland, and Germany." *Med Care Res Rev*, 72(4): 496–509.

Van Ginneken, E. 2015. "Perennial healthcare reforms—the long Dutch Quest for cost control and quality improvement." *N Engl J Med*, 373(10): 885–889.

Van Strien, F. and R. Bhagaloe-Datadin. 2015. *Ontwikkeling en Financiering van de Zorglasten Sinds 2006.* [Financing Dutch Healthcare since 2006]. Voorburg: Centraal Bureau voor de Statistiek.

Visser, J. and A. Hemerijck. 1997. *A Dutch Miracle-Job Growth, Welfare Reform and Corporatism in the Netherlands.* Amsterdam: Amsterdam University Press.

Wammes, J., P. Jeurissen, G. Westert, and M. Tanke. 2013. "The Dutch healthcare system." *International Healthcare System Profiles.* The Commonwealth Fund.

Wilensky, H. 2002. *Rich Democracies: Political Economy, Public Policy, and Performance.* Berkeley: University of California Press.

Zorginstituut. 2016. *Monitor Langdurige Zorg.* [Monitor Long-Term Care].

Zorgkiezer.nl. *Factsheet Evaluatie Zorgverzekering 2006–1012. Trends and Ontwikkelingen in de Zorg Bekeken.* Accessed April 6, 2018.

Zorgverzekeraars Nederland. 2008. www.zn.nl. Accessed October 20, 2008.

Zorgwijzer.nl. 2017a. *Half miljoen Nederlanders raakt zorgtoeslag kwijt in 2015.* April 10, 2017. www.zorgwijzer.nl. Accessed April 6, 2018.

Zorgwijzer.nl. 2017b. *Zorggids 2017.* [Care Guide 2017]. Accessed April 6, 2018.

Chapter 6

Federal Government, Cantons and Direct Democracy in the Swiss Health System

Luca Crivelli and Carlo De Pietro

Introduction

Switzerland is a small land-locked nation in the middle of Europe. It has had a long tradition of political independence and neutrality during the world wars that ravaged the continent. In the late 19th century, influenced by growing international tourism attracted to the Alps, the Swiss economy transformed from an agricultural base to that of manufacturing, financial services and tourism. With that transformation, Switzerland became one of the most prosperous nations in the world. It had about 8.5 million inhabitants in 2018. There are four official Swiss languages: German, spoken by 63 percent of the population, French (23 percent), Italian (8 percent) and Romansh (0.5 percent).

The growing prosperity also allowed for the development of extensive social insurance and welfare support in the 20th century, mostly modeled after the German Bismarckian schemes. This resulted in a mix of public and private insurances and tax-financed welfare services provided by public and private agencies for elderly, handicapped and low-income families.

The Swiss political system combines the tradition of highly decentralized federalism with direct democracy. The 26 cantons have a strong say over fiscal and social policy-making, while the role of the federal government reflects the subsidiarity principle. At the same time, next to general elections at the national and regional levels, referendums and popular initiatives represent a channel for the popular vote to block or enforce policy change. That particular political arrangement gives strong veto power to many well-organized stakeholders. They can use the very threat of organizing a referendum or launching an initiative to support their demands. The new insurance act thus added Hirschman's "exit" in the health insurance to the strong "vote" options as seen later (Hirschman 2008).

In 1996, the federal health insurance (FHI) Act established a universal health insurance mandate (mandatory health insurance [MHI]) for all residents (see Box 1). This reform had three main goals: (1) strengthening the solidarity across different groups of insured; (2) expanding the benefit basket while ensuring high-quality services; and (3) containing the growth of healthcare costs. The FHI followed the so-called managed competition advocated by Alain Enthoven who offers citizens free choice of health insurer and providers (and assumes that both insurers and providers will compete, thus safeguarding good quality and efficient services for all).

While there have been significant improvements in access and in broadening coverage, the same statement doesn't apply to the third reform objective, cost control. In fact, rising health costs appear regularly in political debates as the top concern of families and voters, and rank high on the political agenda at both the national and cantonal levels.

At the same time, the perceived high quality of healthcare and large freedom in accessing health services create major barriers for substantial reforms. In fact, most reform efforts ultimately turn out to be merely incremental. The two abovementioned key features of the institutional and political system—federalism and direct democracy—contribute to the slow pace of health reforms. Other elements hindering major change are the economic traditions of liberalism and private initiative and the high levels of average income and wealth. These elements support the very expensive and highly fragmented institutional framework of Switzerland. There does not seem to be great pressure to improve the current, insufficiently

Box 1. Key Elements of the Swiss MHI, 2018

> Swiss Parliament passed the FHI Act in 1994. The FHI went into effect in 1996. It regulates health insurance and healthcare at the national level. The FHI mandates that all residents acquire health insurance with a comprehensive, standardized benefit basket on par with current medical and technological standards. Each individual must enroll with one of the 50 or so insurers offering the basic contract, and insurers cannot turn down anyone seeking coverage. They have to set the premiums independently from individual health status and income. Premiums can vary according to (1) age (under 19; 19–25; 26 and over); (2) region of residence; (3) size of deductible (for adults: minimum SFr300, maximum SFr2,500); and (4) alternative plans with a variety of conditions, for example, restrictions in the freedom of choice (telephone advice first, gatekeeping family doctor, capitation-based managed care, etc.). Such plans usually combine higher deductibles in exchange for discount premiums. Low-income families can apply for fiscal subsidies for their premiums, and the cantons receive federal co-funding to pay for those subsidies.
>
> The health insurers reimburse the providers with fees for outpatient services and case-based payments (diagnosis-related-group based [DRGs]) for hospital care. The national associations of providers and insurers negotiate over fees and further development of the national tariff structure. Finally, cantons contribute additional financing to hospitals (they pay 55 percent of the DRG-price) and some other health services (De Pietro et al. 2015).

Source: Crivelli and De Pietro.

cost-effective health system. Box 1 presents the key elements of the universal health insurance mandate. The section then analyzes some of the strengths and weaknesses of the present system, followed by the recent health reforms and the main challenges for the future.

Health and Healthcare Performance in Switzerland

Thanks to the country's economic prosperity and extremely favorable socioeconomic conditions, the Swiss health system ranks high in most international comparisons. For example, the (much disputed) 2000 annual report by the World Health Organization (WHO) placed Switzerland second among WHO member states for overall health system results (WHO 2000).[1] Furthermore, Switzerland ranked third in the 2017 Bloomberg Top 50 (Bloomberg 2017) healthiest country index and it had the second best total performance among the 35 countries analyzed by the Euro Health Consumer Index in 2017 (Björnberg 2018).

The health system—together with other social insurances and public policies in other sectors—aims to protect and improve the health of the population, and to protect families from the financial impact of illness and disability. In general, Swiss patients appreciate the short wait times, the ample choice of providers, the widespread availability of new technology (even when not always properly tested for cost-effectiveness) and the comfortable facilities. These elements explain the strong support enjoyed by the health system in public debates, and also the opposition to major reforms in many electoral ballots.

Despite these strengths, there are critical issues such as lack of cost control, equity and inefficiencies. The large amount of out-of-pocket payments (direct patient payments, deductibles and co-payments) and flat insurance premiums led to highly regressive health financing as low- and middle-income families spend a much larger share of their income on healthcare than wealthier ones (Crivelli and Salari 2014a). Those payments also create access barriers to health services.

There is no a priori reason why Switzerland should spend more than comparable countries on its healthcare, both as per capita expenditure and as percentage of gross domestic product (GDP). One reason for this relatively low efficiency originates in the federalist political structure. This traditionally gave the cantons independence over the administration of health insurance and healthcare. It also resulted in wide regional differences in services and reimbursement regimes for inpatient and outpatient care, fragmentation in the provision of services, lack of interoperable data and health technology assessment (HTA). Furthermore, Swiss healthcare comes with high prices and salaries.

---

[1] It should be noted that Switzerland scored worse in terms of performance (ranking 20th), namely, as soon as the overall attainments were put in relationship with healthcare costs.

To assess the performance of Swiss healthcare, this section analyzes four classical dimensions of the system: effectiveness, equity, efficiency and responsiveness.

Effectiveness

The Swiss generally enjoy very good health, as most indicators show (e.g., life expectancy at birth second since 1999 among OECD countries; OECD 2018). Other outcome indicators are potential years of life lost for all causes (ninth among OECD countries for populations aged 0–69 in 2016 or attested data available; OECD 2018a, b), amenable mortality (first in the Eurostat group in 2015) and preventable mortality (fifth in 2015 Eurostat statistics, which include the 28 EU member states plus six other European countries). Finally, it ranked third in 2016 for the share of people over 16 with "very good" or "good" self-perceived health (Eurostat 2018).

As to the quality of the healthcare services, most Swiss (95 percent) consider their care to be good to excellent. According to a recent survey, 30 percent of respondents rated the healthcare they received as good, 49 percent as very good and 17 percent as excellent in 2016 (Merçay 2016). This high satisfaction is mirrored by the low public support for major change. In the same survey, 59 percent of respondents argued that Swiss healthcare needed only minor improvements (Merçay 2016).

The good health of the Swiss is not just the result of good healthcare, however. It results from the complex interaction of several determinants of health. Among them, the non-medical determinants play a major role: high incomes, healthy environment and working conditions, a good education system and strong, stable political institutions.

Equity

Swiss social security offers families and individuals effective financial protection against the risk of accidents, disability and illness. At the core of the system are the well-endowed social insurances developed during the 20th century, largely following Germany's Bismarckian model. The last major step in this development was the 1996 FHI Act with universal, MHI that equalized access to health insurance for all legal residents and dependents by establishing a uniform benefit basket at the national level, and by an ex-post correction of community-rated premiums through earmarked subsidies for households with lower incomes (Crivelli 2020).

The MHI offers all insured virtually unrestricted choice of providers, with a wide availability of health professionals, facilities spread all over the country and very short waitlists. Thus, it safeguards access to all social classes.

The main equity shortfall is caused by the MHI flat-rate premiums. As a result, middle and lower-income households pay a larger percentage of their income on healthcare than higher-income households. Cantons provide subsidies for people with low incomes. Despite a large number of beneficiaries—27.3 percent of the insured in 2016 (OFSP 2018a)—those subsidies do not, in fact, sufficiently redistribute the financial burden across income groups. Middle-income families, who are not the recipients of the subsidies, face the greatest financial burden in many cantons (BAG 2018). Moreover, there is wide variety in the way different cantons apply the criteria for eligibility and subsidize premiums. This aggravates the variation in financial burden depending on the place of residence. For example, the population share that received subsidies varied from 22 percent in Canton Basel-Landschaft to 33 percent in Canton Zurich (OFSP 2018a) in 2016. The subsidies covered on average about 79 percent of the premiums in Canton Aarau, but only 34 percent in Canton Bern (OFSP 2018a).

Another equity issue stems from the high out-of-pocket spending (OOPs) that represented 30 percent of health spending in 2016 (compared with an OECD average of 20 percent; OECD 2018). Most OOPs (around 80 percent) are for services not covered by the mandatory or voluntary health insurances (e.g., routine dental care, co-payment for inpatient long-term care, pharmaceuticals), the remaining mostly concern cost sharing for MHI-covered services. MHI-insured face deductibles (from SFr300 to 2,500 per year for adults) and a 10 percent co-insurance (capped to a maximum of SFr700 per year for adults). Increases in MHI premiums over the years led many insured to opt for the maximum deductible of SFr2,500 (€2,170 or $2,510) for adults in 2016.[2] Almost one quarter of all adults had the maximum deductible that year (OFSP 2018a). Maximum deductibles in combination with managed care can lead to a discount in premiums of up to 50 percent, but they leave the insured with a heavy financial burden.

The high OOPs caused many Swiss patients to skip a visit to the physician or a prescription drug refill. According to a recent survey, Switzerland had the worse score of 10 industrialized nations in 2016, after the United States, for the question "Have any cost-related access problems to medical care in the past year?" (Schneider et al. 2017).[3]

Efficiency

Swiss healthcare is expensive. Total health expenditure (THE) was 12.3 percent of GDP in 2017: the second highest percentage among OECD countries after the United States (the OECD average was 8.9 percent; OECD 2018a). Switzerland also ranked second for the amount of health spending per person ($8,009 PPP, OECD average was $4,069 PPP; OECD 2018a). In addition, the growth rate of Swiss health spending in real terms has been high. Annual growth amounted to 2.5 percent between 2008 and 2017, ranking seventh among the 35 OECD member countries (OECD 2018a).

It is important to note that the total amount of health spending is the result of quantities multiplied by price. The volume of Swiss healthcare services is at, or somewhat above, OECD average but prices are much higher (thus a similar pattern to that of the United States).

Switzerland had 3.7 curative (acute) care beds per 1,000 people in 2016, compared with an OECD average of 3.6 (OECD 2018a). It had 38.9

---

[2] Exchange rates as of July 31, 2018.

[3] The survey included Australia, Canada, France, Germany, the Netherlands, New Zealand, Norway, Sweden, Switzerland, the United Kingdom and the United States. Positive answers to the question ranged from 33 percent in the United States and 22 percent in Switzerland to 7 percent in the United Kingdom and Germany.

computed tomography (CT) scanners per 1,000,000 people, compared with 26.1 in the OECD. There were 4.3 practicing physicians per 1,000 people (compared to the 3.4 OECD average). Switzerland had twice as many hip or knee replacements than the OECD average in 2015.[4] While recognizing the need to use caution when looking at international comparisons (due to differences in definitions and measures used across countries), the Swiss health system clearly emerges as a system with ample availability and use of physical, technological and human resources.

There is little or no routine systematic public data collection on prices and costs. Still, OECD data suggest the "quasi prices" for hospitals services (i.e., the negotiated or administrative prices and tariffs) were 92 percent higher in Switzerland than the OECD average (Lorenzoni and Koechlin 2017). The overall price level for hospitals, outpatient services, pharmaceuticals, medical goods and therapeutic appliances was 71 percent higher (Lorenzoni and Koechlin 2017). Two specific factors contribute to this high price level. The first is the small average size of acute hospitals, which prevents exploitation of economies of scale (OFSP 2018b). The second is the low share of generic drugs (OECD 2017) even while prices of generics tend to be high (DEFR Surveillance des prix SPR 2016).

Responsiveness

The well-endowed Swiss health system is generally able to rapidly address the health needs and demands of the population. Access barriers are low due to the high number of providers across the country. All insured have free choice of accredited providers and they can visit specialists without a gatekeeper (with a few exceptions). There are short wait times.

Federalism and the political history of the country have favored the ample geographical spread of healthcare facilities. For example, over 90 percent of the population lived within 15 minutes driving distance to at least one hospital in 2010 (Christen et al. 2013: 27). Almost three quarters

---

[4]Rates per 100,000 people in the population were 308 for hip replacement and 240 for knee replacement, compared to OECD averages of 166 and 126, respectively (OECD 2017).

of the population lived in municipalities within a 30 minutes drive to at least eight hospitals (Christen et al. 2013).

The FHI confirmed the principle of free choice of provider. Insured can generally access the services without gatekeeping mechanisms. Despite some exceptions or limitations,[5] all MHI-insured can choose their providers, while the insurers cannot exclude any provider authorized to practice by cantonal governments.

A third access element concerns wait times. In 2015, 91 percent of patients with a hip fracture had their surgery within two days of admission to the hospital (OECD 2017). Likewise, there were very short wait times for emergency care and elective surgery in 2016: 57 percent of patients waited less than one hour in the emergency room; 73 percent of patients waited less than one month for an appointment with a specialist (and only 9 percent had to wait two months or longer); 59 percent of patients waited less than one month for elective/non-emergency surgery (and only 7 percent had to wait four months or longer); only one percent of doctors reported that their patients often experience difficulty in getting specialized tests (e.g., CT or magnetic resonance imaging [MRI]); and only 1 percent of doctors reported that their patients often had to wait long to receive treatment after diagnosis (Merçay 2016; Schneider et al. 2017).

The short wait times combined with the comfortable facilities and a service-oriented, pro-market attitude of providers have resulted in the high appreciation and trust of most Swiss patients. No wonder they are reluctant to engage in major reform!

That is not to say there are no problems, for example, the lack of public systemic information on the appropriateness of services and on the quality of professionals and health facilities. Depending solely on patient satisfaction surveys does not seem to be a good substitute for systematic

---

[5]For example, MHI does not reimburse for hospitalizations in facilities not included in the lists of cantonal hospital planning. In case of hospitalization in a canton different from residence, the MHI insurer will not reimburse a higher price than it would have reimbursed in the insured's canton of residence. In ambulatory care, insured who opted for an alternative MHI-plan face some restriction in their choice of provider, for example, by accepting a family physician as gatekeeper, or a managed care plan.

data gathering as a basis for assessing the quality of services and developing useful consumer information on providers. Another weak aspect, as noted earlier, is the high fragmentation and lack of coordination between services across the many healthcare providers. This leads to duplication, waste of resources or, worse, bad health outcomes. We will focus on these problems later.

Recent Healthcare Reforms in Switzerland

The 1996 FHI constituted the most recent fundamental reform of the Swiss health system. It established the national MHI with a population-wide mandate. Swiss health policy since then has aimed to fully implement the mandate, further improve the system and address the new and changing needs of the population. One particular feature of the Swiss political arena is the combination of federalism with general elections, and direct democracy with regular referendums (see Table 1).

Table 1.   Federal Ballots in Switzerland on Health Issues, 2007–2017

Year (and participation rate)	Ballot	Result
PI 2007 (46%)	*For a Single, Social Sick Fund.* Main aim: to establish a single health insurer with income-based premiums.	Rejected by 71% of voters and 21 cantons.
Ref 2007 (36%)	Amendment to the federal social insurance law for the disabled. Main aim: to promote the disabled being able to stay at work and to reduce expenses of the social insurance.	Amendment to the federal law approved by 59% of voters.
Ref 2008 (45%)	Federal government's counter-proposal to the withdrawn popular initiative *On Lower Insurance Premiums.* Main aim: to include the basic principles of the MHI federal law into the Federal Constitution as well.	Amendment to the Constitution rejected by 69% of voters and all cantons.

Table 1. (*Continued*)

Year (and participation rate)	Ballot	Result
PI 2008 (47%)	*For a Reasonable Policy on Cannabis.* Main aim: to decriminalize cannabis consumption.	Rejected by 63% of voters and all cantons.
Ref 2008 (47%)	Amendment to the federal law on drugs and addiction. Main aim: to allow heroin and cannabis use under medical control for specific needs.	Amendment to the federal law approved by 68% of voters.
Ref 2009 (39%)	Federal government's counter-proposal to the withdrawn popular initiative *Yes to Complementary Medicine.* Main aim: to include specific alternative medicines in the MHI coverage—previously only covered by voluntary health insurance.	Government proposal approved by 67% of voters and all cantons.
Ref 2009 (41%)	Federal government's decree to increase the funding of social insurance for the disabled. Main aim: to amend the Federal Constitution to increase the funding of social insurance for the disabled by a temporary increase of the TVA.	Government proposal approved by 55% of voters and 12 cantons.
Ref 2012 (39%)	Amendment to the federal law on the MHI. Main aim: to promote integrated networks of care with budget responsibilities by means of financial incentives for insured (lower co-payment rate).	Rejected by 76% of voters.
PI 2012 (43%)	*Protection Against Passive Smoking.* Main aim: to extend smoking ban to all work places and publicly accessible buildings.	Rejected by 66% of voters and 22 cantons.
PI 2014 (56%)	*Abortion is a Private Affair—Take Out Costs from the MHI.* Main aim: to de-list abortion and related healthcare from MHI coverage.	Rejected by 70% of voters and 22.5 cantons.

(*Continued*)

Table 1. (*Continued*)

Year (and participation rate)	Ballot	Result
Ref 2014 (56%)	Federal government's counter-project to the withdrawn popular initiative *Yes to Family Doctor Medicine.* Main aim: to commit both Cantons and federal government to promoting high quality primary care, easily accessible to all Swiss residents.	Government proposal approved by 88% of voters and all cantons.
PI 2014 (47%)	*For a Public Health Insurer.* Main aim: to replace the current pluralistic system, based on health insurer competition, with a single, public health insurer.	Rejected by 62% of voters and 19 cantons.
Ref 2016 (47%)	Amendment to the federal law on reproductive medicine. Main aim: to authorize—under specified circumstances—pre-implantation genetic diagnosis of embryos obtained by artificial insemination.	Amendment approved by 62% of voters.

Source: Authors' compilation based on https://www.bk.admin.ch/ch/f/pore/va/vab_2_2_4_1.html (accessed on July 31, 2018).

The Rich and Tiresome Workings of Swiss Federalism and Direct Democracy

As noted earlier, Switzerland is a federal state of 8.5 million inhabitants with 26 highly autonomous cantons (or provinces). The federal constitution states: "The cantons are sovereign insofar as their sovereignty is not limited by the Federal Constitution; they shall exercise all rights which are not transferred to the confederation." This strongly decentralized political system, based on federalism and subsidiarity, with shared fiscal and budgetary responsibilities requires continuous negotiations between federal and cantonal governments. These circumstances obviously affect health policies (Crivelli and Salari 2014b).

Despite the traditionally strong decentralization, there has been a remarkable trend of centralization in health policy in recent decades, shifting decision-making power from the cantons to the federal government. This trend gained momentum with the passage of the FHI Act. Three factors stand out that help explain this trend: (1) new information technology enabling greater collaboration between professionals and institutions; (2) greater geographic mobility of people; and (3) the small size of many cantons that forces them to enlarge the scale of their health systems to deal with the challenges of new health technology and specialization of professional skills.

Direct democracy, the second element of Swiss politics, as mentioned earlier, has also been important in the shaping of health policy. Citizens can induce policy change through "popular initiatives." They can stop laws proposed by elective bodies with mandatory or voluntary referendums, grouped into four election days per year. Ballots pass with the majority of voters, but popular initiatives and mandatory referendums require "double majorities" at the federal level, specifically, both the majority of voters and the majority of cantons.[6] It is relatively easy to collect the signatures required for a popular initiative or for an optional referendum. Referendums are often used as a pre-emptive menace or brake on the political process.

To illustrate this process, Table 1 lists the federal popular ballots closely related to health policy in the last decade. It does not include the many ballots on health issues in the same period within the different cantons.

Table 1 illustrates how the combination of direct democracy and federalism affects Swiss health policy-making. The referendums reduce the autonomy of both the central government and the federal administration, and add to the complexity of the already complicated decentralized

---

[6] For calculating the vote of cantons, the 20 (large) cantons have a full vote, and six (small) cantons have half a vote. Therefore, the total of votes is 20 + 3 = 23. Thus, 12 or more votes represent the majority.

political system. This system made the adoption of every legislative reform particularly difficult and slow. The direct democracy allows Swiss citizens to intervene directly in decision-making (by approving or rejecting reform proposals in a popular ballot), while the federalist arrangements encourage the proliferation of widely divergent organizational models and spending patterns at the canton level (Crivelli and Bolgiani 2009). This complex system tends not to approve unbalanced and radical changes, however (as in New Zealand), but rather favors extensive negotiations and consultations with the main stakeholders. This often results in marginal changes at a slow pace.

Reforms in the Insurance Market

The MHI plays a key role in the Swiss health system. It offers financial protection to insured and covers about 40 percent of total healthcare costs.[7] The FHI supports the administrative structure and regulates all main elements of the healthcare system. Since the enactment of the FHI and the MHI, the federal and cantonal governments continue to adjust and improve the legislation.

The cantons acknowledged the need to improve their systems to subsidize premiums, in particular the need for more redistribution. As this implied higher taxes, this posed a challenge for politicians and government. The second issue for cantons was to avoid creating a "poverty trap": families can suddenly lose substantial amounts of financial aid when they start to earn slightly more than the poverty line established for the eligibility of that subsidy (threshold effect).

On the supply side of the MHI, the first main adjustment concerned a further refinement of the risk adjustment mechanism. The risk adjustment compensates MHI insurers for over-representation of costly insured (e.g., older or chronically ill persons). This compensation aims to reduce the

---

[7]The MHI financed directly 36 percent of health expenditure in 2016, families and patients 29 percent, confederation and cantons 17 percent, private voluntary insurance 7 percent, other social insurances 6 percent, other public financing 4 percent and other private sources 1 percent (BAG 2018b).

incentive for insurers to engage in risk selection and allows them to charge community-rated premiums. Until 2011 the formula for risk adjustment was very basic as it only took into account gender and 15 age groups. The MHI expanded the formula by including the previous year's data about hospitalization (more than three consecutive nights spent in an acute hospital or nursing home) and prescription drug consumption to the criteria for the next years.

The rapid diffusion of so-called "alternative" plans led to other problems (Crivelli 2020). These plans differed from the standard ones along two dimensions: (1) higher deductibles, (2) constraints on provider choice, for example, gatekeeping by a family doctor, call center or managed care (health maintenance organization [HMO]) contract. Swiss adults had signed up for a range of plans in 2015: 19 percent had an ordinary insurance contract with the minimum deductible (SFr300 per year), down from 60 percent in 1996 and 40 percent in 2005; 17 percent had a contract with a high deductible (between SFr500 and 2,500 per year); 25 percent had a gatekeeping or HMO plan with a minimum deductible; 39 percent had a gatekeeping or HMO plan that included a high deductible (Interpharma 2018).

In reaction to the changes in the insurance market, the federal government took several measures to enhance surveillance and control. The federal law on MHI surveillance passed in 2014 (in effect since 2016) with three main aims: (1) better separation between standard MHI and the private complementary cover plans; (2) stricter supervision of the insurers by the Federal Office of Public Health (FOPH) for MHI proposed premiums; and (3) the obligation for insurers to provide more data on reimbursements to the FOPH.

The parliamentary debate of the new law started in 2011 but slowed down when faced with mounting lobbying efforts from insurers. The political process regained momentum in reaction to the popular initiative *For a [Single] Public Health Insurer* of 2014 (see Table 1). The federal law on surveillance was used in the debate to convince the population that this regulation would be sufficient to improve the transparency of the health insurance industry and to reject the popular initiative. It passed

Parliament only two days before the popular vote, when 62 percent of voters finally rejected the popular initiative (De Pietro and Crivelli 2015).

Reforms in Healthcare Provision

In the last two decades, Swiss healthcare services faced the pressures of the aging population, new and growing demands of patients and growing public expectations. Most of this pressure was accommodated by steady economic growth in this period. At the same time, there were three main streams of change: specialization of healthcare providers, new rules for reimbursement and integration of care.

An amendment to the FHI in 2007 required the Cantons to participate in national hospital planning for highly specialized (and expensive) medicine. Those were grouped into 39 domains such as cochlear implantation or allogeneic hematopoietic stem cell transplants in adults (FHI, article 39, paragraph 2bis; GDK 2018). Obviously, this collaboration across cantons did not result from bottom-up initiatives, but from federal law. The law states that if cantons do not reach an agreement, the federal government will step in to decide the location of specialty care. This legislation led to acceleration of the ongoing specialization of hospitals.

Another specialization trend was visible in post-acute inpatient care, prompted by an amendment of the federal law on MHI in 2008. This introduced—along with inpatient rehabilitation—new transitional care between acute hospitals, nursing homes and patients' own homes (FHI, article 25a, paragraph 2). This new arrangement became necessary as new DRGs (see below) led to shorter lengths of stay in acute hospitals.

The main change in hospital reimbursement was the introduction of a nation-wide case-based DRG model in 2012. It replaced per diems as the most important mechanism for paying hospitals. SwissDRGs include both investment costs and current cost. Hospitals and insurers negotiate the tariffs for the DRGs. Cantons still bear 55 percent of the cost of each inpatient admission, insurers the remaining amount, minus patient co-payments, if applicable.

The reimbursement of ambulatory medical care is based on a national uniform fee system called TARMED. The cantonal association of physicians and the association of hospitals negotiate with MHI insurers over the monetary values of TARMED points. Cantons do not participate in this reimbursement. The federal government resolved the TARMED structure in 2017 after the negotiating partners (including physicians' association, hospital association and MHI insurers) failed to reach an agreement. This episode represents another example of the increasing role of the federal government in the regulation and administration of Swiss healthcare.

The third important development refers to integration between healthcare providers. Here, too, federal law played a crucial role. The federal law on the electronic patient record (EPR) was passed in 2015 and came into effect in 2017 (De Pietro and Francetic 2017). Hospitals have three years, and nursing homes five, to adopt an interoperable EPR system to facilitate data sharing and cooperation among healthcare providers. Other providers are encouraged but not obligated to adopt interoperable EPRs. In this case, a federal requirement tries to overcome the institutional and political fragmentation of the Swiss health system.

Other Public Health Policies

Two other major new initiatives are changing the direction of the Swiss health system: the federal healthcare strategy *Health2020* of 2013 and national "sector strategies."

With its *Health2020—The Federal Council's Health-Policy Priorities* (OFSP 2013), the federal government aimed to set an important milestone in the development of Swiss health policy. The FOPH prepared this document after intense consultation with the system's main stakeholders. It proposed a general framework for national sector strategies, inter-cantonal actions and cantonal health policy. The report defines four priority areas, each with three objectives and specific measures (see Box 2).

The main stakeholders in Swiss healthcare (including cantons, hospitals, physicians and health professionals, pharmaceutical industry,

Box 2.   Health2020 Priority Areas and Objectives for Policy Action

Priority area 1: Ensure quality of life

Objective 1.1: Promote healthcare innovation: (1) integrate care across providers; (2) adapt long-term nursing care to needs-based care, with sufficient staff levels; and (3) promote health services research.

Objective 1.2: Complement health protection: (1) avoid exposure to radiation and improve monitoring of population health; (2) control antibiotic resistance; and (3) reduce avoidable hospital infections.

Objective 1.3: Intensify health promotion and disease prevention in the areas of: (1) NCDs; (2) mental health; and (3) addiction disorders.

Priority area 2: Reinforce equality of opportunity and individual responsibility

Objective 2.1: Reinforce fair funding and access: (1) reduce risk selection by insurers; (2) protect vulnerable groups; and (3) reduce the financial burden (lower co-payments, no premiums for children) for lower-income households.

Objective 2.2: Keep health affordable by increased efficiency: (1) lower prices of pharmaceuticals and increasing the use of generics; (2) reform provider payment mechanisms; and (3) concentrate highly specialized medicine.

Objective 2.3: Empower insured and patients: (1) include patients and insured in health policy-making processes; (2) increase health knowledge and skills; and (3) place greater emphasis on patient rights.

Priority area 3: Safeguard and increase the quality of healthcare provision

Objective 3.1: Promote quality in services and healthcare delivery: (1) implement the national quality strategy; (2) reduce ineffective and inefficient services, medicines and processes; and (3) increase organ donations.

Objective 3.2: Make greater use of e-health: (1) introduce and promote e-prescription; (2) introduce and promote electronic health records; and (3) support the implementation of digital treatment.

Objective 3.3: More qualified healthcare workers: (1) train a sufficient number of doctors and nurses in relevant disciplines; (2) promote primary care; and (3) introduce a law to regulate non-physician health professionals.

Priority area 4: Create transparency, better control and coordination

Objective 4.1: Simplify the system, create transparency: (1) improve supervision and regulation of MHI insurers; (2) expand and improve data collection; and (3) reduce the number of insurance plans (278,000 in 2013).

Box 2.   (*Continued*)

Objective 4.2: Improve management of health policy: (1) reinforce collaboration between the federal government and cantons, clarify responsibilities; (2) improve planning (e.g., of hospital outpatient care); and (3) make use of new responsibilities to overcome deadlocks in fee negotiations, particularly for TARMED.

Objective 4.3: Reinforce international integration: (1) finalize and implement the health agreement with the EU; (2) implement foreign health policy; and (3) draw inspiration for reforms from comparisons and collaborations with countries that have similar health systems.

Source: Authors' summary based on OFSP 2013.

insurers and patient associations) participated in the development of national health strategies, which were approved by the federal government. Issues dealt with in these national plans include, among others, the control of communicable diseases (e.g., the National strategy for the prevention of influenza—GRIPS 2015–2020) and other health problems like dementia (National strategy on dementia 2014–2019), and the development of electronic capacity (e.g., Strategy e-health Switzerland 2007–2015). Several other national strategies originated from the *Health2020* document.[8]

Challenges in the Current Swiss Health System

As noted earlier, surveys show that the Swiss population generally supports its health system. The outcomes of popular ballots (see Table 1)

---

[8] Other national strategies are, for example, national program on migration and health 2002–2017; palliative care strategy 2010–2015; national program for HIV and other sexually transmitted infections (NPHS) 2011–2021; national strategy against tuberculosis 2012–2017; Action plan *More Organs for Transplant* 2013–2021; national strategy against cancer (NSC) 2014–2017; national vaccination strategy (NVS) 2017–2021; National strategy on addiction 2017–2024. For more information, see https://www.bag.admin.ch/bag/fr/home/themen/strategien-politik/nationale-gesundheitsstrategien.html (accessed on July 31, 2018).

highlight that people do not wish for any radical change. Despite this somewhat conservative attitude, there have been adjustments and changes in the last decade that suggest a certain vitality of health policy-making in the country—but also reveal the challenges it still faces. This section groups those challenges in five main domains.

Lack of Service Coordination and Integration of Care

The federal strategy *Health2020* recognizes the need to "improve integrated management from screening to palliative care for the diseases which have the greatest impact on the population (such as cancer and dementia)." It also states that "integration of services aims to reduce duplication and inefficiency, while increasing the quality of care provided as a result of better coordination of healthcare provision" (OFSP 2013). Poor coordination has several causes, including the political and institutional system based on federalism. The population size of cantons averages 324,000, ranging from 16,000 in Appenzell Innerrhoden to 1,488,000 in Zurich. The great autonomy of cantons in administering and legislating local healthcare represents a natural obstacle to cross-border cooperation. It requires resource-consuming negotiations in order to integrate rules, protocols and services. Another factor explaining the weak coordination is the strong economic liberalism and the principles of economic freedom, as stated in the federal Constitution.[9] This liberal attitude explains the high value many Swiss citizens attach to the freedom to choose their provider (and health plan). It also explains the limits of public regulation and the institutional fragmentation of a healthcare system with many autonomous actors.

The weak coordination is exemplified by the lack of universal gatekeeping mechanisms. Family doctors play a key role in primary care, but they have little leverage over secondary and tertiary care. In addition,

---

[9]Article 27 of the Constitution states: "1. Economic freedom is guaranteed. 2. Economic freedom includes in particular the freedom to choose an occupation as well as the freedom to pursue a private economic activity."

170

there is no easily available, operational medical information. Despite the recent federal law on EPRs, most medical information is still paper based. Most information and communication technologies are not interoperable. The local actors in the system are aware of the weaknesses in the functioning of recognized clinical pathways but the cantonal administrations usually do not interfere with care pathways. Moreover, reimbursement systems (e.g., TARMED or the SwissDRG) do not promote coordination across providers.

Health Expenditure

The continuous growth of total health spending, per capita health expenditure and MHI subsidy amounts have raised concerns about the long-term financial sustainability of Swiss healthcare. Healthcare costs ranked first among 19 urgent political problems in Switzerland for 70 percent of all adults in a recent survey in June 2018 (Tamedia 2018).[10] Another recent poll revealed growing awareness of the difficulty in curbing health spending (Interpharma 2018) as 81 percent of interviewed declared that "healthcare costs will continue to increase." Only 18 percent thought that "healthcare costs can be stabilized" (1 percent expected costs would decrease). The annual announcement of insurance premiums for the following year by the FOPH usually prompts media headlines about the inevitability of rising premiums and leads to widespread public debate.

Figure 1 presents the trends in total health expenditure (THE), MHI reimbursements, out-of-pocket spending (OOP), and nominal GDP, from 1995 (the year before the implementation of the MHI) to 2016. In that period, health expenditure grew twice as fast as GDP (114 vs. 63 percent) and more than six times the rate of the population (18 percent). The growth of OOPs was lower than THE, but has accelerated in recent

---

[10]The major problems mentioned were health costs (70 percent of interviewed) followed by pensions (57 percent) and relations with the European Union (47 percent; Tamedia 2018).

Figure 1. Population, GDP, Health Expenditure, MHI reimbursement and OOPS, 1995–2016 (1995 = 100).

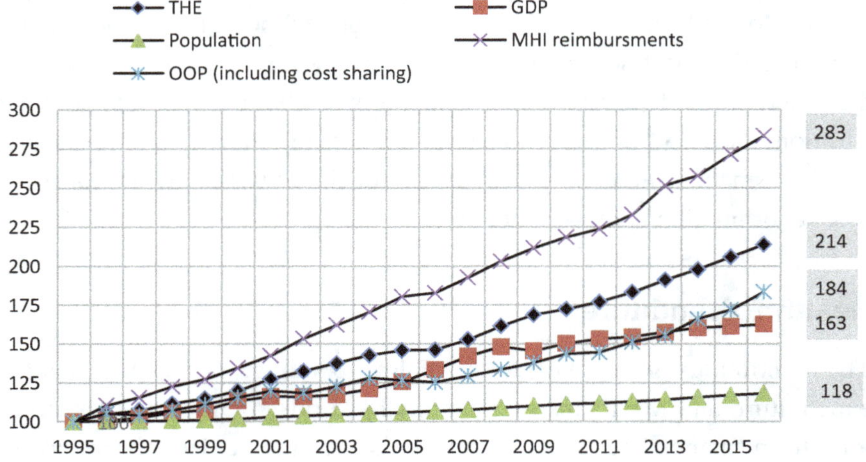

Source: Authors' compilation based on https://www.bfs.admin.ch/bfsstatic/dam/assets/5046326/master (accessed July 31, 2018).

years. Finally, MHI reimbursements (as well as premiums) had the highest growth rate (183 percent).

Subsidized Premiums for the Middle Class

The increase in MHI reimbursements shown in Figure 1 reflects the substantial growth in subsidized premiums for low-income households. This redistribution requires additional fiscal subsidies. Obviously, this represents a major challenge for cantonal parliaments (and can add to the fiscal competition among cantons). It can also exacerbate the differences produced by formulas defined in each canton for determining the amount of the subsidy (see above).

MHI subsidies increased three-fold, from 1.47 to 4.31 billion SFr, between 1996 and 2016 (OFSP 2018). That meant that by 2016 the Swiss government had spent more than SFr500 per resident on MHI subsidies (OFSP 2018). This redistribution especially affected middle-class

172

families. Low-income households and individuals are generally the beneficiaries of subsidies and other social protection schemes. For middle-income families, however, MHI premiums can represent one of the main household expenditures, often much higher than, for example, rent. As a general result, Crivelli and Salari (2014a) found that "the subsidy policy adopted by the state does not succeed in making the financing of [MHI] progressive or proportional." In terms of public consensus, the large number of middle-income families not receiving subsidies for their premiums represents a real menace for the political sustainability of the current MHI in Switzerland.

To cope with these difficulties, the Canton Vaud added a general rule to the ordinary system of cantonal subsidies in 2018. It set a ceiling of 12 percent as the maximum share of available income that families would have to pay for MHI premiums.[11] The canton will compensate families if costs exceed that level.

Control of Demand and Appropriateness

The high density of medical doctors, the institutional fragmentation, the absence of systematic gatekeeping and the fee-for-service payment for ambulatory care are all factors that have contributed to the high volume of Swiss health services. Some critics have claimed misuse and overtreatment, but there have been cases of underuse as well, as suggested by the variation in the rate of child immunization across cantons. For example, the two-dose measles vaccination rate at age 2 varied between 81 percent in Sankt Gallen (in 2015) and 95 percent in Geneva (in 2016: BAG 2018c). Those differences cannot be attributed to "vaccine hesitancy" alone, they are also the result of federalism (with its inter-cantonal differences) and direct democracy (with its lack of mandatory immunizations for children in some cantons). Hospital care is another area with high

---

[11] The "unified available income" considered by this policy is based on revenues (labor, financial investments, MHI subsidies, scholarships, other financial public aids for families) and on 1/15th of net assets owned by the family. More information is available on www.vd.ch/rdu (accessed August 30, 2018).

regional variation, as shown in the small area analysis of the Swiss Atlas of Health Utilization. This Atlas documents hospitalization rates for surgical procedures (www.versorgungsatlas.ch; Chmiel et al. 2015; Zechmann et al. 2018). In ambulatory care, differences are presumably even larger but those have not been documented.

Two additional factors contribute to the weak control of appropriateness of health services. The first is the obligation of MHI insurers to contract with all providers. The FHI mandates that insurers reimburse all healthcare providers authorized to practice by the cantonal authorities or, for inpatient care, all facilities included in cantonal planning. The federal law does not permit selective contracting by insurers, except in the case of the so-called "managed care" plans. Only few insured have chosen PPO or HMO plans. The second factor refers to the high number of MHI insurers and independent health providers. There were about 50 MHI insurers by 2018. They had to contract with and reimburse a large number of independent providers dispersed across the country. This did not encourage the development of shared knowledge and trust.

In fact, Swiss managed competition never became effective, as public information about healthcare has remained very scant. Insurers had no means to control or steer the quantity and quality of health services. Neither could they engage in more active risk management of over- or underuse, or the quality of care through shared adoption of clinical pathways, specialization of healthcare providers and other issues like the definition of minimum caseload volumes and minimum structural requirements.

Health Promotion and Prevention

Recent reports on the Swiss health system have highlighted the need to improve the coordination of policies and programs for health promotion and prevention. One report stated "the fragmentation of responsibilities … favored dispersed and largely un-coordinated activities. Policy coordination would benefit from a framework law governing policies in this area" (OECD/WHO 2006). An update of this report in 2011 recognized that there had been progress (especially in the communicable diseases programs), but it still saw room for improvement (OECD/WHO 2011). The report considered Swiss federalism and the highly decentralized health system as major factors to explain the lack of coordination.

Another cause of the relatively weak health promotion is the institutional architecture of the system itself, based on health insurance and freedom to change insurer. These elements favor a curative approach and tend to neglect prevention.

The Swiss federal government has tried to address this problem. It requested that the federal administration draft a law on disease prevention and health promotion. The public consultation process on this legislative proposal started in 2008. Parliament debated the revised draft in 2011 and 2012, but finally rejected the proposal (De Pietro et al. 2015).

The poor coordination and governance of prevention activities is responsible for the uneven regional distribution of screening programs. Only 13 out of 26 cantons offer breast cancer screening programs with routine mammography for target populations with no patient cost sharing. Only two cantons have a program for colon screening in place.[12] In other cases, the pattern is more erratic, at the initiative of patients, with patient cost sharing and without systematic quality control or cancer registries.

Despite these shortcomings, health promotion in Switzerland benefits from the very favorable social conditions of the country. On average, there are high income and levels of wealth, good education and low unemployment. As foreign tourists will testify, the roads are in excellent condition due to continuous maintenance. So are houses, workplaces and other infrastructure. There is limited pollution and an accessible and effective administrative and justice system for all. All these non-medical determinants contribute to healthy living and working conditions for the population.

---

[12] An updated picture of cantonal programs is available on https://www.swisscancerscreening. ch/fr/offres-dans-votre-canton (accessed July 20, 2018).

Conclusions

The Swiss are generally both healthy and happy people (Helliwell et al. 2018). They also have a health system that shows good or excellent results in effectiveness (i.e., the contribution to the health of the population) and in responsiveness (i.e., the ability of the healthcare system to address the needs of patients). These two elements helped to solidify social consent and contentment, with over 85 percent interviewed in a recent poll evaluating the Swiss health system as good or very good (Interpharma 2018).

At the same time, there are still major challenges, especially in the areas of equity and efficiency. The Swiss social security system protects the income of individuals and families against several risks (disability, illness, old age, death, unemployment and other social protection). Social insurance schemes cover medical expenses and related costs. MHI premiums are community-rated but not income-related, however. Low-income insured can apply for earmarked subsidies for their premiums. Despite those subsidies, healthcare financing remains regressive. Middle-income families often spend a substantial share of their household income on MHI premiums and other healthcare costs. Moreover, there are large regional differences in healthcare costs as the cantons are responsible for determining the MHI subsidies. Finally, out-of-pocket payments have been rising rapidly in recent years and that can create access barriers to healthcare, as we have seen in other countries.

The high and rising level of health spending is a main challenge for health policy-makers. Per capita health expenditures reached SFr 9,612 in 2016, and it is expected to exceed SFr 10,000 in 2018 (BFS 2018). The level of MHI premiums remains among Swiss families' main concerns. Rising health expenditure has become a top priority on the political agenda. Nevertheless, the institutional characteristics of the Swiss political system appear to be a major barrier to action. The system lacks effective tools to control the appropriateness of health services and to avoid misuse. This also applies to prices. The system is largely based on multi-source financing (e.g., MHI, federal and cantonal taxation and OOPs) with fee-for-services reimbursement. It accommodates spending increases in a reactive way. The fragmentation of provision, together with federalism and the obligation for MHI insurers to contract with all providers (with few exceptions) hinder competition.

The Swiss case reflects a high degree of professional power (with their interest in keeping payment levels high). In fact, health professionals and insurers have successfully defended their mutually reinforcing interests in the federal system. Insurers do not appear to put much pressure on providers, as they have to contract with all hospitals and providers in their region. In this system, it has become easier to shift costs to another payer than to cut expenditures or improve efficiency.

The reforms of the last decade, summarized in this chapter, represent incremental change rather than wholesale reform. The changes aimed to improve the functioning and the sustainability of the system. For the first time in Swiss political history, a national health policy emerged as a new element in the mid-1990s. Swiss Parliament passed the FHI Act, the federal law establishing the MHI in 1996. Over time, the FHI strengthened the role of the national government, and in parallel, gradually decreased the responsibilities of the cantons. The stronger role of national politics subsequently became visible in the national strategy *Health2020* of 2013 and in the national sector strategies (e.g., for dementia, NCDs or palliative care). Given the small size of the country and its population (and its regional constituent units), a more substantial and legitimate role of the federal government in the long term would give greater leverage to steer the system than in the current state of affairs.

Apart from the role of the federal government, we presented how three other elements of the Swiss institutional system are important to health policy-making. First, the political principles of federalism and direct democracy undermine the power of federal authorities. Second, the dominant liberal economic culture emphasizes individual freedom of choice and consumer-driven economic decisions. Third, historical development of the healthcare sector, with a high degree of institutional fragmentation provides well-organized interests and strong lobbying groups veto power to block or influence policy decisions. The interaction between these three elements represent a terrific challenge for health policy development—but also an interesting laboratory for analyzing the role of government and public opinion in shaping the future of health systems in advanced democratic countries.

References

BAG. 2018a. *Bundesambt for Gesundheit.* https://www.bag.admin.ch/bag/fr/home/themen/versicherungen/krankenversicherung/krankenversicherung-versicherte-mit-wohnsitz-in-der-schweiz/praemienverbilligung/monitoringpraemienverbilligung.exturl.html/aHR0cDovL3d3dy5iYWctYW53LmFkbWluLmNoLzIwMTZfdG-FnbG/FiLzIwMTZfbXB2L3BvcnRhbF9mci5waHA_cD12aWV3XzImbGGFu/Zz1mcg==.html. Accessed July 31, 2018.

BAG. 2018b. https://www.bfs.admin.ch/bfs/fr/home/statistiques/sante/cout-financement.assetdetail.5006749.html. Accessed July 31, 2018.

BAG. 2018c. https://www.bag.admin.ch/dam/bag/fr/dokumente/mt/i-und-b/durchimpfung/tabelle-durchimpfung.xlsx.download.xlsx/tabelle-durchimpfung-fr.xlsx. Accessed July 31, 2018.

BFS. 2018. https://www.bfs.admin.ch/bfs/fr/home/statistiques/sante/cout-financement.assetdetail.5006749.html. Accessed July 31, 2018.

Björnberg, A. 2018. *Euro Health Consumer Index 2017 Report.* Health Consumer Powerhouse. https://healthpowerhouse.com/publications/. Accessed on November 24, 2018.

Bloomberg. 2017. https://www.bloomberg.com/news/articles/2017-03-20/italy-s-struggling-economy-has-world-s-healthiest-people. Accessed July 31, 2018.

Chmiel, C., O. Reich, A. Signorell, et al. 2015. "Appropriateness of diagnostic coronary angiography as a measure of Cardiac Ischemia Testing in non-emergency patients—a retrospective cross-sectional analysis." *PLOS ONE,* 10(2): e0117172. doi:10.1371/journal.pone.0117172

Christen, A., P. Hänggi, C. Kraft, et al. 2013. "Système de santé suisse 2013." *Le marché hospitalier en mutation,* Credit Suisse Group AG. https://www.credit-suisse.com/media/production/pb/docs/unternehmen/kmugrossunternehmen/gesundheitsstudie-fr.pdf. Accessed July 31, 2018.

Crivelli, L. (2020). "Consumer-Driven Health Insurance in Switzerland, where Politics is Governed by Federalism and Direct Democracy." *International*

Experience with Private Health Insurance: History, Politics, Performance. S. Thomson, A. Sagan, and E. Mossialos (eds). Cambridge: Cambridge University Press.

Crivelli, L. and I. Bolgiani. 2009. "Consumer-Driven Versus Regulated Health Insurance in Switzerland." *Six Countries, Six Reform Models? The Health Care Reform Experience of Chile, Israel, the Netherlands, New Zealand, Singapore, Switzerland and Taiwan, Singapore.* K.G.H. Okma and L. Crivelli (eds). Singapore: World Scientific Publishers: 137–170.

Crivelli, L. and P. Salari. 2014a. "The inequity of the Swiss health care system financing from a federal state perspective." *Int J Equity Health*, 13: 17.

Crivelli, L. and P. Salari. 2014b. "The Impact of Federalism on the Healthcare System in Terms of Efficiency, Equity, and Cost Containment: The Case of Switzerland." *Health Care Provision and Patient Mobility. Health Integration in the European Union, Developments in Health Economics and Public Policy 12*, R. Levaggi and M. Montefiori (eds). Milan: Springer Italia: 55–178.

De Pietro, C., P. Camezind, I. Sturny, et al. 2015. Switzerland: Health system review. *Health Syst Transit*, 17(4): 1–288, http://www.euro.who.int/__data/assets/pdf_file/0010/293689/Switzerland-HiT.pdf?ua=1. Accessed July 31, 2018.

De Pietro, C. and L. Crivelli. 2015. "Swiss popular initiative for a single health insurer... once again!" *Health Policy*, 119(7): 851–855. doi:10.1016/j.healthpol.2015.05.004

De Pietro, C. and I. Francetic. 2017. "E-health in Switzerland: the laborious adoption of the federal law on electronic health records (EHR) and health information exchange (HIE) networks." *Health Policy*, 122: 69–74, doi:10.1016/j.healthpol.2017.11.005

DEFR–Surveillance des prix SPR. 2016. *Comparaison avec l'étranger du prix des génériques et des médicaments originaux dont le brevet a expiré: vu le caractère excessif des prix suisses, des mesures de régulation s'imposent d'urgence.* Berne: Département fédéral de l'économie, de la formation et de la recherché. https://www.preisueberwacher.admin.ch/dam/pue/fr/dokumente/studien/Auslandpreisvergleich%20von%20Generika%20und%20patentabgelaufenen%20Originalmedikamenten.pdf.download.pdf/27_10_16%20Bericht%20APV%20Generika%20und%20patentabgelaufene%20Originale_d.pdf. Accessed July 31, 2018.

Eurostat. 2018. http://ec.europa.eu/eurostat/statistics-explained/index. php?title=Self-perceived_health_statistics and http://ec.europa.eu/eurostat/ statistics-explained/index.php?title=File:Amenable_and_preventable_mortality,_ standardized_deaths_rates,_2014_and_2015_(per_100_000_inhabitants). PNG. Accessed July 31, 2018.

GDK. 2018. https://www.gdk-cds.ch/index.php?id=822&L=1. Accessed July 31, 2018.

Helliwell, J., R. Layard, and J. Sachs. 2018. *World Happiness Report 2018*. New York: Sustainable Development Solutions Network.

Hirschman, A.O. 2008. "Exit and Voice." *The Palgrave Dictionary of Economics* (2nd ed.). S. Durlauf and B.L. Basingstoke (eds). New York: Palgrave Macmillan.

Interpharma. 2018a. *L'essentiel en bref sur le Moniteur de la santé 2018. Pas d'expériences souhaitées, mais plus d'exigences vis-à-vis de la prise en charge*. Bâle, Suisse: Interpharma. https://www.interpharma.ch/sites/default/ files/gesundheitsmonitor_2018_f_final.pdf. Accessed July 31, 2018.

Interpharma. 2018b. https://www.interpharma.ch/fr/faits-et-statistiques/2944-forte-augmentation-des-modeles-alternatifs-dassurance. Accessed July 31, 2018.

Lorenzoni, L. and F. Koechlin. 2017. *International Comparisons of Health Prices and Volumes: New Findings*. Paris: OECD Publishing. https://www. oecd.org/health/health-systems/International-Comparisons-of-Health-Prices-and-Volumes-New-Findings.pdf. Accessed on July 31, 2018.

OECD. 2017. *Health at a Glance 2017*: OECD Indicators. Paris: OECD Publishing.

OECD. June 2018a. *Health Statistics*. https://stats.oecd.org/index.aspx?DataSetCode= HEALTH_STAT. Accessed July 31, 2018.

OECD. 2018b. *Potential Years of Life Lost* (*indicator*), doi: 10.1787/193°2829-en. https://www.oecd-ilibrary.org/content/data/193a2829-en. Accessed July 31, 2018

OECD/WHO. 2006. *OECD Reviews of Health Systems: Switzerland*. Paris and Geneva: OECD Publishing and WHO.

OECD/WHO. 2011. *OECD Reviews of Health Systems: Switzerland 2011*. Paris: OECD Publishing, doi:10.1787/9789264120914-en

OFSP. 2013. *Santé2020—Politique de la santé: les priorités du Conseil fédéral*, Berne, Office fédéral de la santé publique. https://www.bag.admin.ch/dam/bag/fr/dokumente/nat-gesundheitsstrategien/gesundheit2020/g2020/bericht-gesundheit2020.pdf.download.pdf/rapport-sante2020.pdf. Accessed July 31, 2018.

OFSP. 2018a. *Statistique de l'assurance-maladie obligatoire 2016*. Berne: Office fédéral de la santé publique. https://www.bag.admin.ch/dam/bag/fr/dokumente/kuv-aufsicht/stat/publications-aos/STAT%20AM%202016%20pdf.pdf.download.pdf/C_STAT%202016%20full_v2%20pp%20f%20180720.pdf. Accessed July 31, 2018.

OFSP. 2018b. *Statistiques de l'assurance-maladie. Chiffres-clés des hôpitaux suisses 2016*. Berne: Office fédéral de la santé publique http://www.bag-anw.admin.ch/2016_taglab/2016_spitalstatistik/data/download/kzp16_publikation.pdf?v=1522921400. Accessed July 31, 2018.

Schneider, E.C., D.O. Sarnak, D. Squires, et al. 2017. *Mirror, Mirror 2017: International Comparison Reflects Flaws and Opportunities for Better U.S. Health Care*. The Commonwealth Fund. https://www.commonwealthfund.org/sites/default/files/documents/___media_files_publications_fund_report_2017_jul_schneider_mirror_mirror_2017.pdf. Accessed July 31, 2018.

Tamedia. 2018. https://www.tamedia.ch/tl_files/content/Group/PDF%20Files/Franzoesisch/20180629_MM_Tamedia-Wahlumfrage_FR.pdf. Accessed July 31, 2018.

WHO. 2000. *The World Health Report 2000. Health Systems: Improving Performance*. Geneva: World Health Organization. http://www.who.int/whr/2000/en/whr00_en.pdf. Accessed July 31, 2018.

Zechmann, S., N. Scherz, O. Reich, et al. 2018. "Appropriateness of bone density measurement in Switzerland: a cross-sectional study." *BMC Public Health*, 18: 423. doi:10.1186/s12889-018-5305-0

Section IV

Health Reforms in Eastern Europe and the Middle East: The Czech Republic, Slovenia and Israel

The healthcare systems of Eastern Europe share the legacy of decades-long central state control from the mid-20th century. The systems reflected the principles of universal coverage, income-related payment and a particular emphasis on mother and child care resulting in low infant and maternal mortality rates. At the same time, fiscal and budget pressures had led to underfunded public facilities, low pay for health professionals, widespread dissatisfaction and unofficial payments across the systems.

The end of Communism, the independence of nations in the early 1990s and the promise of accession to the European Union (EU) all created windows of opportunity for major change. Policy-makers embraced capitalist values and favored market-oriented health policies. They mostly rejected private healthcare financing, however, in several cases opting instead to return to the Bismarckian model of social health insurance they had in the mid-20th century. The urge to act rapidly sometimes led to failure, however, and reform outcomes did not always meet expectations.

The Czech Republic gained independence by separating from Slovakia in 1993; Slovenia became independent in 1991 after the breakup of the former Yugoslavia. The healthcare services and health status of their populations have generally ranked well internationally. The health reform experiences of both nations illustrate how long-lasting legacies of values, interests and institutions are important factors in the shaping and outcome of social policies. In both nations, shifting toward market-oriented healthcare turned out to be more complicated and time-consuming than expected. Strong popular support for traditional values of solidarity, as well as veto powers of core actors, created barriers to the efforts to introduce market competition in health insurance and to increase co-payments for patients (that were never popular to start with). Medical traditions, in both countries, included free choice of healthcare provider and a wide range of entitlement under the social health insurance.

The return to the social health insurance model as a means for generating additional financial resources was based on the expectation that competing health insurance funds (HICs) would improve the efficiency of the healthcare services, but the reality was more complex. Rather than competing, health insurers engaged in mergers to strengthen their market position (an experience not unique to the region, see e.g., the chapters about the Netherlands and Switzerland). If anything, the transformation required more rather than less government intervention and subsidy to bail out failing insurers and health facilities.

Moreover, the accession to the EU brought new issues to the health policy agenda, like e-health, patients' rights, alcohol and tobacco control and other public health measures. Those issues, as well as aging populations and new disease patterns of obesity and chronic illness, required an active stance of government.

Israel, also, has had a long practice of social insurance. In fact, as shown in that country's chapter, that tradition predates the establishment of the State of Israel.

Map 7. Eastern Europe and the Middle East (The Czech Republic, Slovenia and Israel): Population, Income per Capita and Health Expenditure, 1960–2015.

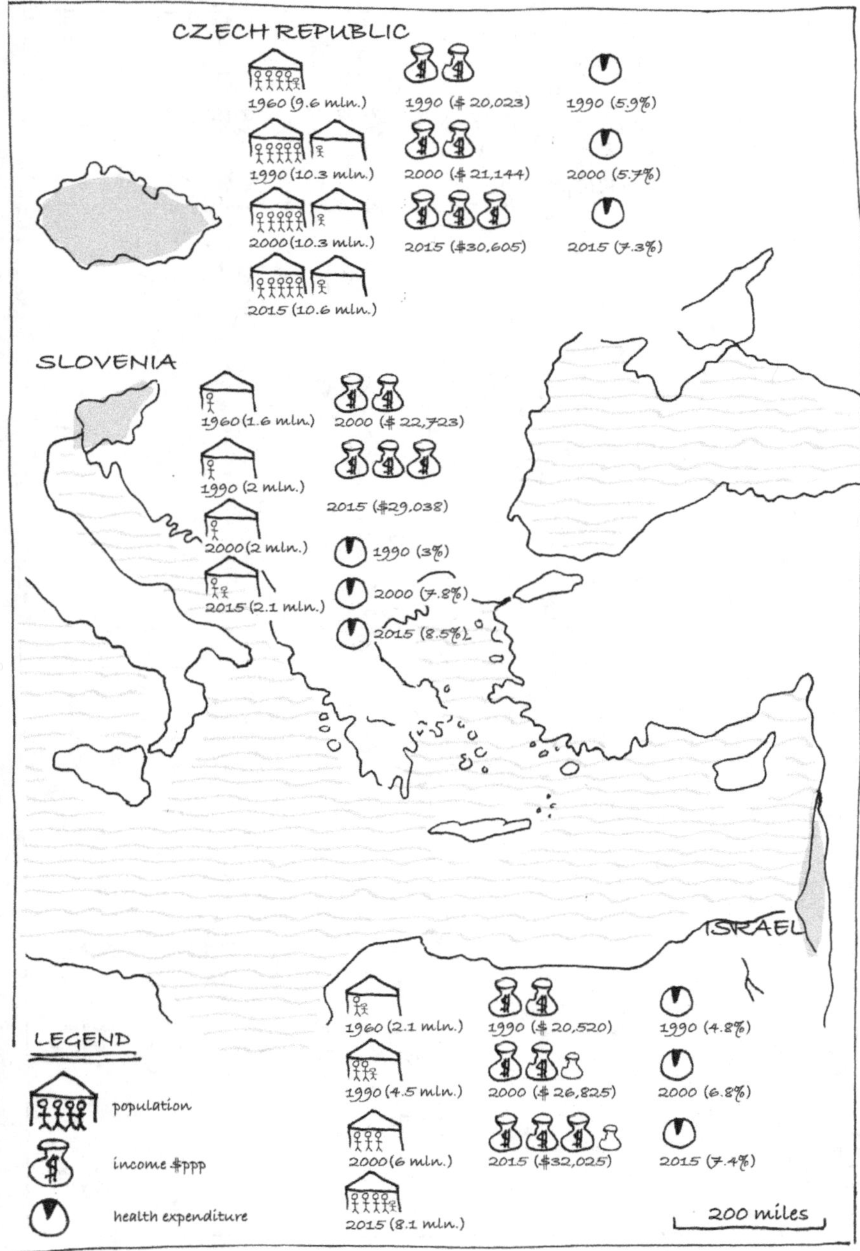

Map 8. Eastern Europe and the Middle East (The Czech Republic, Slovenia and Israel): Number of Physicians, Infant Mortality and Life Expectancy, 1960–2015.

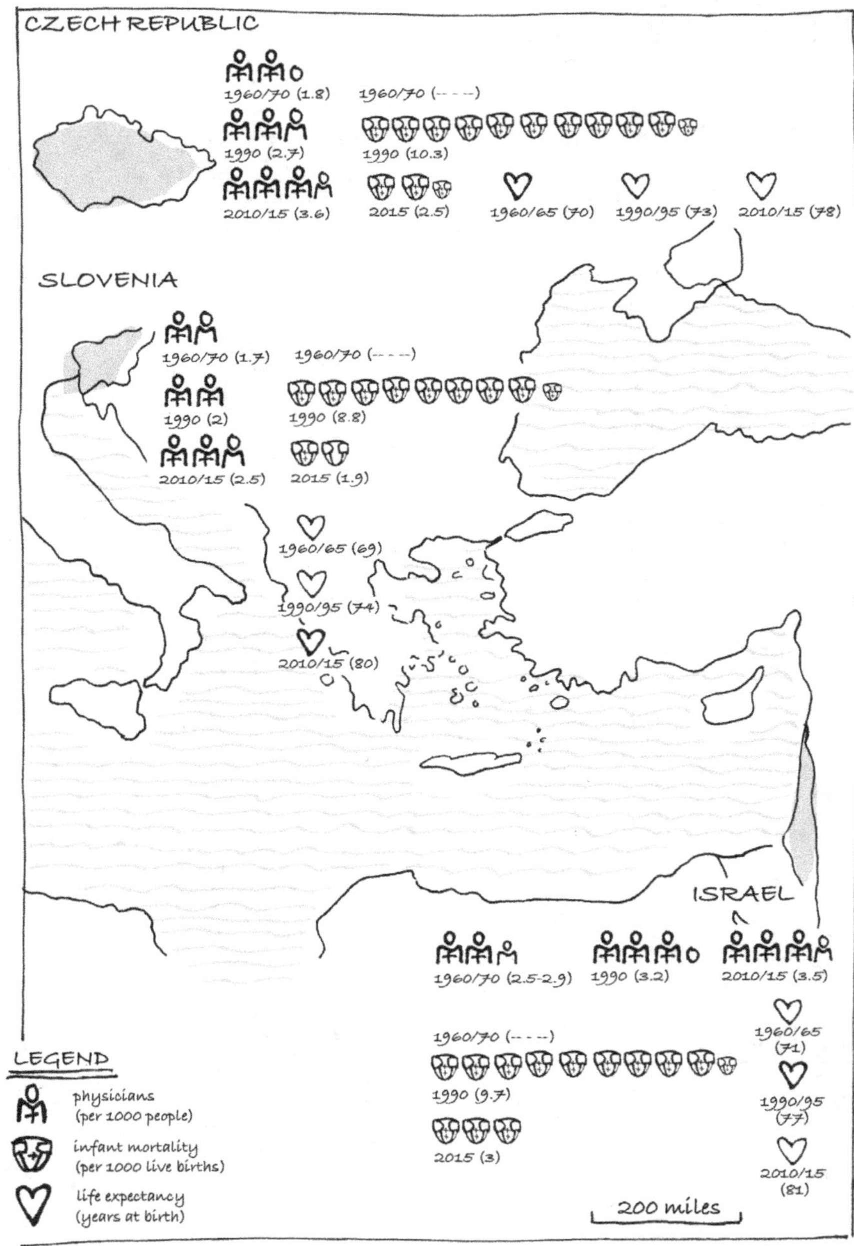

186

Chapter 7

Czech Healthcare: Its Past, Present and Future Challenges

Marek Pavlík and Zuzana Kotherová

Introduction

The Czech Republic is a small land-locked nation in Central Europe, with a population of about 10 million in 2017. It is a relatively young country, having gained independence by separating from Slovakia in 1993. The Czech healthcare services, as well as doctors' skills, generally rank well in international tables. Health indicators, such as infant and maternal mortality and life expectancy, have continuously improved in the past two decades. Shedding its Communist legacy, the country moved from a non-market system towards partial markets, and then (back) towards a system with more limited market principles and a stronger role of the government. Like any country, the healthcare system faces the challenges of rapidly expanding possibilities of medical treatment and research with restricted public resources. Balancing between maintaining open access to healthcare and the need to improve efficiency has kept the country in constant debate about the future of its healthcare. The last three decades saw semi-permanent changes through small, and sometimes contradictory, steps.

The Czech case provides another interesting illustration of how values or ideas, interests and institutions (see Klein and Marmor 2006) are important factors in the shaping and outcome of social policies. The major political transformations after the shift from Communism to a market economy, the separation from the Slovak Republic in 1993 and the accession to the EU in 2004, all served in one way or another as windows of opportunity (Kingdon 1984) for change in policy directions. Despite the dramatic political turnover that prompted a sense of urgency in shedding the Communist legacy, the shift towards market-oriented health policy turned out to be more complicated and more time-consuming than expected. Strong popular support of solidarity (as well as the veto powers of some of the core actors in the system) created barriers to government efforts to introduce competition in the health insurance market.

At first, in its search for new health financing models after independence, the government considered the 19th-century Bismarckian social health insurance model as an appealing alternative that promised to combine additional financing with competing insurance agencies. In practice, however, the model did not quite work out as envisioned. As Palmer and Short noted (1989), policy as formally stated in government documents is not always the same policy as ultimately implemented.

The Czech Healthcare System, 2018

The Czech health insurance entails compulsory membership for all legal residents. All insured have free choice of one of the health insurance companies and pay wage-based contributions. Health insurance is the largest source of healthcare financing. The government pays the insurance contributions for economically inactive people (almost 60% of population). Population coverage is virtually universal, and the range and depth of benefits are unusually broad. Insured may freely choose their health insurer.

Total health expenditure remained relatively low as compared to Western Europe (7.3% of GDP), but the public share remained high (82%) in 2016 (OECD 2017). While still low compared with other European nations, out-of-pocket spending has risen in the last decade and is expected to increase further. Private expenditure includes over-the-counter pharmaceuticals, some dental procedures, as well as co-payments for medical aids, certain prescription drugs and emergency care.

Primary care physicians usually act as solo practitioners, providing an estimated 95 percent of primary care. They do not play a true gatekeeping role. Patients are free to visit specialist directly, and they do so frequently. Private specialist clinics, health centers, public polyclinics and hospitals provide secondary care services. After a variety of reforms in the 1990s, the ownership and management of hospitals that formerly belonged to the state shifted to a range of sectors, including central government ministries, regional municipalities, private entities and churches.

The Ministry of Health (MoH) is a key player in the system. It is responsible for setting the policy agenda, supervising the health system and preparing legislation. The Ministry administers a variety of healthcare institutions and bodies like the public health network, the State Institute for Drug Control (SÚKL) and the General Health Insurance Company (GHIC). The regional authorities and the HICs play an important role in ensuring access to healthcare, the former by registering providers, the latter by contracting and paying them. There were only seven HICs in 2017. HICs are quasi-public, self-governing bodies that act as payers and purchasers of care. They must accept all legal applicants; risk selection is not permitted. The HIC funds serve as the main purchasers of healthcare services, usually based on long-term contracts.

Recent health reforms sought to address the chronic financial instability that marked the system since its inception in the early 1990s. Other reforms focused on issues of hospital ownership and management, purchaser–provider relations, compliance with EU law and the coordination between health and social care. One key challenge is how to maintain access to high-quality care for all, given economic and fiscal pressures, aging populations and the capacity of the health insurance system. Other issues are the codification of patient rights, the clarification of purchaser–provider relationships and the refining of the health insurance system.

Origins and Evolution of Czech Health Financing

The Czech healthcare system originated as part of Bohemia under the Austro-Hungarian Empire. It followed Germany's model of social insurance established by Councilor Otto von Bismarck in 1883. After Czechoslovakia's independence in 1918, it expanded the Bismarckian health system. The new Republic consolidated the fragmented system of social insurances into one institution, the Central Social Insurance Company in 1924. It relabeled the sickness funds as health insurance companies (HICs) and limited their number to approximately 300. The new direction marked a significant shift in expenditure from an emphasis on sick pay to healthcare benefits. The compulsory health insurance covered over half the Czechoslovak population by 1938.

Czechoslovakia came under the Soviet sphere of influence after World War II. In February 1948, the Communist Party became the only autonomous political entity in the country. It unified the social security and health insurance into one compulsory scheme for all citizens, paid entirely by employers with a 6.8 percent wage charge. Next, the state assumed responsibility for healthcare provision and financing (through general taxation), based on the Semashko model of healthcare, in 1952. It proclaimed healthcare free of charge for all citizens.

The Velvet Revolution of 1989 ended the Communist era and brought a new stimulus to every part of the national economy. Politicians opted for a return to the Bismarckian tradition of healthcare financing as a transition toward more market-oriented mechanisms and institutions. They saw this step as a way to diversify health financing, apart from general taxation, while maintaining solidarity and universal coverage as the core values of the system. Two key groups of actors in the system supported the changes: the Ministry of Finance (which was preparing tax reform and did not want to increase taxes) and health professionals, in particular physicians as the proposals included an increase in their remuneration. The changes were very quick, sometimes even chaotic. Some key health financing laws coincided with the implementation of other health policy. The consequences are still visible in the Czech system today. Table 1 shows the long list of changes in health financing between 1991 and 2018.

Table 1.   Changes in Czech Health Financing, 1991–2018

1991–1994

— General Health Insurance Authority (GHIA) established to manage the health insurance under responsibility of MoH.

— MoF and MoH responsible for preparing the new system of healthcare financing.

— Parliament approves General Health Insurance Act and the Act on the General Health Insurance Fund; gradual move towards compulsory health insurance with multiple insurers (HICs) contracting with healthcare providers.

— GHIC replaces GHIA.

— Government approves rules for reimbursement.

— Act on departmental, professional, corporate and other HICs approved.

— Chamber of Deputies approves HIC financing plan.

— Many healthcare laws negotiations approved rapidly.

— Government decides that state budget will cover shortfalls in GHIC financing.

1995–1999

— First problem in financial stability.

— Financing reports of five HICs not approved.

— Direct payment of basic dental services introduced.

— MoH and MoF rejected financial plans of nine HICs because of financial instability.

— MoH and MoF approved rules for HIC mergers and abolishment.

— MoH instructs HIC to increase the value of each point (every medical procedure corresponding to certain number of points).

— The MoH introduces a reimbursement ceiling for services by the healthcare facilities managed by the Ministry (110% of cost in a reference period of time).

— Any new contract between HIC and a healthcare facility must be approved by regional or national government.

— Profit margins for drugs sellers and pharmacies decreased.

— Providers and patients encouraged to increase the use of healthcare.

— First phase of financial solution: government approves the possibility for HIC to get a bank credit, with state guarantees.

— The MoH announced reduction of provider network, including large state hospitals.

— Effort to solve the problem of health premium debtors.

— Four HIC financing reports not approved by the MoH; three HICs abolished or merged.

— MoF authorized to cover the financial instability in the healthcare system.

— Special agreement between the president of the Medical Chamber and the director of GHIC: the provider network without any change.

— The government required hospitals to take measures to maintain financial stability.

— After the financial report of a HIC was not approved, it was abolished.

— Government approved financial stability strategy and stronger GHIC control.

(Continued)

Table 1. (***Continued***)

2000–2004

— One HIC merger.
— Consolidated Bank takes over HIC losses (about five trillion CZK, or 3.5% of total health expenditure in 2001), covered by state budget.
— MoH to prepare a Health System Strategy aimed to assure financial stability in the medium term.
— Czech Consolidated Agency (former Consolidated Bank) undertakes HIC assets (approximately three trillion CZK, or 1.7% of total health expenditures in 2003). State budget covers losses of the Agency.
— GHIC debt increases due to system failures and weak management.

2005–2008

— Chamber of Deputies sets up Special Committee to analyze GHIC's debt problem.
— Czech Consolidated Agency undertakes HIC assets (about 4 trillion CZK, or 2% of total health expenditures in 2005).
— MoH takes over GHIC administration temporarily because of financial and management problems.
— Drug price ceiling introduction (start of HIC financial reserve increase).
— First contribution increase for state insured.
— Economic crisis seems to have little or no impact on healthcare system (drug ceilings from 2006 and increased state contributions from 2007).
— Despite plans to increase contributions for state insured, amounts to remain the same till 2013.
— Introduction of regulatory fees.

2009–2013

— Health expenditures continue to increase.
— After physicians protest because of low salaries, MoH signs a Memorandum guaranteeing increased remuneration.
— Financial problems of GHIC and some other HICs.
— The MoH reallocates reserves of smaller HICs to solve GHIC's financial problem.

2014–2018

— Government announces annual increases in state contribution.
— Government announces annual increases in health workers' salaries, unrelated to quality of care.
— Regulatory fees abolished, inconsistent with the Constitution ("healthcare free of charge for all").
— Despite higher economic growth, no discernible savings by HICs—due mainly to salary increases.
— Smaller HICs remain passive (their strategy is to stay in the market), mostly following VZP (state) decisions.

Source: Darmopilová 2012, and authors' update.

Outcomes of the Czech Health Insurance Reforms

The decision to return to the Bismarckian tradition was based on the expectation that competition among payers would increase the efficiency of the system. There were about 27 HICs by the early 1990s. Rather than competing, however, they engaged in mergers and acquisitions. Some were abolished because they had financial problems or did not meet legal requirements. This caused a sharp drop in their numbers, from 27 to 7 HICs in 2017.

One particular factor that restrained competition was the unusually broad range of entitlements, which all insurers had to offer (the MoH also forbade HICs from offering benefits above this standard package). Furthermore, while GHIC was formally independent, the MoH repeatedly shored up GHIC's precarious finances. Smaller HICs, often in better financial positions, felt the consequences of those measures, and in reaction, again engaged in mergers. Political interference in the insurance system as well as poor management and lack of transparency over the contracting of care providers were also problematic issues. Critics regarded HICs as powerful institutions that in fact undermined the position of patients. At the same time, several government policies appeared to hinder the proper management of HICs.

These facts re-opened the discussion over the appropriate role and optimal number of health plans. The debate over the number of HICs is not new but became one of the evergreens of the Czech health policy (see e.g., Darmopilová 2012). In fact, the debate centers on the question: plural or unitary system. The government favored the plural model of HICs based on the earlier experience of the period between the two world wars. As a new element (encouraged by the EU and other external agencies), the government assumed that independent insurers would compete for contracts with healthcare providers.

Healthcare had become a significant focus for political fights between left- and right-oriented political parties (see below). Reform efforts in 2006, again aimed to strengthen market competition, led to the creation of two new HICs. This created more uncertainty, however, and fueled exit behavior and political gaming. Physicians went on strike for higher salaries. Some left the public system and others tried to use their political relations to gain advantage. The General HIC, once again, received extra support, and was perceived as a threat to the other HICs.

The Czech experience provides an interesting case of the differences between policy intentions, as stated in formal government documents, versus actual outcomes (Palmer and Short 1989). While the government maintained that HICs were competing, in reality, the system appeared to shift towards monopolistic structure with greater state control. People's trust in the HICs decreased and there did not seem to be a clear vision of the future role of the insurance system. In 2012, about two-thirds of respondents polled perceived the role of the HICs as one of the biggest problems in Czech healthcare.

Healthcare and Health Policy in the Czech Republic, 2000–2018

Generally, good health in the population is a precondition for higher productivity. It is thus useful to distinguish between policies focused on providing healthcare services and policies oriented towards improving the health of the population. The latter entails a range of health policies with direct or indirect effects on health (e.g., road safety, food regulation, consumer protection). It is hard to create a simple framework for these policies as well as a catchall for their economic impact.

The health policy documents of the WHO, as well as the EU, mention a broad spectrum of health aims, like access to drinkable water or access to basic care. While such broadly formulated policy goals are usually generally accepted, the way they should be implemented, including the healthcare sector organization involved, is often a matter of dispute. The health ministry is usually considered a key agency for policy formulation under his leadership. This raises the issue of (dis-)continuity. Despite elections every four years, the average survival rate of Czech health ministers (and many of his or her counterparts in other countries) is about two years. Many ministers do not have the chance to prepare or implement their strategic plans, and consequently, many changes in the healthcare system are ad hoc interventions rather than thoughtful parts of an overall policy design.

The administrative reform in Czech healthcare of 2000–2003 took place before the entrance to the EU. Most public hospitals transferred from the central state (controlled by the MoH) to regional and municipal bodies (Rokosová et al. 2005). Many of these hospitals had budget deficits, so the regional municipalities had to solve those problems. This affected the Czech Cabinet's 2006 plans to optimize the network of providers. The proposal to re-structure regional hospitals had failed because regional municipalities preferred local, if not always high-quality health facilities for their populations.

In the period 1998–2006, the Social-Democratic Party held a majority. This period was characterized by financial instability of the healthcare system and a rapid turnover of health ministers. At the same time, access to the EU in 2004 required new legislation to harmonize with existing EU law. The EU membership also brought new focus on health policy goals as framed in the plan Health 21.

Despite earlier bailouts, the GHIC ran deficits again in 2005 and 2006. Opinions differed about the cause of those deficits. Some argued that GHIC had an over-representation of insured with contributions paid by the government (who on average had higher costs but lower payments than other insured). Others pointed to the inefficient administration and low payment collection of GHIC. The debt problems of the GHIC were partly transferred to large hospitals that already had financial problems due to late payments by the GHIC.

During this period, Health Minister Rath refused to publish his healthcare policy ideas, claiming the need to "surprise" other actors and prevent them from taking action against the plans. The Cabinet's main priorities were centralization of financial flows (to prevent debt problems), an increase in the salaries of physicians and other health workers and an increased focus on the quality of healthcare.

The Cabinet increased physicians' pay by increasing point values (each doctor's activity is awarded some number of points). Higher point values thus increased physician revenues. At the same time, the MoH set revenue limits. After physicians protested, the MoH softened the limits again. Next, it took on the debate over hospital ownership: should the ownership of state hospitals shift to regional and local authorities, or be privatized? And would private hospitals be non-profit or for-profit? Unfortunately, Rath was in office less than a year, so he was not able to finish those issues.

One specific issue in the Czech healthcare system concerns the geographical regions. Regional municipalities traditionally had a strong role in healthcare. Many regions, for example, had founded healthcare facilities. Opinions diverged widely about the future role of regions in health policy, depending on which political party was in power (Pavlík 2016). In the first decades of the 21st century, regions were regularly politically opposed to the central Cabinet (i.e., a right-oriented Cabinet but majority of left-oriented regions; Nemec et al. 2015).

General elections in 2006 brought a new right-wing coalition into power, led by the Civic Democratic Party. The coalition had a very small majority in the Chamber of Deputies (102–98 seats). The new Health Minister Julinek introduced an ambitious health reform plan. This plan had two parts: (1) stabilize the system and reform institutions; (2) secure long-term stability in health financing. While the reform was considered pro-market, it also emphasized the principles of solidarity and open access to healthcare.

The first part of the reform had four specific goals: (1) to increase choice for the insured and strengthen individual responsibility; (2) to increase the responsibility of HICs; (3) to modernize a network of providers; and (4) to rein in prescription drug expenditure. The reforms were publicly presented and extensively discussed (more so than any other reform in the previous decades). Proposals to increase user fees were hotly debated. After the MoH implemented modest amounts of co-payments in 2007 (€1 for physician visits and €3 for a visit to emergency services, with an annual limit of €166), the opposition became very strong. The main stated purpose of the fees was to prevent the overusing of physician services, like visiting more than one doctor for the same problem or visiting a doctor just to chat.

User fees became a contested political issue (as in many other countries, see e.g., the chapter on Ghana in this volume). During the next regional election in 2008, it contributed to the victory of opposition (left-oriented) parties that gained majority in all 13 regions. Soon almost all regions started to boycott the fees, and hospitals and facilities stopped charging them. The position of the Health Minister became very fragile. He ultimately had to resign, followed by the demission of the entire Cabinet. That case illustrates how politically sensitive health issues can become.

After the general elections of 2010, another right-oriented coalition gained (a small) majority. Health Minister Heger announced no new reform plans but limited his agenda to activities already in the pipeline and some non-market interventions (Medical Tribune 2010). Parliament accepted his new laws on public health and emergency services. It did not even discuss the previous financing reform plans.

His successor, Rath, was able to stave off a financial crisis in 2007 by adjusting the contributions paid by the state and covering shortages in the reserve funds of HICs. Health expenditures continued to rise, however, and physicians went on strike (again) under the slogan "Thank you we are leaving," adding to the pressure for change. The memorandum signed between former Health Minister Heger and the then-striking physicians led to higher salaries, but also to higher deficits for the HICs, and that problem was aggravated by the economic crisis. To address this problem, Rath took the reserve funds from all HICs in 2012 and redistributed them between the HICs according to their financial need. Critics called this redistribution theft of private property. Supporters emphasized that all resources should be considered to be public money. This intervention fueled new debate about the optimal number of HICs and the position of employers.

The next (left-oriented) Cabinet declared an interest in increasing efficiency, especially within health facilities (the EU Council had also suggested this as a priority). The Cabinet presented its *Health 2020— National strategy for Health Protection and Promotion and Disease Prevention* (Ministry of Health 2014a). It also implemented DRG payments for hospitals in 2014 (Ministry of Health 2014b). It required HICs and providers to publish their contracts and introduced a new control mechanism for the HICs.

Parliament passed the law about public health insurance in 2015. Under influence of the EU and other international organizations, there was a shift in focus of the health policy agenda, with the new law on tobacco control in 2016 (in effect in 2017). The Cabinet adopted the national strategy "Health 2020" in 2015 (Ministry of Health 2015a, b). Its action plan for 2016 involved support for young doctors and nurses. It also published an extensive description of the Czech healthcare system (Alexa et al. 2015).

The Cabinet further proposed an e-health agenda. One particularly contentious issue turned out to be electronic prescriptions. At first, a minority of physicians participated in the voluntary arrangement for e-prescriptions. As soon as the Cabinet suggested obligatory participation, however, it faced strong protests, especially from general practitioners and ambulatory physicians. These physicians refused to use e-receipts and threatened to shut down their ambulances.

The union of HICs contributed to the discussion about the healthcare system orientation and published four recommendations for the public health insurance (Friedrich 2017). Thus far, none have been implemented, however. These were the following:

(1) A clear (basic) standard of care and set rules for above-standard prices (e.g., so that patients can pay the difference between standard and higher services such as a two-person instead of a four-person room). The debate over standards has been ongoing for over two decades and it is not likely to end soon;

(2) A two-part health insurance, with (1) a mandatory tax-based part and (2) a voluntary individual part. For the supplemental insurance, the premium serves as a price signal;

(3) Effective cooperation between patients and doctors, with programs for managing chronic illness. HICs should be allowed to develop their own price policies and contracting;

(4) Price competition among HICs to improve efficiency and transparency.

After the general elections in 2017, attempts to create a new coalition failed, so the current Cabinet remained in demission (announcing there might be new elections later in 2018). Despite the lack of mandate, the Health Minister presented an ambitious reform plan for healthcare organizations and HICs (increasing HIC autonomy and implementing quality indicators into the reimbursement mechanisms). The Cabinet also announced that it would consider further decreasing the number of HICs.

Czech Health Policy and the Influence of the EU

Despite some of the abovementioned problems (e.g., the physicians' strike and the HIC deficits) in the early 21st century, Czech healthcare remained functional. Longer-term problems, however, remained unsolved (Nemec et al. 2015). For example, the chronic financial shortages of the HICs, the pressure of aging populations, reimbursement methods, co-payments, the role of individual responsibility for health, physician remuneration and the brain drain of physicians and other qualified staff were all important issues. Furthermore, based on evaluation by the EU (Council of EU 2015), there is a clear need to shift healthcare from hospitals to ambulatory services, improve public health and pay more attention to the cost-effectiveness of services.

The influence of the EU is apparent in the 2002 document "Health for All," which was inspired by EU strategy (Czech Government 2002). EU recommendations were stated in the document *Together for Health—A Strategic Approach for the EU* that outlines a policy agenda for the years 2008–2013 (EU 2007a). This included three strategic aims: (1) promoting good health throughout the lifespan of aging populations in Europe; (2) addressing health threats, including communicable diseases and bioterrorism, and patient safety; and (3) developing medical technologies and innovation.

Similarly, the EU paper "A Strategy for Europe on Nutrition, Overweight and Obesity" inspired Czech policy-makers (EU 2007b). The Czech government implemented some of the recommendations from this paper, for example, sports activities in primary schools or replacing unhealthy foods in school vending machines with fruits and other healthy snacks. It built new public sports facilities and reconstructed old ones with EU support during the past ten years. The EU tobacco control agenda inspired several measures like the prohibition of smoking in restaurants and warning labels on tobacco products. Unfortunately, the prices of tobacco still remain quite low in comparison with other EU countries (KPMG 2017).

The EU document *Health for Growth 2014–2020* (EU 2013, 2014) succeeded the abovementioned publications. It emphasized the need to make healthcare services more sustainable and encourage innovation in health, improve public health and provide protection from cross-border health threats, such as flu epidemics. Another problematic area is the legal distribution of drugs and prevention against illegal or faked drugs (see e.g., Návrh Směrnice Evropského parlamentu a Rady 2008).

Finally, the influence of EU legislation can be seen in the area of patients' rights and mobility, as well as mobility of health professionals.

Conclusion

The Czech Republic is an example of a relatively successful state, where health indicators as well as quality of healthcare are considered good. However, its healthcare has faced the effects of recurrent economic crises. The last decades have seen ongoing debates about the need for significant change. Looking at factors important in the current quality of care, it seems that patients and (older) physicians tend to prefer traditional standards of care. In contrast, younger physicians increasingly prefer to set up their own practices appear more likely to favor managerial methods that emphasize short-term economic results rather than long-term population health. The Czech healthcare system is still in danger of future change shaped by unwise or populist political pressure. More optimistically, the system has a potential to shift towards increased efficiency.

References

Alexa, R., V. Ginneken, and S. Wittenbecher. 2015. "Czech republic, health system review." *Health Syst Transit*, 17(1): 1–165. www.euro.who.int/__data/assets/pdf_file/0005/280706/Czech-HiT.pdf.

Council of EU. 2015. *Council Recommendation on the 2015 National Reform Programme of the Czech Republic and Council Opinion on the 2015 Convergence Programme of the Czech Republic.* https://ec.europa.eu/info/sites/info/files/file_import/csr2015_czech_en_0.pdf. Accessed November 20, 2017.

Czech Government. 2002. *Dlouhodobý program zlepšování zdravotního stavu obyvatelstva ČR–Zdraví pro všechny v 21. století. Usnesení vlády č. 1046.* (in Czech). http://www.mzcr.cz/Verejne/dokumenty/zdravi-pro-vsechny-v-stoleti_2461_1101_5.html. Accessed November 20, 2017.

Darmopilová, Z. 2012. *Role plátce ve zdravotním systému. Zdravotnictví v České republice.* 3–4/XV/2012. ISSN 1213-6050.

EU. 2007a. *Together for health–a strategic approach for the EU, 2008–2013.* europa.eu/rapid/press-release_IP-07-1571_en.pdf. Accessed November 20, 2017.

EU. 2007b. *A strategy for Europe on nutrition, overweight and obesity related health issues from 2007.* https://eur-lex.europa.eu/legal-content/EN/TXT/?uri=LEGISSUM%3Ac11542c. Accessed November 20, 2017.

EU. 2013. *Proposed EU Health for Growth Programme (2014–2020) Citizens' Summary.* https://ec.europa.eu/health/sites/health/files/programme/docs/summary-prog_en.pdf. Accessed November 20, 2017.

EU. 2014. *Health for Growth Programme 2014–2020.* Online http://eur-lex.europa.eu/legal-content/EN/TXT/PDF/?uri=CELEX:32014R0282&from=EN). Accessed November 20, 2017.

Friedrich. 2017. O výši úhrad na rok 2018 musí rozhodnout ministerstvo. *Medical Tribune.* June 6, 2017. https://www.tribune.cz/clanek/42040-o-vysi-uhrad-na-rok-musi-rozhodnout-ministerstvo.

Háva, P. 2002. Vývoj institucionálního rámce veřejného zdravotního pojištění. *Institucionalizace (ne)odpovědnosti: globální svět, evropská integrace a české zájmy.* L. MlČoch and J. Kabele (eds). 1 vyd. Praha: Karolinum s. 400–418. ISBN 80-246-0431-0.

Kingdon, J.W. 1984. *Agendas, Alternatives, and Public Policies.* New York: Longman.

Klein, R. and T.R. Marmor. 2006. "Reflections on Policy Analysis: Putting it Together Again." *The Oxford Handbook of Political Science.* R. Goodin (ed.). Oxford: Oxford University Press: 982–912.

KPMG. 2017. https://assets.kpmg.com/content/dam/kpmg/uk/pdf/2017/07/project-sun-2017-report.pdf. Accessed November 20, 2017.

Medical Tribune. October 11, 2010. *Heger o reformě zdravotnictví*. https://www.tribune.cz/clanek/19500-heger-o-reforme-zdravotnictvi. Accessed November 20, 2017.

Ministry of Health. 2014a. *Health 2020—National Strategy for Health Protection and Promotion and Disease Prevention*. http://www.mzcr.cz/Verejne/dokumenty/zdravi-2020-narodni-strategie-ochrany-a-podpory-zdravi-a-prevence-nemoci_8690_3016_5.html. Accessed November 20, 2017.

Ministry of Health. 2014b. *Projekt DRG Restart (in Czech)*. http://www.mzcr.cz/dokumenty/ministerstvo-zdravotnictvi-predstavilo-projekt-drg-restart-_9803_3030_1.html. Accessed November 20, 2017.

Ministry of Health. 2015a. *Čeho chceme dosáhnout v roce 2016*. http://www.mzcr.cz/dokumenty/ceho-chceme-dosahnout-v-roce-2016_11132_3237_1.html. Accessed November 20, 2017.

Ministry of Health. 2015b. *Jaké změny jsme zavedli*. http://www.mzcr.cz/dokumenty/jake-zmeny-jsme-zavedli/prosadili-v-roce-2015_11131_3237_1.html. Accessed November 20, 2017.

Návrh Směrnice Evropského parlamentu a Rady. 2008. *kterou se mění směrnice 2001/83/ES, pokud jde o zabránění vstupu léčivých přípravků, které jsou padělané, pokud jde o identifikační údaje a údaje o jejich historii či původu, do legálního dodavatelského řetězce*. KOM. 2008. 668. http://eur-lex.europa.eu/LexUriServ/LexUriServ.do?uri=COM:2008:0668:FIN:CS:PDF. Accessed November 20, 2017.

Nemec, J., M. Pavlík, I. Malý, and Z. Kotherová. 2015. "Health policy in the Czech Republic: general character and selected interesting aspects." *Central Eur J Public Policy*, 9(1): 102–125.

OECD. 2017. *Health at a Glance 2017*. https://www.oecd-ilibrary.org/health-at-a-glance-2017_5jfqgv50kpjk.pdf?itemId=%2Fcontent%2Fpublication%2Fhealth_glance-2017-en&mimeType=pdf. Accessed November 20, 2017.

Palmer, G.R. and S.D. Short. 1989. *Healthcare and Public Policy—An Australian Analysis*. Melbourne, Australia: The Macmillan Company of Australia.

Pavlík, M. 2016. "Comparison of Health Care Policy among Czech Regions during 2000–2015." *Proceedings of the 20th International Conference Current*

Trends in Public Sector Research 2016. Brno: Masarykova University, 8 s: 344–351. ISBN 978-80-210-8082-9.

Rokosová, M., P. Háva, J. Schreyögg, and R. Busse. 2005. *Health Care Systems in Transitions, Czech Republic.* Copenhagen: WHO European Observatory on Health Systems and Policy.

Chapter 8

Healthcare in Slovenia: Progress, Stagnation and the Need for Further Reform

Stanislava Setnikar Cankar and Dalibor Stanimirović

Historical Development

The modern social and health security arrangements in Slovenia originate from the early 19th century. Rules enacted in 1820 and 1837 required employers to see to the treatment of their employees during the first four weeks of illness. Volunteer organizations provided care for the elderly, ill and disabled, widows and orphans—fulfilling a public social security function. In the second half of the 19th century, growing demand from organized labor pressured governments to take action and introduce the first mandatory health insurance for specific trades, followed by mandatory insurance for miners and refinery workers in 1854, and one for iron workers in 1869. Workers in other fields founded their own societies for illness and mutual support, sometimes supported by employers (Toth et al. 2003).

During World War II, from 1941 to 1945, German, Italian and Hungarian forces occupied different parts of Slovenia (at the time part of the Kingdom of Yugoslavia) and each brought its own approach to social security. The Germans and Hungarians arranged for social security in line with their own regimes, while the Italians left the existing rules in place. In all three cases, both the mandatory and supplemental voluntary social insurance schemes faced severe financial shortages.

The Democratic Federative Republic of Yugoslavia, established after the World War II, passed a law on social security for workers and employees in 1946. The new Republic and the end of World War II had created a window of opportunity (Kingdon 1984) for reshaping social security. While the law kept the classic Bismarckian model of financing by workers' and employers' contributions based on workers' total earnings (with contributions flowing directly into the state budget), centralized social security administration replaced local self-management. The law introduced the principle of equivalence, where all groups of insured persons are treated equally, yet it still excluded some occupational groups, such as lawyers, farmers and the clergy. Healthcare splintered off from social security and became part of the public health services. In all other regard, the system could best be described as state-run social security (Toth et al. 2003).

The Yugoslav government reestablished the former, quasi-independent institutions administering social security in 1952. Those institutions had independent administrative boards consisting of workers and other insured persons. Economic organizations (quasi-independent enterprises) and state organizations paid contributions for workers, officials and other insured persons. The general level of contributions for health insurance was the same for all insured, but the institutes could charge higher fees. The contributions flowed into a central social security fund that consisted of two parts: a fund for pension and disability insurance, and a separate health insurance (Toth et al. 2003).

The 1945 Health Insurance for Workers and Officials Act laid out uniform regulations for health insurance, based on solidarity[1] among contributors. It outlined two sets of rights: basic health security and expanded

---

[1] "Solidarity" is a term widely used but rarely defined in any operational way (Okma and Marmor 2013). In the context of social insurance, it often means that all insured pay a certain percentage of their income (sometimes with a ceiling); but, in other cases, it means that all insured are in the same risk pool but they pay flat-rate premiums, sometimes with government subsidy for low-income families. Then it is also important to define the population to which the term applies: specific groups such as industrial workers, farm workers, elderly or the entire population (including or excluding non-documented aliens).

health security. The 1970s saw the rise of workers self-management and autonomy for republics and provinces. As a Yugoslav Republic, Slovenia basically operated its own health insurance since 1972 (Nikolić 2015).

The mandatory health insurance covered nearly the entire population. It expanded the tax base for contributions to include gross salaries and pension incomes. The contributions also depended on the form of insurance. The 1974 Health Security Act instituted health insurance based on solidarity and strong social security. It regulated user rights, the function and organization of healthcare services and self-management by healthcare communities. It did not affect healthcare financing, however. This law was in place until 1989, when Slovenia passed a constitutional law that again centralized the administration by terminating healthcare communities and transferring their tasks to the Republic Administration for Health Security. Contributions were redirected directly into the state budget.

Economically, this transition period was one of the most difficult chapters in the post-war development of health security in Slovenia (Toth et al. 2003). Incomplete legislation and unclear rules on healthcare financing and a freeze on infrastructure investments created major problems. While improved living conditions and healthcare services had led to a marked drop in child mortality, it had also caused a steady rise in average life expectancy between 1980 and 2016 from 67 to 78 for men and from 75 to 84 for women, further aggravating the burden on public health spending.

Health Insurance and Healthcare in Slovenia, 2018

The independence of Slovenia in 1991, with the promise of European Union (EU) membership, created another window of opportunity (Kingdon 1984) for change. Policy elites eager to shed the legacies of communism embraced capitalist values, enabling a shift towards market-oriented health policies. Policy-makers rejected the model of private healthcare financing: They opted instead for the German model of social health insurance returning, in fact, to the earlier legacy of the mid-19th century.

The government enacted four major laws as a framework for health security and health insurance (Toth et al. 2003): (1) The Health Care and Health Insurance Act (ZZVZZ or Health Care and Health Insurance [HCHI]); (2) The Health Services Act (ZZDej), The Official Gazette of the Republic of Slovenia; (3) The Pharmacy Practice Act (ZLD); and (4) The Health Institutes Act, covering public services and public institutes, nationalized hospitals, health clinics and pharmacies.

The HCHI Act of March 1992 reintroduced the Bismarckian model of health security and completely abandoned self-management. The HCHI mandated that all Slovenian citizens and permanent residents register with one of the sickness funds. Payments come from contributions from insured persons, their employers and the state or municipality. The state budget covers healthcare for prisoners and active military. The Employment Service of Slovenia picks up the contributions for the unemployed. The Pension and Disability Insurance Institute deducts the income-related contributions for health security for its beneficiaries. The Financial Administration of the Republic of Slovenia collects these contributions (Toth et al. 2003). The Health Insurance Institute (HII) administers the mandatory health insurance, considered a non-economic public service, throughout the territory of Slovenia. The board of the HII consists of 20 employer representatives and 25 representatives for the insured (including representatives for pensioners and persons with disabilities). The National Assembly must approve the appointment of the board's managing director (Toth et al. 2003), who serves a four-year term.

Contributions depend on income level and employment status of the insured (e.g., full-time employee, self-employed, tradesman, pensioner, farmer or unemployed). The insurance covers dependents like spouses, children under the age of 18 and students. Dependents do not make contributions. The mandatory health insurance covers the costs of illness and injuries at work and off the job (Toth et al. 2003: 476). The government, after advice from the HII, submits proposals for adjusting the contribution rate to the National Assembly. The contribution rate declined from 18.3 percent in 1992 to 13.5 percent in 2002—the latter is still in effect today. Other types of insurance cover a more limited range of risks, with accordingly lower contributions, and contribution payments are split between employers and employees (Nikolić 2015). Until 2002, these contributions were divided 50:50 between employers and employees, but today employers pay a somewhat larger share.

According to the 1992 HCHI law, the mandatory health insurance guarantees the insured two sets of rights: the right to health services and the right to monetary compensation. All insured persons are entitled to health services. The mandatory insurance provides complete coverage for certain services outlined in the national program. For most services, patients face co-payments they must settle directly with their provider (or they can seek supplemental coverage from private insurance). The share of services covered by health insurance varies between 10 and 90 percent, depending on the area of treatment or the specific type of service. Co-payments for emergency operations, treatment in an intensive care unit, radiation therapy and dialysis cannot exceed 10 percent of the total cost; 50 percent of the costs of orthodontic services for adults are covered, while only 10 percent of the price of medications on an intermediate list is covered by the mandatory insurance.

The legislation implemented in the early 1990s aimed to provide all Slovenes with access to quality healthcare, based on principles of solidarity among all insured. Mandatory universal insurance replaced the former state-provided national health security (Farkaš 2017). The newly created HII was charged with administering the mandatory as well as the voluntary health insurance. Health insurance became compulsory for all legal residents (and their dependents). Additionally, there was also the option for supplemental insurance, either private or through the state. Co-payments replaced participation fees (the latter was phased out). Physicians could establish private medical practices and provide services as an integral part of public healthcare. The government introduced a partnership approach to determine the extent and content of programs and the pricing elements of health services.

Some of the tasks previously handled by the state shifted to professional organizations that became responsible for monitoring the qualifications, training and continued education of medical staff. The new legislation also fueled a rapid rise in the number of private healthcare providers. This trend was particularly noticeable in primary care and specialist health services. Most care is still provided by facilities owned by the central state (hospitals, most specialty and tertiary care providers) and the municipalities (community centers for primary care). The state and municipalities still employ over 75 percent of the country's medical workforce (Zimšek 2016).

Private healthcare finance and provisions have gained ground. Expecting that increased competition among private practitioners would lead to higher efficiency and better results, governments encouraged physicians and other medical staff to establish their own practices (Albreht et al. 2009).

The supplemental insurance remains a contentious issue, especially the regressive effect of the flat-rate insurance premium. In 2017, all insured paid €28 per month; therefore, those with minimum wages pay a higher percentage of their income (Mekina 2018). Despite decades-long debate and promises from a long line of governmental parties and ministers to address this inequality, the issue remained unresolved. Policy-making in healthcare, as political scientists have observed, often faces opposition from well-organized and well-connected shareholders with strong veto powers who can thwart or block measures of governments.

Healthcare Governance: Federal and Local Levels of Government and Other Stakeholders

There are three levels of decision-makers in the Slovenian healthcare system. At the macro level, the main actors are the central government, including the Ministry of Health (MoH), the National Assembly, the Medical Chamber of Slovenia, the Slovenian Association of Health Institutes, the HII of Slovenia and the National Institute of Public Health. A second intermediate group is made up of the directors or boards of health institutes, and private health institutes or private healthcare workers. This level includes the national associations of physicians, nurses and other healthcare workers. At the local level, the individual healthcare facilities and workers, patients and local communities are the main actors (Yazbeck 2012).

There are only two administrative government levels: the state and the local (municipal) levels. Local self-governing communities therefore also take part in the implementation of health policy. Local authorities are responsible for awarding concessions to private health service providers who wish to work in the public, primary healthcare system. Most of the funds provided by the municipalities go to programs for basic health security and to autopsy units (Zimšek 2016). Only about 30 percent of all local self-governing communities (mostly larger, economically prominent ones) provide investments into infrastructure and equipment for primary medical care (Albreht et al. 2009).

There are other stakeholder groups that seek to influence policy-making at the national and the local level, for example, the pharmaceutical industry. International organizations like the EU and World Bank have influenced recent policies as well.

Despite recent efforts to reestablish the Bismarckian insurance model with independent sickness funds, the healthcare system, including the mandatory health insurance, has remained very centralized. All administrative decisions and regulatory functions take place on the national level. The power at the intermediate level and the local communities is limited mostly to carrying out administrative responsibilities within the rules set on the national level. Local governments have limited autonomy in planning healthcare.

The central government is responsible for safeguarding a healthy environment and for preventive health programs promoting general well-being. The state, through its legislative and executive bodies (ministries, state agencies and offices), conducts regulatory functions. It passes and enacts laws and implements standards and other mechanisms to protect the population against infectious diseases and ensure a health-friendly environment and healthy workplaces.

The Health Ministry (MoH) participates in policy design and the development, administration, monitoring and supervision of public health services (Farkaš 2017). The MoH administers and finances the public hospitals and other healthcare institutions on a national level. It has an active role in appointing directors at healthcare institutions. The National Assembly has a standing Health Committee that discusses legislation pertaining to public health.

The National Institute of Public Health is responsible for research on the protection and promotion of the population's health. It analyzes trends as a base for determining policy priorities and supports the development of health information technology (IT). It administers healthcare databases and runs the Health Care Data Center and is involved in national IT projects such as ePrescription, eAppointment, electronic health records, health portal and Telestroke. Decision-makers appear increasingly aware that modern IT affects the safety and quality of healthcare and provide management support at all levels of the system.

The HII of Slovenia, founded in 1992, administers the mandatory health insurance. It has the status of a public institute, governed by public law and overseen by the state. The HII drafts rules, consults other stakeholders in the design of health services, collects and distributes insurance revenues (Zimšek 2016). HII meets annually with its partners (including the MoH, the Medical Chamber of Slovenia, the Slovene Chamber of Pharmacy) to draft programs, and determine fee schedules and standards for health services.

Non-governmental organizations are taking on a larger role, advocating for certain changes or reforms (e.g., patient rights groups) and providing self-help to members. The latter include Alcoholics Anonymous of Slovenia and groups of patients with diabetes or cancer. The next group of stakeholders is the health service providers, including public health institutes and private practitioners (who can work in the public system). Agreements with the HII of Slovenia allow private providers to work on equal terms with public ones, but they do not give access to public funding for infrastructure or equipment.

Health services are divided among three levels of care. The primary level incudes basic healthcare and pharmaceutical services provided by community health centers, health stations and private health workers. Special public institutes and private businesses are in charge of the sale and distribution of pharmaceutical products. In 2017, there were 57 community health centers founded by municipalities (Farkaš 2017). General and specialized hospitals, sanatoriums and private specialists in individual fields provide the secondary level of care. Specialized clinics, clinical institutes and clinical departments provide tertiary care. There were 27 secondary- and tertiary-level public hospitals in 2017 (Farkaš 2017). Slovene citizens have the right to choose a personal physician, dentist and gynecologist anywhere in the country (Turk and Albreht 2008). Patients can switch physicians, obtain a second opinion and contact other health experts.

The Office of the Human Rights Ombudsman began its work in 1994, handling complaints and patient rights. Among the complaints filed with the Ombudsman, restricted access to medical documentation, inappropriate conduct of medical staff and long wait times stand out. The Consumer Association is also engaged in issues of patient rights, quality of healthcare, patient's right to information, confidentiality and consent. Citizens are particularly critical of long wait times and complicated administrative procedures (Farkaš 2017).

Economic Crisis and Public Finance: Consequences for Health Financing

Fluctuations in the general economy and employment levels affect both the level of social contributions (the revenues of the social funds) and the demand for social services contributions (spending of the funds). The 2008 financial crisis and the concomitant strategy of reducing public spending across EU member states (the Washington Consensus) created enormous pressure on Slovenia's healthcare system. Poor economic conditions, increased unemployment, lower wages and higher capital expenditures affected public finances. Government debt ballooned from around 30–80 percent of gross domestic product (GDP) since 2008. The budget deficit grew (from 1.4 to 5.9 percent of GDP between 2008 and 2009, and then to 14.9 percent in 2017), largely due to recapitalization of the country's banks, totaling over €3 billion.

Annual economic growth averaged 4.2 percent between 2000 and 2008, while real GDP fell by 7.8 percent in 2009, one of the largest declines in the EU. GDP further dropped by 2.6 and 1.0 percent, respectively, in 2012 and 2013 (Thomas et al. 2015). The recession dragged on until 2014. Since 2014, economic growth has picked up again, largely due to exports, and in 2017 the economy grew by 5 percent, one of the highest rates in the EU (Finance 2018). The crisis impacted the labor market. As the available healthcare finances depend on income-related contributions, it is highly sensitive to the number of employed persons and wage fluctuations. Unemployment rose sharply during the crisis: from 4.4 to 10.1 percent between 2008 and 2013 (still, it remained below the EU average). In 2014, unemployment began to fall again, and it was under 7 percent by 2017 (Finance 2018; Eurostat 2018).

Average wages per employee also declined. In the private sector, this was the result of a drop in production, while austerity measures in the public sectors affected all types of payments (salaries, additional pay, travel costs, bonuses for length of service, etc.) At first, the additional pay- ments above the basic incomes remained unchanged, but eventually they declined too. Wages stagnated everywhere, much more so in the public than the private sector (Bole 2017). The changing employment composi- tion, with a marked rise of short-term and part-time contracts, further reduced the total wage bill and consequently the amount of health contri- butions (Bole 2017). The active population (employees, the self-employed and farmers) declined from 2008, while the number of people with health insurance financed by the government (pensioners, unemployed) and fam- ily members who do not pay contributions have risen.

Public health expenditure as a share of total government spending fell, from about 14 percent in 2003–2004 to 11.6 percent in 2013. Public health spending per resident continued to decline by almost 1 percent per year between 2010 and 2014 (Thomas et al. 2015). There were some changes in the relative shares of the contributions by employers, employees and others between 2013 and 2016, as shown in Table 1. Employers and employees paid over 77 percent of the total, farmers less than 0.3 percent. Differences in contribution rates led to substantial differences in monthly

Table 1. Health Insurance Revenues by Categories of Insured in Slovenia, 2013 and 2016 (Percent share of total)

Categories		2013	2016
1.	Employers	38.01	40.10
2.	Employees	37.69	37.03
3.	Pension and Disability Institute contributions for pensioners	15.78	14.85
4.	Other contributions	6.02	5.44
5.	Other revenue	2.24	2.32
6.	Farmers' contributions	0.26	0.26

Source: Zavod za zdravstveno zavarovanje Slovenije 2017.

Table 2. Health Insurance Contribution Rates and Average Monthly Amounts in Slovenia, 2016

Categories	Contribution Rate (Percent)	Monthly Amount per Insured Person (Euros)
Employers	7.09	107
Employees	6.36	98
Self-employed	13.45	138
Farmers	6.36	45
Pension and Disability Institute contributions for pensioners	5.96	57
Unemployed	11.92	89

Source: Zavod za zdravstveno zavarovanje Slovenije 2017.

payments by those groups, ranging from €45 to €138 in 2016, as shown in Table 2.

Total health financing consists of contributions for mandatory health insurance, general taxation, premiums for voluntary insurance and out-of-pocket payments. Table 3 shows the changes in the composition of the health financing between 1995 and 2016.

As shown in the earlier data, the last three decades witnessed a growing share of private financing, encouraged by a government that expected increased competition among private practitioners to lead to greater

Table 3.   Total, Public and Private Health Spending, 1995–2016 (Percentage of GDP or Total Health Expenditures)

Year	All Public Spending (Percent GDP)	Total Health Spending (Percent GDP)	Public Health Spending (Percent of Total Health Spending)	Private Health Spending (Percent of Total Health Spending)
1995	52.6	7.5	77.7	22.3
2000	46.7	8.3	74.0	26.0
2005	45.3	8.7	71.9	28.1
2010	50.3	9.1	71.9	28.1
2011	50.9	9.0	71.4	28.6
2015	47.7	8.5	71.7	28.3
2016	45.1	8.6	71.8	28.2

Sources: OECD 2018a, b.

efficiency and better results. The share of public financing (general taxation and social health insurance contributions) declined from 77.7 to 71.8 percent between 1995 and 2016. Private financing, including out-of-pocket spending and voluntary insurance, went up from 22.3 to 28.2 percent. The latter, originally seen as an emergency measure and source of additional finance, arose out of the financial uncertainty confronting the new state. Co-payments and voluntary premiums amounted to 14 percent of total health financing in 2017 (Keber et al. 2003; Keber 2017).

The voluntary health insurance has a largely supplementary function. It covered 71 percent of the population or 95 percent of insured persons (Albreht et al. 2016). Before 2008, about 1.5 million insured had supplementary health insurance, but that number declined between 2009 and 2011. Three insurers offered supplementary health insurance but their products were almost identical. Since 2006, premiums have been the same for all insured persons, regardless of age, gender or risk level. To compensate insurers with a disproportionally large share of pensioners, a risk equalization scheme has been in place since that year.

Private insurers collect around half a billion euros in premiums each year. Of this amount, about €50 million or almost 10 percent (in some years even more) remains in the coffers of the insurers to cover administrative and other costs (Mekina 2018). Even in the hard times following the crisis, the supplementary health insurance remained profitable. Administrative costs for private health insurance amounted to 1.8 percent of total healthcare spending. That is nearly half the total administrative costs of healthcare in Slovenia, even though private insurance represents only 15 percent of total healthcare spending (Thomas et al. 2015).

The supplemental insurance remained a contentious issue, especially the regressive effect of the flat-rate insurance premium. All insured paid €28 per month in 2017. That meant that insured with minimum wages paid a higher percentage of their income (Mekina 2018). This issue has been debated for decades. It remains unsolved, despite a multitude of pledges by various political players to tackle this disparity. As noted earlier, powerful stakeholders can often thwart or derail policy change that they consider harmful to their position.

Effective coverage of co-payments through the supplementary insurance reduces the out-of-pocket costs. Between 2008 and 2014, households spent about 12 percent of their budget on healthcare. Nearly two-thirds of out-of-pocket spending went to medication and medical devices, one-fourth to dental services. Poorer households spent an average of €232 out-of-pocket, while wealthier households spent €728 in 2012 (Thomas et al. 2015).

Austerity Measures and Health Reforms

The financial crisis of 2008, with its substantial economic downturn, as noted earlier, also cut into resources available for healthcare. Belt-tightening and cost-cutting government measures resulted in declining funds and human resources, while the healthcare needs of the population continued to grow. This led to visible cracks in the system. It prompted further cost-cutting and efforts to generate additional revenue (Ministry of Health 2016). The MoH increased co-payments, contribution rates for the self-employed and students, curtailed some free services and reduced the reimbursement rates for prescription drugs and other health services. To avoid running deficits (prohibited by law), health insurers, too, engaged in cost-cutting strategies (Thomas et al. 2015). They lowered reimbursement to providers (who maintained the same level of service), further increased co-payments, postponed some payments and sought to reduce administrative costs.

Lowering reimbursements for medication and health services did result in savings at the HII. Hospital's revenues dropped by €1.28 billion in 2011 and €1.24 billion in 2014. The nominal level of health spending in 2014 was equal to the level of spending in 2010. Some hospitals incurred financial losses and increased wait times for certain services. The following year they received partial compensation for the extra work, after widespread action by dissatisfied physicians and patients. Hospitals were forced to seek internal solutions. They redirected patients to outpatient care and specialty clinics and reduced the number of beds (see Table 4; Setnikar Cankar and Petkovšek 2011). The reduced payments to hospitals sometimes caused longer wait times. According to the National Institute of Public Health, the number of patients who had to wait for health services rose in 2014, from 155,862 to 182,498, while the cases exceeding the maximum wait time norm increased from 14,770 to 24,815 patients.

The austerity measures also affected wages for healthcare workers. The government rolled out a new salary system for the entire public sector

Table 4. Hospital Beds and Occupancy Rates in Slovenia, 1980–2016

Year	Hospital Beds	Occupancy Rate (Percent)	Beds/100,000 Inhabitants
1980	13,183	88	695
1985	12,496	85	633
1990	12,081	82	605
1995	11,411	77	574
2000	10,745	71	540
2005	9,666	70	483
2009	9,389	71	459
2010	9,367	71	457
2015	9,315	76	451
2016	9,266	76	449

Source: National Institute of Public Health 2017.

in 2008. Physicians' salaries rose by 15.3 percent in 2008 and another 11.2 percent in 2009, but that growth rate hovered around 1 percent per year until it rose again by 6.1 percent in 2013. General practitioners and specialists earned roughly 2.3 times the average salary in Slovenia. In contrast, nurses, who represent the majority of the medical staff, earned only 97 percent of the average salary. The austerity measures also limited overtime pay. Nearly half a million hours of overtime work went unpaid in January 2015, over half of which was for nurses (Thomas et al. 2015). In response, the unions for physicians and dentists demanded a raise and staged several general strikes.

The 2012 Fiscal Balance Act led to an average decrease of 5 percent in reimbursements for health services. It reduced the compensation for periods of leave by 10 percent and lowered prices for medical aids and technical devices. As a next step in austerity, in 2014, the government reduced the number of employees financed from public funds (with certain exceptions) by 1 percent each year. Austerity also meant a drop in the level of healthcare investments from about 5.5 to 4.5 percent of all health spending, with particularly high cuts in new infrastructure investment, by 63.3 percent in 2013, and by 25.5 percent in 2014 (Thomas et al. 2015). Most investment financing came from the state budget, with the private sector accounting for about a third. Hospitals curtailed spending on new equipment between 2011 and 2014 and the austerity measures ultimately resulted in longer wait times, delayed replacement of worn-out equipment and a decrease in medical research.

Slovenia's Unfinished Health Reform Agenda: Governance, Finance and Other Issues

While the MoH is the formal bearer of healthcare policy and strategies, it relies on the professional support of other bodies and outside experts. The Ministry does not have the necessary capacity to carry out active healthcare policy and lacks expertise in various areas. In the early 1990s, the government decided to set up independent agencies to deal with specific tasks, for example, the HII (850 employees), the National Institute of

Public Health (470 employees) and the Agency for Medicinal Products and Medical Devices (136 employees). The MoH saw its own position reduced to an administrative role, while functions dealing with the content of healthcare were handled externally. This led to split responsibilities and a high degree of instability. The MoH is still formally responsible for health policy, but it has limited power to enforce it. In fact, many issues remain unresolved, for example, conflicts over the size of the healthcare budget and the financing of the deficits of health insurers and providers. There is mounting criticism of the lack of coordination and accountability (Kranjec 2015). The two-track administration of the healthcare system, whereby the MoH and the National Assembly enact formal legislation while the HII is responsible for the material side of things—namely, the money—is clearly not particularly effective. Ministers and governments come and go too quickly to finish any reforms they commence.

Modernizing the governance of the general hospitals has been another long-standing issue faced with many barriers. Earlier proposals to limit the number of specialized departments of general hospitals but broaden their range of outpatient services met with fierce opposition from local communities. In that proposal, each hospital would develop a high level of excellence by focusing on a handful of fields available to all patients in the country. This would also help improve the financial position of the hospitals and shed their reputations for sub-par services. The local communities rejected the plan, however, preferring proximity of healthcare infrastructure, even while that might not be of highest quality (Zupanič 2015; Zwitter 2018).

Another major challenge has been the need for diversification of revenue sources. Contributions vary sharply with cyclical economic circumstances, as illustrated by the experience after 2008. Moreover, within the social insurance, there is large variation in contribution rates by different population groups. It seems appropriate—if not politically easy—to harmonize payments across all insured. Solidarity would be further improved by the termination of voluntary insurance and replacement of flat-rate premiums with income-relative contributions (earmarked tax), as proposed by the MoH in 2017 (Keber 2017). Another alternative financing source to replace the supplemental insurance would be (higher) co-payments or user fees. By paying into the participation scheme, some experts expect that people would be made aware that healthcare is not free, and patients would be more frugal in using healthcare services, as they have skin in the game (Zwitter 2016).

As in other countries, patients and insured in Slovenia are reluctant to face higher payments for their healthcare and health insurance. While acknowledging that they cannot have everything for the current amount of money, only a minority (38 percent) of respondents in a recent poll expressed willingness to pay more (11 percent would be willing to pay for visits to physicians and medications, 11 percent for non-emergency services, 10 percent for health insurance contributions and 6 percent for additional insurance; Zupanič 2015).

Reducing the range of insurance entitlements is another venue to cut (or rather, shift) costs. Historically, Slovenia's social health insurance covered a (very) wide range of entitlements. Efforts to base the selection of health services and medical practice on more rational criteria, like evidence-based medicine and cost-effectiveness studies within the limits of overall available budgets, have thus far met with fierce resistance. At the same time, long wait times undermined the right to healthcare (Nolte et al. 2015). Politicians generally avoided such steps, not wanting to be seen as curtailing certain rights, which will almost certainly evoke angry reactions from providers and patients alike. Nor can healthcare providers be expected to look favorably upon changes that affect their incomes and practice style.

Apart from the abovementioned two major issues of healthcare governance and finance, a range of other policy issues remain on the unfinished agenda. Most of these are not unique to Slovenia. Other countries struggle with the same problems, and many of the issues are fraught with high expectations and common failures. For example, several EU countries (and other industrialized nations) announced a rapid introduction of a countrywide system of electronic patient records (EPRs). After almost two decades of intensive debate and substantial government subsidy, however, there is hardly any nation in the world that has actually implemented such a system. The decentralized decision-making nature of healthcare, with many individual actors (e.g., hospitals and health professionals, insurers and other agencies and NGOs) in charge of developing separate information systems, and the unresolved issues of ownership of medical data, privacy, and effective data protection are among the common barriers in implementing national systems.

Reforming healthcare (or perhaps just gradually changing and adjusting, as part of the regular health policy process) involves many other issues, like the remuneration of physicians, nurses and other health workers, in addition to manpower planning, improving the organization and management of health facilities, strengthening primary care and the gatekeeper function of family physicians, and further development of eHealth and other electronic applications. All of these are time-consuming, and require substantial investments and government commitment, and all involve many stakeholders, both within and outside of government (and often, outside of the country as well). The same applies to other efforts to improve the healthcare system in Slovenia: establishing a national system for evidence-based medicine, cost-effectiveness studies and the evaluation of healthcare technology, introducing rewards for employee excellence, developing the digital platform for healthcare users and putting in place a system for long-term care.

Conclusion

Slovenia is a fairly prosperous middle-income country in Central Europe. Its healthcare resources came under great pressure after the economic crisis of 2008 and its aftermath. Despite this, Slovenia has a good public health record. The under-five mortality rate of 2.4 deaths per 1,000 live births in 2016, down from 17.5 in 1981, is one of the lowest in the world. There are extensive public information campaigns to inform citizens about the importance of a healthy lifestyle. Combined with greater access to advanced heart procedures, this has helped to cut the number of deaths due to heart disease in half. Likewise, programs for early cancer detection have improved patient outcomes. Until recently, wait times were getting shorter. For example, in the early 2000s, the wait time for heart surgery was a year and a half; today it is three months (Keber 2017). Slovenes can expect to live 80 years on average: 77 for men and 83 for women. There has been marked improvement in the area of patient rights and information, although patients still have no access to systematic information about the quality of different providers (Björnberg 2016). Patient rights advocates, located in the district offices of the National Institute of Public Health, are accessible to everybody. In short, the system has improved considerably since Slovenia's independence, but it began to stagnate after the economic crisis of 2008.

The long legacy of social insurance based on strong popular support for solidarity-based financing, combined with recent efforts to strengthen the role of private players within healthcare, has created tensions and dilemmas. The balancing of interests in public–private partnerships and the need to improve the efficiency of healthcare pose major problems for government and healthcare institutions. Political decisions in the past created institutional legacies of systematic inefficiencies in investments and spending patterns. The recent shift to privatization, and cuts in public spending, has created new access barriers to healthcare and caused mounting dissatisfaction from patients and healthcare staff alike (Kranjec 2015; Tajnikar 2016).

The history and reform efforts of Slovenia's health insurance and healthcare provides an interesting case of strong institutional legacies with stakeholders resistant to change, major political upheaval opening windows of opportunity but governments hesitant or unable to implement major change rapidly. The state-controlled central government agencies remained largely centralized (and in some cases, took on even more responsibilities), and efforts to privatize healthcare and health insurance failed to deliver on promises of major efficiency and quality gains. The newly created specialized healthcare institutions took over tasks and responsibilities from the Health Ministry but the MoH remains (with Parliament) formally in charge of overall policy-making. At the same time, there is mounting pressure from patients, citizens and healthcare providers (well-organized physicians in particular), to reduce waitlists and improve the quality of services (and income of providers). Adding to those demands are the external pressures of EU membership that bring new issues to the health policy agenda like health IT, quality assessment and patient rights.

References

Albreht, T., R. Pribaković Brinovec, D. Jošar, et al. 2016. "Slovenia: health system review." *Health Syst Transit*, 18(3): 1–207.

Albreht, T., E. Turk, M. Toth, et al. 2009. "Slovenia: health system review." *Health Syst Transit*, 11(3): 1–168.

Björnberg, A. 2016. *Euro Health Consumer Index 2015*. Report. Health Consumer Powerhouse.

Bole, V. 2017. Gospodarska rast, inflacija in "nova paradigma." *Gospodarska gibanja*, 500: 9–17.

Eurostat. 2018. *Total Unemployment Rate (Percentage of Active Population)*. http://ec.europa.eu/eurostat/web/labour-market/overview. Accessed March 30, 2019.

Farkaš A. 2017. *Analiza regulacije zdravstva v izbranih državah*. Master Thesis. University of Ljubljana.

Finance. 2018. *Finance*. https://www.finance.si/danes?op=danes&date=29.03.2018. Accessed March 29, 2018.

Keber, D. 2017. "Zdravstvo v Sloveniji." *Mladina*, April 21, 2017.

Keber, D., B. Leskovar, K.V. Petrič, et al. 2003. *Zdravstvena reforma: pravičnost, dostopnost, kakovost, učinkovitost*. Vlada Republike Slovenije, Ministrstvo za zdravje, Ljubljana.

Kingdon, J.W. 1984. *Agendas, Alternatives, and Public Policies*. New York, NY: Longman.

Koechlin, F., P. Konijn, L. Lorenzoni, et al. 2014. *Comparing Hospital Prices and Volumes Across Countries: A New Approach*. Paper Prepared for the IARIW 33rd General Conference, Rotterdam, Netherlands.

Kranjec, M. 2015. "Zdravstveni sistem je dober, a se ne uresničuje." *Sobotna priloga Dela*, March 7, 2015.

Mekina, B. 2018. "Finančna ministrica zaščitila superbogate." *Mladina*, January 5, 2018.

Ministry of Health. 2016. *Resolucija o nacionalnem planu zdravstvenega varstva 2016–2025 "Skupaj za družbo zdravja."* Ljubljana: Ministrstvo za zdravje.

Ministry of Health. 2017. *Povečala se bodo sredstva, namenjena izboljšanju kakovosti zdravstvenih storitev.* Ljubljana: Ministrstvo za zdravje.

National Institute of Public Health. 2017. *Zdravstveni statistični letopis 2016.* Ljubljana.

Nikolić, B. 2015. *Pravna ureditev sistemov financiranja zdravstvenega varstva.* PhD Diss. University of Ljubljana.

Nolte, E., J. Zaletel, A. Robida, et al. 2015. *Optimizing Service Delivery,* Final Report. Copenhagen: European Observatory on Health Systems and Policies, WHO regional office for Europe. Ministrstvo za zdravje Republike Slovenije.

OECD. 2018a. *General Government Spending.* https://data.oecd.org/gga/general-government-spending.htm. Accessed April 6, 2018.

OECD. 2018b. OECD.stat. *Health Expenditure and Financing.* http://stats.oecd.org/index.aspx?DataSetCode=HEALTH_STAT. Accessed April 6, 2018.

Okma, K.G.H. and T.R. Marmor. 2013. "Comparative studies and healthcare policy: learning and mislearning across borders." *Clinical Medicine,* 13(5): 487–491.

Setnikar Cankar, S. and V. Petkovšek. 2011. *Review and analysis of the health-care system in Slovenia 1980–2010.* Public administration of the future: 19th NISPAcee Annual Conference, Varna.

Tajnikar, M. and P. Došenović Bonča. 2010. Kritična analiza organiziranosti zdravstva v Sloveniji. *16. strokovno posvetovanje o sodobnih vidikih analize poslovanja in organizacije.* T. v Čater (ed.). Slovenia: Portorož.

Tajnikar, M. 2016. "Javno, zasebno ali državno zdravstvo." *Delo,* September 24: 8–10.

Thomas, S., E. Tamás, and S. Thomson. 2015. *Evaluating Health Financing,* Final Report. Copenhagen: WHO regional office for Europe, European Observatory on Health Systems and Policies/Ministrstvo za zdravje republike Slovenije.

Toth, M., B. Kramberger, M. Premik, et al. 2003. *Zdravje, zdravstveno varstvo, zdravstveno zavarovanje.* Ljubljana: Zavod za zdravstveno zavarovanje Slovenije.

Turk, E. and T. Albreht. 2008. "HTA in Slovenia-New Developments." *Health Policy Monitor.* http://www.hpm.org/survey/si/a11/4. Accessed July 25, 2016.

Yazbeck, A.M. 2012. *Ekonomika zdravstva.* http://img.ivz.si/janez/1926-4854. pdf. Accessed July 25, 2016.

Zakon o zdravstvenem varstvu in zdravstvenem zavarovanju (ZZVZZ). Ur. list RS, št. 72/06–UPB3, 91/07, 76/08, 87/11, 91/13.

Zakon o zdravstveni dejavnosti (ZZDej). Ur. list RS, št. 23/05–UPB2, 23/08, in 14/13.

Zavod za zdravstveno zavarovanje Slovenije. (2017). *Poslovno poročilo Zavoda za zdravstveno zavarovanje Slovenije za leto 2017.* Ljubljana.

Zimšek, J. 2016. *Revizije smotrnosti poslovanja v zdravstvu.* PhD Diss. University of Ljubljana.

Zupanič, J. 2017. "Milojka Kolar Celarc, ministrica za zdravje, intervju." *Večer,* October 28, 2017.

Zupanič, M. 2015. "Slovensko zdravstvo: miti in dejstva." *Delo,* May 9, 2015.

Zwitter, M. 2016. "Čakalne vrste lahko odpravimo." *Delo,* June 29, 2016.

Zwitter, M. 2018. "Zdravstvo kot predvolilni golaž." *Delo,* March 24, 2018.

Appendix

Municipalities
Ministry of Health
Capital investments
Capital invest ments
Health Insurance Institute of Slovenia (HIIS)
Voluntary health insurance (for co-payment coverage)
Line item budget
National Institute of Public Health (NIPH)
Providers of primary healthcare (healthcare centers, concessionaires)
Capitation, fee for service
Providers of outpatient specialist care (hospital ambulances, concessionaires)
Fee for service
Providers of inpatient care (hospital clinics, concessionaires)
Diagnosis-related group, bed day, case, fee for service
Pharmacies (public, concessionaires)
Fee for service
Providers of dental practices (health care centers, concessionaires)
Fee for service
Social institutions
Fee for service, day of nursing care
Health resorts, Spa
Fee for service
Private providers without concession
Out-of-pocket payments
Voluntary health insurance premiums (e.g., for co-payments)
Compulsory health insurance contributions
Taxes
Citizens

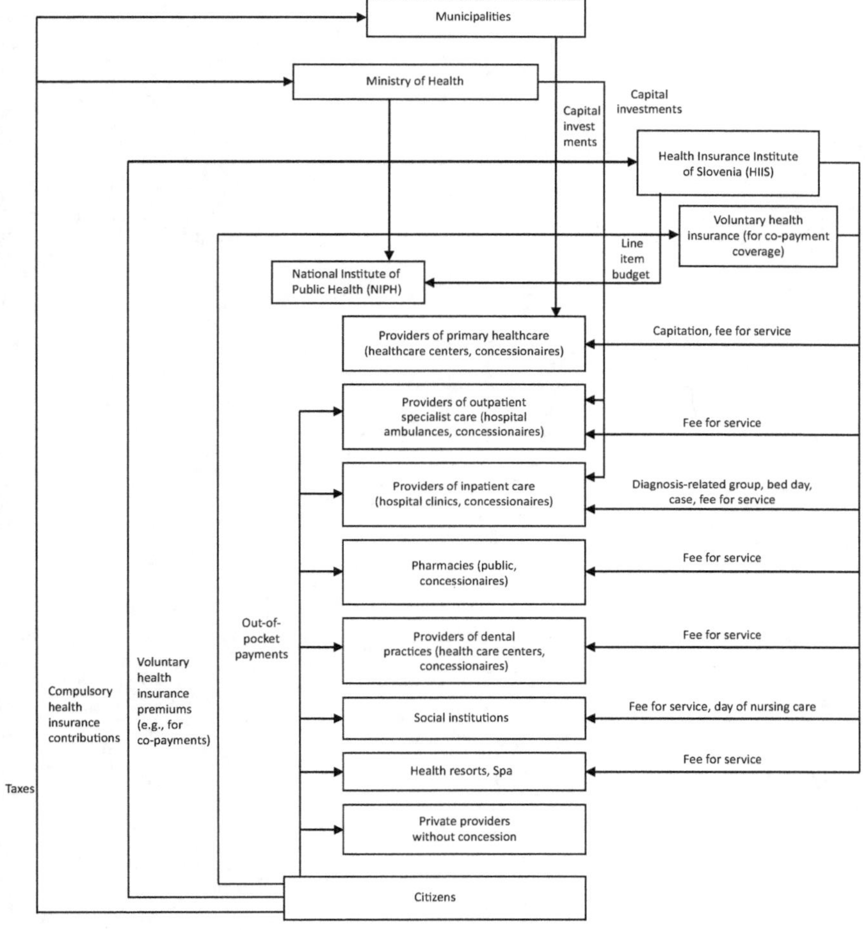

Chapter 9

Israel's Healthcare Reforms: From Big Bang to Incremental Change

David Chinitz

Historical Background

Israel is a small country (nearly nine million inhabitants) at the Eastern shore of the Mediterranean bordered by Lebanon, Jordan and Egypt that followed the Western European tradition of public health insurance managed by independent sick funds. Seventy years after the creation of the State of Israel, current trend analysts of the country's geopolitical and political economy refer to the impact of the institutions that were in place while the State was "in waiting" (Chinitz 1995).

The General Sick Fund (GSF) and the Histadrut Labor Federation were among the most important of such institutions. At the time of Israel's major health reform, the enactment of the National Health Insurance (NHI) in 1995, Histradut owned the GSF. The GSF actually preceded the Histradut, as it has been in existence since 1912, while the Labor Federation started some years later. In 1911, labor unions established the first mutual sick fund, followed by other funds in the 1920s and 1930s (Rosen 2015). The health insurance started as an employment-based scheme modeled after the German Bismarckian social health insurance. After the establishment of the state of Israel, it gradually expanded to cover almost the entire population. The importance of this point is that historically, some health arrangements with grassroots origins were later taken over or organized by higher governing entities. This introduced, from the outset, a dynamic and sometimes tense relationship between health as a progeny of civil society and health as a policy realm for government (Anderson 1989).

With the creation of the State, stakeholders harbored different assumptions about the fate of the pre-State institutions. Israel's first Prime Minister, David Ben Gurion, envisioned that the new apparatus of the State would incorporate the activities of these institutions. At the same time, their decades-long existence had created strong path dependency and limited room for the expansion of government sovereignty. Israel's governing apparatus featured competing giants, both public and civil society institutions dating from the pre-State era. They competed in several areas for control over the activities of the new State. This competition affected styles of governance and shaped attitudes towards mechanisms such as exit, voice, loyalty and their corollary: accountability. With unclear assignment of responsibility for the financing and provision of services, nested within an ownership structure, which had many blurred lines; accountability for financial and benefit outcomes of public services never became Israel's strongest point. In fact, the Hebrew language spoken in Israel today has no widely accepted word for accountability (Maor 2010).

Nowhere were these patterns more evident than in the health arena. After the creation of the state, the number of sick funds dropped from eight to four. By the early 1980s, the GSF enrolled 80 percent of the population. The three smaller funds enlisted another 15 percent. The GSF had strong ties with both the Labor Federation and the Labor Party, which ran Israel's governing coalition from 1948 until 1977. In this "iron triangle," the GSF competed with the Ministry of Health (MoH) for dominance. They both engaged in the planning and operation of health services. Since the GSF could count on friendly governmental support, it did not need to worry about the makeup of its membership or financial losses. The GSF expanded health services at its own discretion and used its political leverage to escape accountability for deficit spending. At the same time, it was beholden to the Labor Federation, and obligated to enroll any of the Federation's members. Moreover, the dominant position of the Labor Federation (with membership of up to 60 percent of all workers) meant that the GSF had little incentive to be responsive to the needs of its insured.

By the late 1980s, 95 percent of the population had (voluntarily) enrolled with one of the four (not-for-profit) funds. Despite this nearly universal coverage, the system was plagued by financial instability, public and provider dissatisfaction, hospital overcapacity and fragmentation of services. Finally—at least in the eyes of the Israeli public and politicians—there were too many uninsured (as in the Netherlands, even a small number of uninsured can cause political pressure on government to take action, see below).

Forces Leading to Reform

Outside forces caused pressure on the government to take action. The Herut Party (the predecessor of today's Likud) unseated its archrival, the Labor Party, in 1977 and formed the governing coalition. Likud remained in power, sometimes in coalition governments with Labor until the early 1990s. This power shift changed the rules of the game for the GSF and Histadrut. Likud's policy agenda included the dismantling of the iron triangle, and reduction of government subsidies in areas such as health. It tried to introduce reforms, restrict the autonomy of the GSF and encourage the smaller sick funds to become more active.

The Macabbi Sick Fund advertised greater freedom to choose one's physician as a vast improvement over GSF. Perhaps the notion of "exit" (Hirschman 1970) came into play for the first time in Israeli healthcare. Younger, wealthier—and healthier—populations, not encumbered by employment ties to the Histadrut, shifted to Macabbi. As both members' and employers' contributions were based on income, Macabbi built up a membership that generated higher revenues but with lower costs than other funds. The perception of a two-tier system became palpable in Israeli society and fueled significant public debate during the 1980s.

Israel introduced its NHI in 1995. The mandatory health insurance required all legal residents to register with a sick fund.[1] It is a

---

[1] The NHI covers Israeli Palestinians (an estimated 1.5 million people). The Palestine Authority is responsible for providing healthcare for the Palestinians living in the West

population-wide social health insurance, administered by four major (competing, not-for-profit) sick funds. The passage of the HI was due to a confluence of factors. The first was the weakening of the Histadrut and its ties with the Labor Party and GSF. Some Labor members began to view the ties with the Histadrut as a burden rather than a boon. The second was the increased consumerism in Israeli society. The third was the world-wide trend of reinventing government that affected public policy-making, and the fourth was the wide-spread dissatisfaction with the lack of respon-siveness and long wait times (especially for GSF members), a sense of inequality in the system, and bureaucratic arbitrariness regarding the rights of sick fund members. Finally, increased technocratic know-how and posturing by health professionals, including the experts at the MoH, contributed to the climate for change. The emphasis on patient choice in the NHI reflected the principles of New Public Management and turned the health system into a change leader in the political economy.

The NHI was part of a three-pronged reform proposed by the 1990 Netanyahu Commission, a state commission of inquiry. Two other spheres of the reform—transforming government hospitals into public trusts and reorganizing the MoH—never materialized because of too much resist-ance from the (hospital) labor unions. From a rational planning point of view, the partial implementation of the reform is a recipe for frustration. From a policy-learning point of view (Helderman et al. 2005), however, NHI's enactment set in motion a chain of events worth looking at. First of all, the NHI led to one radical change that in itself did not depend on the full implementation of the envisioned reform: a process for defining the universal standard basket of services. Previously, each fund determined its own entitlements. While other countries like the Netherlands (Berg et al. 2004) and New Zealand (Chinitz 1999) abandoned the idea of (explicitly) defining a core basket of health services, Israel went quite clearly, if not always resolutely, down this road. Additionally, in the longer term, the NHI led to organizational change within the system (see next page).

Bank and Gaza territories (about 4.5–5 million people). This chapter does not discuss that part of the healthcare system.

Israel's Healthcare System, 2018

The major funding sources for healthcare in Israel are social insurance contributions, tax subsidies and modest, if growing, amounts of patient co-payments and private insurance premiums. In the early 21st century, co-payments for specialist encounters prescription drugs had risen, but there were many exemptions and caps on the total amount families pay each year, with lower caps for elderly. The mandatory social health insurance offers a wide range of entitlements. It covers the cost of private physicians, treatment in private clinics and complementary medicine.

Supplemental insurance plays an growing role. The share of household spending went up, from 0.2 to 1.3 percent on supplemental insurance, from 0.2 to 0.9 percent on private insurance and from 0.8 to 2 percent on out-of-pocket payments (OOPs) for drugs and medical items. Total household OOPs for healthcare thus increased from 1.2 to 4.2 percent in the last two decades (Ministry of Health 2017). Still, as a proportion of total health spending, total OOPs actually declined, from 29.5 to 24.4 percent between 2000 and 2017 (WHO/World Bank Database).

Israeli citizens can choose the fund they want to register with, and can change up to four times per year. The first year they had this option, in 1995, about 4 percent of the population switched plans. After that, the rate of change went down to about 1 percent. The largest fund, the GSF, covered 60 percent of the population (down from 80 percent in the 1980s, see above), the other three covered about 36 percent by 2018. The NHI explicitly lists its entitlements in the appendix. It specifies procedures, pharmaceuticals and provides guidelines for applications. If a physician prescribes off-label or outside of the guideline use for a particular drug, the sick fund is within its legal rights to refuse to reimburse.[2]

The government set up an expert public committee to assess the addition of new services in 1998 (Chinitz et al. 1998). The committee meets

---

[2]This causes endless disputes. Qualitative research by Chinitz indicates that Israeli physicians spend up to 10 percent of their time engaged in quarrels with sick fund managers over these points. The physicians often win the argument, but the organizational consequences in terms of efficiency and morale are significant.

several times a year. It ranks potential new services, based on health technology assessment by the MoH's Health Technology Unit. In a typical neo-corporatist mode, the committee is made up of 24 physicians, experts from the MoH, representatives of health plans, and public representatives. It applies ethical, economic and social criteria to decide which services should be included. Based on the recommendations of the committee, Parliament adds (or de-lists) entitlements within the available public budget (the Ministry of Finance [MoF] agreed to expand the annual budget by about 1 percent for this expansion). There is regular media coverage on the committee's activities. Not surprisingly, the list of services seeking entrance into the basket, mainly pharmaceuticals, usually exceeds the available funding. An interesting phenomenon is that pressure from high-profile lobbying and patient groups is less powerful than might be expected. Colon cancer patients, for example, conducted a hunger strike to receive Avastin, but did not get their way. It appears that the Israeli public and decision-makers accept the sad truth that not all drugs that might be of benefit will be financed out of public means.

Insured citizens can seek supplementary insurance offered by both sick funds and private health insurance. In the early 2000s, some funds expanded their supplemental coverage for drugs and other services not covered under the basic insurance. The MoF opposed this move, as it would increase national health expenditure and create a two-tiered system.

Despite population growth, there has been a decrease in density of medical personnel in recent years, and the number of hospital beds decreased from 6.3 to 3.5 per 1,000 population between 2010 and 2015 (World Bank Health Nutrition and Population Statistics). Healthcare providers include hospitals owned by the government or health plans, clinics owned by health plans, self-employed physicians who have contracts with insurers and private for-profit hospitals, laboratories and institutes. Mother-and-child healthcare, mental health care (till 2015) and long term care were not originally included in the NHI and are subject to different arrangements. All insured can select a primary care physician who works in a nearby clinic owned by their fund, or a self-employed physician who has a contract with their fund. Access to non-emergency care generally requires a referral from a physician or pre-approval from the fund. While Israelis can, and do, exercise free choice of hospital, the referrals generally include direction to a specific provider.

Hospitals receive capped budgets, though the funds typically reimburse 50 percent of budget overruns. Emergency care and outpatient clinics receive fee-for-service payments. Community-based physicians usually receive salaries, often combined with a capitation payment for each individual on their patient list. Independent physicians receive a capitation payment for their patients. The capitation payments are generally a form of capped fee-for-service, and do not involve risk-bearing on the part of the physician. The MoH sets the per diem rates and fee schedules for hospitals.

National professional associations of hospital physicians, nurses and other providers negotiate salaries on behalf of their members. In Jerusalem, physicians are permitted to work privately in hospitals under strict regulation. Elsewhere, ad hoc rules had allowed physicians to work privately in hospitals, but the State Attorney General halted these arrangements and the issue has not been resolved. Many physicians based in public hospitals have private practices after-hours and perform procedures at private hospitals.

The health plans are legally independent entities, but the MoH has the overall responsibility. It sets hospital budgets and defines benefits. It is involved in the planning and allocation of budgets, imposing limits on public spending as well as on the numbers of physicians. The National Health Insurance Institute (NHII) is responsible for the administration of the NHI. It allocates the contributions collected via the tax system to healthcare funds based on a risk equalization scheme (see below).

The collective bargaining and active participation of the main organized stakeholders resembles the traditional neo-corporatist style of social policy-making in Western European nations. In general, this gives providers a strong veto position. Wage negotiations often lead to strikes by health professionals.

The NHI Regulator, a branch of the MoF, regulates private health insurance. Recently, it ruled that private insurers cannot refuse payment for pharmaceuticals if an equivalent exists in the national standard basket of services. In addition, it required insurers to limit choice of provider to closed panels of physicians, and to standardize benefits baskets.

Traditionally, the MoH was responsible for monitoring both the basic insurance and supplemental coverage. The MoH had the reputation of an ineffective regulator, however. It owned two-thirds of general hospital beds. This created a conflict of interest and, on occasion, an inability to focus on forward-thinking planning and regulation instead of the day-to-day management of hospitals. In recent years, the MoH strengthened its role as a financial regulator. It took firmer control over reimbursement rates to stabilize hospital expenditure. As of 2006, by and large, health plans were working within balanced budgets for the standard basket of services, although they have all since accrued deficits due to population growth and aging.

At first, the MoH was less adept at regulating the quality of care. Facing a lack of resources and unwillingness to cooperate on the part of physicians' associations, the MoH was unable to create a framework for ongoing quality assurance in healthcare provision and insurance. In recent years, however, the health plans and the associations of hospitals and physicians have participated in benchmarking and other quality assurance efforts. These include the publication of quality indicators at the institutional level. After frequent critical media coverage of medical errors and malfeasance, the MoH set up investigative and disciplinary committees to deal with these concerns.

Israeli health policy-making thus provides an interesting example of a radical big bang reform, namely, the implementation of the NHI, followed by incremental change. Faced with stakeholder opposition, lack of popular support and specific budget constraints, the government has been able to make bold changes in some areas but not in others. For example, when the MoH sought to expand hospital capacity and increase physicians' salary to reduce the tendency of physicians to engage in private practice, the MoF placed financial restrictions that blocked these measures. Likewise, efforts to give state-owned hospitals more autonomy in hiring and firing were limited by national labor relation agreements to which the MoF is party.

The same applies for changing employment relations between hospitals and physicians. At the same time, the government has increased its weight in the regulatory sphere, by taking an active role in the development of health indicator programs as well as the increased regulation of supplemental and private health insurance markets. This suggests that should the government eventually decide to increase public health spending, it will be able to use the additional resources more effectively in terms of quality, efficiency and perhaps even equity.

The Continuing Evolution of the 1995 Health Insurance Reform: From Big Bang to Incrementalism?

Perhaps the most important result of the 1995 NHI was improved regulation of the existing sick fund system, which already covered 95 percent of the population. The preamble of the NHI law states that it is based on "justice, equity and mutual aid." Its major provisions are open enrollment, freedom to switch sick funds, a uniform income-based health tax (replacing the former member dues paid directly to the sick funds) and a standard basket of services for all insured. The wording in the law of the "cost of the standard basket" basically implies an overall budget for the system set and provided for by government. General taxation covers any shortfall between revenues from health taxes and expenditures. The funds are allocated to the health plans through a capitation formula weighted for age and geographical residence.

As noted earlier, the NHI was a main component of the 1995 health reform. The NHI dealt mainly with finance and rights to health. The adoption of NHI was a radical change, as it shifted and universalized the base for insurance from membership to citizenship. The two other facets of the reform aimed to decentralize general hospitals and other health facilities and change the role of the MoH. Government-owned hospitals were to become trusts, and mental health and long-term care services provided for directly by the MoH were to shift to the NHI. These proposals were only partially implemented by 2018, however.

Notwithstanding the reform shortfall, there has been (more gradual) change across the system. The implementation of the NHI itself had, predictably, fueled new forces of change. The interesting point for policy learning is that here the big bang reforms transformed into an incremental process of ongoing change. The original design of the NHI with competing sick funds survived and adapted to the new challenges.

The Shift to Incrementalism

Since the implementation of the NHI, the Israeli health system continued to change but in a more incremental and less organized way. The changes did not always follow the logic intended by NHI's creators, the Netanyahu Commission and Parliament. The following list of changes illustrates that incrementalism does not always mean change in one particular or coherent direction.

The Israeli Parliament passed a patients' rights bill soon after implementing the NHI. Patients' rights seemed more salient in care settings (especially in hospitals) than in the relationship between insured and their health plan. After the first year, there was a marked drop in the share of insured switching funds (an experience in common with Switzerland and the Netherlands). With no price competition over the standard basket, and with registration located in post offices, where the sick funds cannot engage in risk selection through targeted marketing, perhaps the low number of transfers was to be expected. A reasonable alternative assessment appears to be that the health insurance market is contestable. The very threat of losing members keeps insurers on their competitive toes; and, their activities are focused as much on preventing losing members as on attracting new ones.

Despite concerns about the unsophisticated capitation formula for allocating money to the health plans (not adjusted for the health status of the insured), there has not been evidence of significant quality skimping, for example, by undertreating chronically ill patients. Some critics argued that the plans do not provide enough care in underserved areas with costly insured, however (Shmueli 2011).

Since the annual Omnibus Budget Arrangement Act in 1998 (initiated by the MoF), the insurers may charge user fees. In the first year after the introduction of co-payments, over 30 percent of the population mentioned that they had delayed obtaining certain health services and goods, especially pharmaceuticals; this percentage had declined to about 15–20 percent by 2011 (Chinitz and Grau 2015).

The MoH regularly adjusts the standard basket of services (mainly prescription drugs), but the MoF does not always provide enough financing for additional entitlements. Nonetheless, as mentioned earlier, pressure from patient groups is not always effective.

Insurers may offer supplemental coverage for services not included in the standard basket. Supplemental plans are regulated in a pro-competitive manner, but risk-rating is prohibited, and premiums are flat rate by age group. The supplemental policies serve increasingly as a marketing device and strategic tool in the hands of insurers. For example, after the MoH failed to increase the budget for the standard basket in 2007, the Macabbi and GSF offered supplemental insurance covering "life-saving drugs" not included in the standard basket. The MoF opposed these expanded supplemental policies on the grounds of inequity and the risk of expanding national health expenditure. The MoH at first supported the supplemental policies but agreed to roll them back when the MoF promised larger budgets for updating the standard basket, in exchange for taking life-saving drugs out of the supplemental policies. This debate recurs every few years, especially as advances in medical science produce new, experimental (and expensive) drugs that show promise but only limited gains in survival (Efrati 2015).

Both the MoH and MoF stepped up their regulation of private commercial health insurance to reduce duplication, externalities and uncertainty for insured.

While the insurers shy away from alienating members by restricting freedom of choice in provider, they sometimes engage in efforts to channel patients. One incentive for this is the hospital budget regulation by the MoH. Each plan pays general hospitals a combination of case-based payment, fee-for-service and per diem amounts. Based on estimates of expected volume, the funds pay full prices up to a budget cap, and only 50 percent for services above the cap. The funds thus have an incentive to channel patients to hospitals that have exceeded the cap (as their prices are lower).

Choice is less of a salient issue for patients, however, as they can still insist on going to the hospital of their choice. There was extensive media coverage on a dispute between a major hospital and the GSF concerning its efforts to channel patients. In the end they reached a compromise, and in recent years such conflicts seem to have abated (Waitzberg and Merkur 2017).

Health inequality has become another major concern, especially regarding the Arab population and other minority groups such as Ethiopian Jews (Epstein et al. 2006). The Maccabi fund initiated a program aimed at closing the gaps in access to care, primary prevention and cultural competency (Epstein et al. 2006; Macabbi Health Services 2016).

As noted earlier, in the early 2000s, the four insurers collaborated in developing measures for quality of care in the community, under the auspices of the MoH and in conjunction with a health services research group. It is up to each fund how they use the measures and publicize their own activities in quality assurance, but the very participation in the collaboration turned out to be a convergent source of consensus targets based on evidence-based medicine. By 2012, this collaboration had become a national program, with a national body that conducted studies and published the results for each health plan. The MoH instituted a similar program for hospitals in 2012.

All insurers and hospitals developed electronic patient records (EPRs) to improve the appropriateness, coordination and continuity of care. The EPRs reside with each constituent of the system. While the MoH advocates unifying the data sets, it faces—as in many other countries—the expected obstacles of proprietary ownership and lack of interoperability.

The MoH and MoF started to transfer mental health care to the sick funds in 2015. Parliament only passed part of the legislation necessary to allow for that transfer and there is still discussion in a parliamentary subcommittee. Controversy persists over whether the transfer implies privatization of services, whether the sick funds will provide adequate quality care in this realm, and the future employment status of those currently working in the public mental health system.

The two sick funds with dominant labor union affiliations reduced the role of unions in their governing boards. The question of who governs the sick funds (a major issue in the early years of the western European sick funds, see the chapter about the Netherlands) arises periodically in various contexts, as well as the high-profile coverage of well-paid sick fund managers.

Theoretical Implications of the Israeli Case: The Role of the State and the Dominant Cultural Orientation

The introduction of Israel's NHI in 1995 is a case of health insurance reform that started as a big bang reform, but after partial implementation, fizzled out and transformed into a process of incremental change.[3]

The MoH still has overall responsibility for policy-making. While the MoF plays its usual role in restraining public and national health expenditure—it also became more accountable for the perception that despite increasing budgets, Israel's health system is underfunded and over time, becoming increasingly privatized in terms of finance. The MoH is now struggling to combine its new role as regulator with the traditional one as the owner of public hospitals and provider of health services.

Social solidarity remains a prominent value in Israeli society. This value orientation has created barriers to any structural measures, such as introducing a for-profit sick fund or allowing private practice in government hospitals. Critics perceive these steps as privatization that may undermine equitable access for all.

As mentioned, payments for supplemental and private health insurance have risen. This has not been perceived as a major threat to solidarity,

---

[3] Carolyn Tuohy's book *Remaking Policy* (2018) mentions four health reform strategies: blueprint, big bang, mosaic and incremental reforms. It designates the Dutch reform as blueprint. In fact, one might argue that the Israeli case, similar to the Dutch one, started as a blueprint but became much more incremental (see the chapter about Holland in this volume). The Dutch and Israeli experiences illustrate the difficulty in categorizing or labeling systems into fixed categories.

thus far, especially as the supplemental policies (held by the majority of citizens) are bound by the prosocial conditions of no risk-rating and community-rated premiums.

Policy debates indicate that "voice" (Hirschman 1970) is very much at work in holding governments and other players accountable in Israel's healthcare system. Choice and exit is a value, too, but it appears to play a greater role in healthcare services than in the choice of health plan—an experience not unique to Israel (see, e.g., the chapters on Chile or Holland in this volume).

Overall, the Israeli health system has evolved in terms of increased financial accountability, with a broad range of social health insurance entitlements subject to explicit rationing of new technologies. While the Health Ministry is a major player in the policy arena, its role is also shaped by the institutional legacy of the early pre-State political economy. The results of this legacy were social systems with blurred lines of authority and responsibility. The path dependency of this inheritance seemed particularly strong in the ownership and regulation of healthcare. Cutting the cord between the largest sick fund and the Labor Party opened the way for more (continuous) change in the organization and management of health insurance.

One could argue that the incremental changes reflected the need to manage the mix of public–private responsibilities. The changes aimed to find a viable balance among exit, voice and choice. The changes included a stronger role for government, for example, in increasing regulation of the health insurance market, and also in increasing autonomy for public hospitals and other actors.

At the same time, the overall policy framework is bound by centralized control, especially the MoF's effective fiscal control, which blocks the emergence of a more sophisticated regulatory approach.

References

Anderson, O. 1989. *The Health Services Continuum in Democratic States*. Aspen: Health Administration Press.

Bentur, N., A. Berg, and D. Chinitz. 1998. "Health system reform and the elderly: the case of Israel." *J Aging Soc Policy*, 10(2): 85–104.

Berg, M., T. van der Grinten, and N. Klanzinga. Fall 2004. "Technology assessment, priority setting, and appropriate care in Dutch health care." *Int J Technol Assess Health Care*, 20(4): 564.

Chinitz, D. 1995. "Israel's health policy breakthrough: the politics of reform and the reform of politics." *J Health Polit, Policy Law*, 20(4): 909–932.

Chinitz, D. 1999. "The Basic Basket of Health Services under National Health Insurance" (Vol. 54). *Social Security*: 53–68.

Chinitz, D. and I. Grau. 2015. "Privatization in the Israeli Healthcare." *Privatization and the Boundaries of the State Jerusalem*. I. Galnoor and A. Paz Fuch (eds). Van Leer Institute and Kibbutz Hameuchad.

Chinitz, D. and A. Israeli. 2015. "Not everything is black or white. Commentary on Filc D and Cohen N, blurring the boundaries between public and private health care services as an alternative explanation for the emergence of black medicine: the Israeli case." *Health Econ Policy Law*, 11(02): 215–221, *L*.

Epstein, L., R. Goldwag, M. Greenstein, and S. Ismail. 2006. *Reducing Health Inequality and Health Inequity in Israel: Towards a National Policy and Action Program Summary Report*. Jerusalem: Myers JDC Brookdale Institute.

Gross, R., B. Rosen, and D. Chinitz. 1998. "Evaluating the Israeli health care reform: strategies, challenges and lessons." *Health Policy*, 45(2): 99–117.

Plotknik, R. and N. Keidar. 2017. *Twenty Years of the National Health Insurance Law*. Jerusalem: Ministry of Health.

Macabbi Health Services. 2016. *Reducing Health Inequalities*. https://www.youtube.com/watch?reload=9&v=xSGT1IvoIl8 video. Accessed January 15, 2019.

Maor, R. 2010. "There is no hebrew word for accountability." *Jerusalem Post*, December 21.

Nisanholtz, R., D. Chinitz, and S. Rosenbaum. 2018. "What should health insurance cover: a comparison of US and Israeli policies towards essential health benefits." *J Health Econ, Policy Law*, 13(2): 189–208.

Rosen, B. 2015. *HiT Israel*. Copenhagen: European Observatory on Health Care Systems, World Health Organization.

Shmueli, A. 2011. "Switching sickness funds in Israel: adverse selection or risk selection: some insights from an analysis of the costs of switchers." *Health Policy*, 102(2–3): 247–254.

Tuohy, C. 2018. *Remaking Policy Scale, Pace and Political Strategy in Health Care Reform.* Toronto: University of Toronto Press.

World Health Organization. 2017. *Health Statistics Data Base.* http://apps.who.int/gho/data/node.main.GHEDOOPSCHESHA2011?lang=en. Accessed January 15, 2019.

Waitzberg, R. and S. Merkur. 2017. "Policy efforts to strengthen public hospitals in Israel." *Eurohealth*, 23(4): 34–37.

Section V

Oceania and Asia: New Zealand, Singapore and Taiwan

Asia and Oceania are vast and heterogeneous continents, including the two largest nations of the world, China and India, and many smaller ones, with widely divergent income levels, economic growth rates, levels of health spending and health status of their populations. They also vary in political regimes, administrative capacities and cultural and institutional legacies, and those factors are reflected in the direction and pace of their health reforms.

The three nations of this regional section are robust capitalist states, with quite different traditions of governance, ranging from New Zealand's Westminster "winner takes all" politics, which allow for relatively rapid change (perhaps more rhetorically than in reality), to the more autocratic leadership traditions of Singapore and Taiwan. Over time, the latter two have become less exclusive as organized stakeholders and civil society groups successfully push for greater voice in the political arena. The different political traditions are also reflected both in the healthcare arrangements and in the reform efforts analyzed in this regional section. The nations share the policy goal of providing their population universal access to good quality healthcare at an affordable cost; they consider the healthcare sector as an important economic sector that provides employment and industrial innovation opportunities. At the same time, the populations of all three nations feel strongly that their governments have a responsibility to safeguard access to healthcare for all and protect vulnerable groups, such as the elderly, the low-income families or the disabled.

In all three cases, governments took the lead role in changing the financing, administration and regulation of healthcare.

The two Asian "tiger economies," Taiwan and Singapore, saw major improvements in the health of their populations following the very high economic growth rates of the 1970s and 1980s, which lifted the majority of their population out of poverty and also allowed for substantial investments in their healthcare systems. Their income levels now surpass those of most European nations, and their health indicators are among the best in the world, even with (still) relatively modest levels of health spending. They both looked at experiences abroad but ultimately took strikingly different pathways to realize the goal of universal coverage.

Despite those major differences in historical development, political structures and financial and administrative arrangements of their healthcare systems, the health reforms of the three nations show many similarities. There is widespread policy rhetoric about individual responsibility and the need for more competition in healthcare as a means to enhance efficiency, but in practice, governments did not step aside to let "markets" do the job anywhere. User fees, for example, are seldom popular and governments commonly exempt large population groups from such payments—thus, basically defeating the purpose of the measure in the first place. Also, despite fiscal and budgetary pressure, healthcare budgets tend to expand more easily than contract. As another example, high hopes for information technology (IT) as a means to transform healthcare into a modern industry often did not realize. The introduction of electronic medical records, for example, turned out to be very complicated. The healthcare system, in most countries, entails decentralized decision-making. It also involves many actors in the financing and provision of healthcare services, who have often developed their own IT systems.

In all cases of this regional section, with aging populations and epidemiological change, we have also seen a shift in emphasis from acute medical care for individual patients to issues of population health, health prevention and health promotion. These developments also led to a more activist stance of governments in health policy.

Map 9. Asia and Oceania New Zealand, Singapore and Taiwan: Population, Income per Capita and Health Expenditure, 1960–2015.

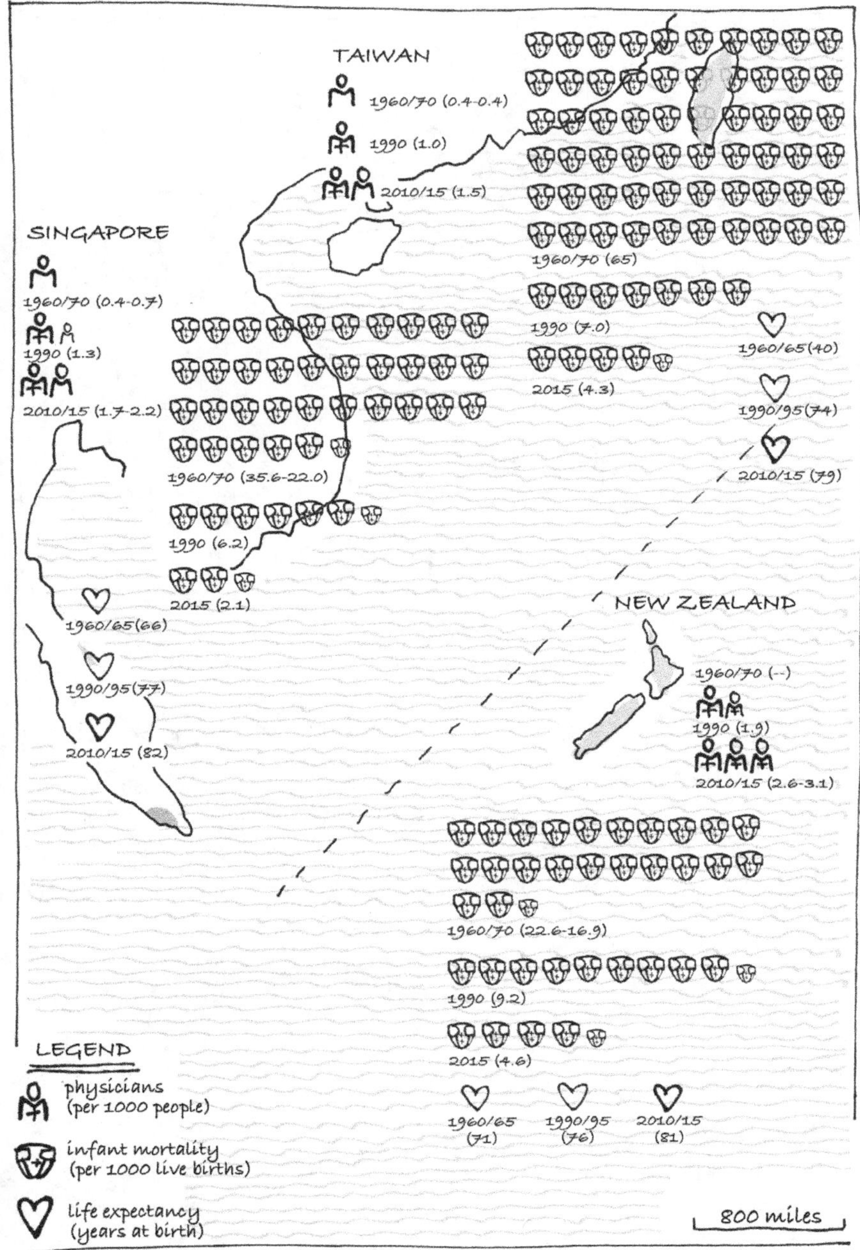

Map 10.   Asia and Oceania New Zealand, Singapore and Taiwan: Number of Physicians, Infant Mortality and Life Expectancy, 1960–2015.

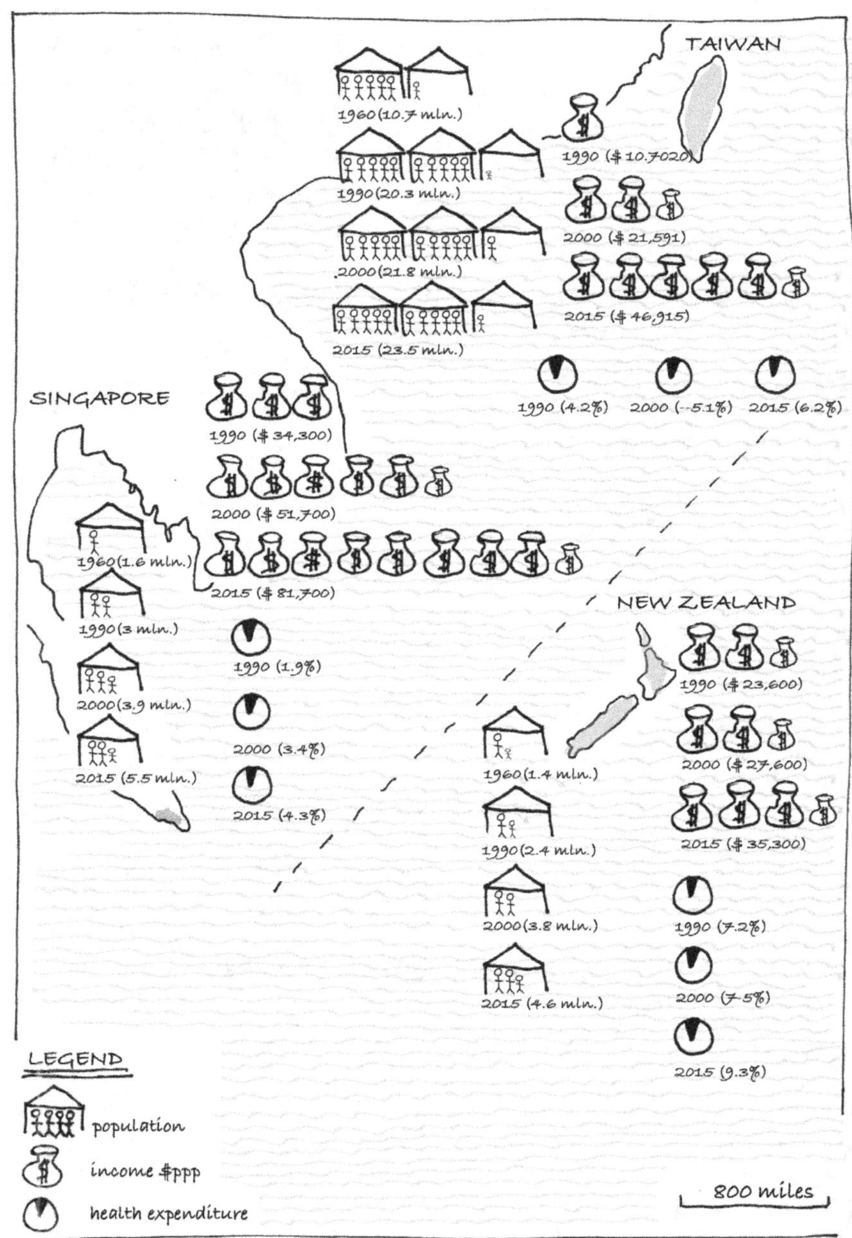

Chapter 10

New Zealand's Healthcare System: Rapid Reform and Incremental Change

Tim Tenbensel and Toni Ashton

Introduction

In the 1990s, New Zealand attracted widespread attention with its highly ambitious and seemingly radical health reform. Less well known but equally significant were the attempts to "re-reform" the health system in the 2000s. Both sets of reforms were largely driven by the ideology of the major political party in government at the time. Despite these waves of reform, some key aspects of the system remained remarkably stable (Gauld 2009; Ashton et al. 2005). The New Zealand experience provides a fascinating case study in the politics of healthcare, the resilience of institutions and the rhetoric and reality of health sector reform.

The next sections discuss the structure of the New Zealand health system, the waves of reform in recent decades and the theories and ideas that underpinned them. We then explore some of the drivers who shaped those reforms. Finally, we consider how the reforms affected various dimensions of the system including efficiency, equity, competition and governance.

New Zealand's Healthcare

New Zealand lies at the bottom of the world in the southwestern Pacific Ocean, approximately 2,000 kilometers southeast of Australia. Its land area is similar in size to that of Japan, yet its population is only

4.8 million. About 70 percent of the population lives in the main urban areas, one-third in the largest city, Auckland, and only 10 percent in remote rural regions. Almost three-quarters (74 percent) of the population are of European descent, while 15 percent identify themselves as Māori (the indigenous people of New Zealand), 12 percent as Asian, and 7 percent as Pacific Islander (New Zealanders can identify with more than one ethnic group; Statistics New Zealand 2018).

The country has a unicameral parliamentary system with representatives elected via a system of mixed member proportional (MMP) representation. A unique feature of New Zealand's constitution is the Treaty of Waitangi, signed between the British Crown and Māori tribes in 1840. Although largely ignored by governments until the 1970s, the Treaty now has great influence over both the direction and the process of social policy.

The Social Security Act of 1938 laid the foundation for New Zealand's public health system as the government of the day sought to introduce a universal, tax-based national health system as part of a broader set of welfare reforms. Resistance from primary care medical practitioners, who did not wish to become government employees, blocked this plan. As a consequence, a dual system emerged, with state-owned hospitals providing services free of charge and general practitioners (GPs) acting as self-employed physicians, only partly publicly funded. The basket of services covered by public funding expanded significantly over time, but this dual structure of funding and provision has remained relatively unchanged.

New Zealand spent about 9.0 percent of gross domestic product (GDP) on healthcare in 2017 (OECD 2018). Most (79 percent) came from public sources: 5 percent from private insurance and 16 percent was out-of-pocket spending. The public funding consists largely of general taxation (89 percent) plus about 11 percent contribution by the Accident Compensation Commission (ACC). ACC is a state-owned insurance fund providing compulsory, comprehensive no-fault insurance for accident-related injuries. ACC revenues consist of levies paid by employers, employees, self-employed people and motor vehicle licensing. It also receives some government subsidy to cover non-workers (Treasury 2014).

All permanent residents in New Zealand are automatically covered by the public health system. They receive most services free of charge. This includes inpatient and outpatient healthcare (usually in the state-owned hospitals), maternity services and many community-based services. Co-payments apply for general practice consultations and pharmaceuticals, while access to some disability support (such as home care and long-term residential care) is means tested.

Most GPs work in group practices with three or more GPs, at least one practice nurse, and other support staff. Citizens can choose their own primary care provider but they need GP referral to access secondary care. Patients usually have little or no choice of specialist or hospital within the public system, and waitlists for elective surgery are prioritized according to need (Gwynne-Jones and Iosua 2016). There is a parallel private system where patients can chose their own specialist or hospital, and pay for their own care either through voluntary private health insurance or directly out-of-pocket. About one-third of the population holds private health insurance. Private insurance is not subject to any special regulations, and premiums are not tax-deductible.

The Ministry of Health (MoH) distributes the vast majority of tax funding to 20 District Health Boards (DHBs) via a weighted population-based funding formula. The MoH retained responsibility for public health, maternity care and disability support services for people under 65. The MoH purchases this care directly from providers.

DHBs are responsible for improving, promoting and protecting the health and independence of their populations by either providing or purchasing services for the people residing in their geographically defined region (New Zealand Public Health and Disability Act 2000, s22). The so-called DHB "provider arms" own public hospitals and some community-based facilities. DHBs, the ACC and the MoH purchase all other services—including most primary care—from private providers through contracts or "Service Agreements" (see Figure 1).

Figure 1. Financing and Provision of New Zealand Health and Disability System.

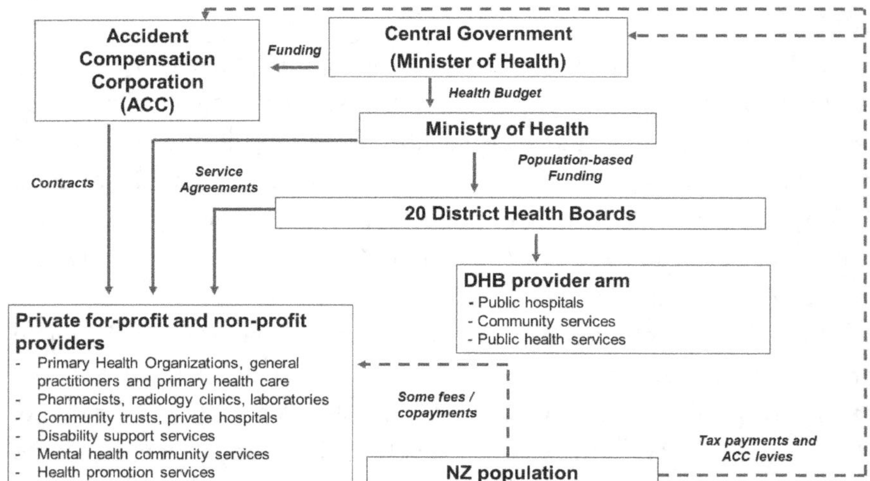

Source: New Zealand Ministry of Health 2016c.

Health Reform Waves in New Zealand

New Zealand's economic policy and public sector management underwent enormous changes between 1984 and 1996, instigated by both major political parties while in government. Many commentators considered these economic and public sector reforms to be the "purest" laboratory of neo-liberal policy prescriptions and new public management ideas (Boston et al. 1996; Pollitt and Bouckaert 2000). Initially, the Labour government of the 1980s did not support such reforms into the areas of health and social services, perhaps to avoid deepening rifts within the party. After Labour lost power in the 1990 election, the incoming National Party (NP) government had fewer qualms about extending the neo-liberal reform agenda to healthcare. In 1996, however, this government's capacity for radical reform was weakened by the need to coalesce with minor political parties following the first election under MMP proportional representation. The first coalition government watered down the reforms of the early 1990s and shifted to incremental adjustments instead. From 2000, the incoming Labour-led (center-left) government finally reversed

Figure 2.   Major Health Reforms in New Zealand, 1939–2018.

Year(s)	Type of Reform
1938	Social Security Act introduced universal tax-funded healthcare.
1940s	Full public financing for hospital and mental health services, and partial financing for a range of primary healthcare services.
1993	Contract model: four Regional Health Authorities (RHAs), public hospitals commercialized and renamed Crown Health Enterprises (CHEs).
1997	Purchasing centralized under Health Funding Authority (HFA). CHEs restructured and renamed Hospital and Health Services (HHSs). Free GP consultations and prescription drugs for children under 6.
2000	HFA abolished. Return to a mix of contract and integrated models. 21 locally elected DHBs established to purchase or provide services for their district populations.
2001–2007	Development of 82 Primary Health Organizations (PHOs). Universal (and higher) subsidies for GP consultations and pharmaceuticals.
2007–2018	2 DHBs merged (reducing total number to 20). Number of PHOs reduced (to 32 in 2017). Development of district alliances (DAs) between DHBs and PHOs; free GP consultations and pharmaceuticals for all children under 13 (2015), children under 14 (2018).

Source: Authors.

many of the 1990s reforms and embarked on its own program of restructuring the health system, with a focus on primary healthcare (Figure 2).

Early 1990s: The Big Bang

The (center-right) government led by the National Party announced plans for a radical restructuring of the public health system, after its election in late 1990 (Upton 1991). The proposals reflected the market-oriented ideas that had inspired reform in other sectors of the economy during the 1980s. The new government announced the reforms in July 1991. At the same time, it dismissed the elected and appointed board members of 14 area health boards, replacing them with commissioners to oversee the implementation of the new proposed structure.

Apart from a few, relatively minor modifications (Finlayson 2001), on July 1, 1993, the government implemented the new structure, as announced two years earlier. The new structure came with high hopes of improved access "to a health system which is effective, fair, and affordable … encourage efficiency, flexibility, and innovation in health care delivery … reduce waiting times for hospital operations … widen the choice of hospitals and health services for consumers," and "enhance the working environment for health professionals." In addition, it expected that the changes would lead to greater recognition of the importance of public health in preventive illness and injury, and in promoting health to the changing needs of society (Upton 1991).

The 1993 reforms represent a perfect example of a big bang style of reform (Tuohy 2018). The central feature of these reforms was the switch from an integrated model towards a contract model that separated the purchasing and provision functions. The financing for all personal primary, secondary and tertiary healthcare and disability support was channeled into a single purse. The MoH distributed this money to four newly established RHAs, whose role was to purchase services for their regional populations. On the provider side, the old public hospitals became for-profit businesses, with the Ministers of Health and Finance as shareholders. Now renamed CHEs, the hospitals were to compete with private providers for contracts to supply health services. The CHEs were to run as commercial enterprises and many hired chief executives from the private sector to import "best business" practice. The theory behind this quasi-market was that the actors would behave like buyers and sellers in a competitive market, with providers responding to the preferences of the RHAs, and the most efficient providers winning the contracts.

There was little evidence of any major efficiency gains accruing from the new system, however, by the time of the next general election in 1996 (Cumming and Salmond 1998; Ashton 2002; Easton 2002). This was not altogether surprising, given the short time period, and the depth and breadth of disruption the reforms had caused.

The restructuring had been costly in terms of money and eroding trust. Many health professionals felt quite alienated working in a system that encouraged competition (Malcolm et al. 1996). There was also widespread media coverage of anecdotes wherein patients did not receive adequate care in public hospitals, and of public dissatisfaction with the new system after some services were terminated because service providers failed to win contracts.

Modifications in the Late 1990s

A new coalition government stepped into office after the 1996 election, with the NP in the senior role. The populist junior coalition partner, New Zealand First, was ideologically opposed to market competition in healthcare. The first health policy statement of the new coalition indicated a withdrawal, at least from the rhetoric, of a competitive system and so a new round of restructuring began. While keeping the contracting model, the government centralized the purchasing responsibilities of the four RHAs under a single national organization, the HFA. The HFA was to move away from competitive tendering and collaborate with providers in the planning of service volumes and in establishing benchmark prices. The new direction also included higher subsidies for GP consultations and pharmaceuticals to facilitate free services for young children. CHEs underwent another round of restructuring into not-for-profit publicly owned entities called HHSs. The coalition agreement limited the scope for the HFA to contract with private hospitals, favoring the publicly owned HHSs.

A Return to Community Governance and Regional Collaboration in the 2000s

A new Labour-led government came into power at the end of 1999. The Labour Party (the senior coalition partner) had at that point returned to a more traditional social-democratic identity and opposed the competitive system. It argued that the previous government had allowed the health system to become "run down, privatized, and corporatized" and that the reforms had resulted in an "overwhelming alienation of the public" (New Zealand Labour Party 1999). It proposed a restoration of the non-commercial system, with "full involvement of representatives of local communities" in the planning and management of health services.

This led to yet another round of major reforms. The central feature this time was the establishment of 21 DHBs with locally elected boards. The government disbanded the central purchasing agent (the HFA) and distributed its purchasing roles between the DHBs and the MoH. DHBs became responsible not only for hospital financing but also for primary healthcare and disability support. As the latter were mostly provided by private sector organizations, DHBs became both providers *and* purchasers of services. This brought the responsibility for community-based and hospital services within a single organization, and required a strategic planning framework for most publicly funded health services within the district. The New Zealand Health Strategy served as guidance for DHBs. It set out fundamental principles, goals and objectives for the sector (King 2000; Ministry of Health 2016a).

The reforms also included restructuring primary healthcare. The 2001 Primary Health Care Strategy announced plans for a primary health system that would "focus on the health of populations as well as individuals, was community-oriented and would encourage a team-based approach to care" (King 2001). The plans included substantial financial support by DHBs for networks between GPs and other primary health providers: Primary Health Organisations (PHOs). PHOs are non-government organizations set up to provide a range of primary health services to their enrolled populations. Their workforce composition varies. In addition to GPs and practice nurses, a PHO may include physiotherapists, dentists, sexual health workers, health promotion workers and other allied health professionals. To encourage enrollment in PHOs, the MoH increased subsidies significantly so that patients who joined faced lower co-payments. More than 80 PHOs started within five years, with most GPs and over 95 percent of the population belonging to a PHO (Ministry of Health 2018b).

Structural Stability, Incremental Change and Austerity in the 2010s

Following another change of government (from Labour-led to National-led) in 2008, the incoming Health Minister commissioned a major review of the organizational arrangements of the public health system in 2009 (Ministerial Review Group 2009). This review did not recommend any major health reforms, but set the stage for more incremental, often bottom-up rather than top-down, policy changes.

One important development since 2009 has been the emphasis on greater collaboration among DHBs and between DHBs and PHOs, especially in the planning of regional services and efforts to reduce duplication of administrative functions. Two DHBs merged in 2010, reducing the total number to 20. The number of PHOs also fell significantly (many of the early ones were very small). Mergers and restructuring reduced their number to around 30 (New Zealand Ministry of Health 2018b).

As part of this new direction, the MoH required DHBs (government organizations) and PHOs (non-government organizations) to form District Alliances (DAs) with Alliance Leadership Teams. DAs are responsible for joint planning of services at the local level (Gauld 2017). Many DAs created project teams (known as Service-Level Alliance Teams, or SLATs) to focus on specific issues such as urgent care, rural health services and child healthcare. DAs can include other organizations like Māori providers.

The reform also led to increased emphasis on health sector performance measurement and quality improvement since the early 2010s. National health targets became an important mechanism for measuring the performance of DHBs and PHOs. Primarily defined in terms of outputs or processes, the targets focused on activities such as child immunizations, elective surgery, referral rates to specialist services, time to treatment and discharge or hospital admission for emergency care. These dimensions of performance were largely within the control of health sector organizations. Official reports of target performance indicated significant improvement, but it is not clear to what extent this was at the expense of other, unmeasured aspects of health system performance. Some targets were partly met by organizations engaging in behavior that ensured they "hit the target, but missed the point" (Tenbensel et al. 2016).

The revised version of the New Zealand Health Strategy of 2016 reflected the MoH's desire to make the system more "people-powered," shift services from hospitals into the community and to improve service integration (Ministry of Health 2016b). The performance measurement efforts by the DAs of DHBs, PHOs and other organizations shifted towards "outcomes-based" or "system level measures" (SLMs), including amenable mortality and ambulatory sensitive hospitalization for children under age 5 (Chalmers et al. 2017). This approach, built on local efforts to define and measure health system performance, moved the focus towards service quality and patient outcomes. Such a shift brings the particular challenge of attribution: how are the outcomes at the district level attributable to the activities and investments of health sector organizations?

This SLM approach is also important for quality-related policies. The Health Quality and Safety Commission, established in December 2010, monitors and reports on quality and patient safety, and supports other organizations in these areas (Health Quality and Safety Commission 2016a).

In another important incremental development, the MoH extended the free visits to GPs and free prescriptions to all children under 13 years of age in 2015, and to all those under 14 in 2018.

Throughout the 2009–2017 period, the center-right government kept a tight rein on government expenditure generally, and health spending specifically. Average annual increases in real per capita health expenditure dropped from an average of over 3.5 percent in 2002–2009 to below 0.25 percent in 2010–2017 (Cumming 2017). As government funds almost 80 percent of health expenditure, this change reflects a significant shift to austerity. As a consequence, health system issues became prominent in the 2017 election campaign. Many DHBs were running significantly larger deficits, and some were openly challenging the Minister and MoH (Meier 2017). Although the National Party maintained a high percentage of the vote in the election (over 44 percent), it lost office to a coalition of Labour and two smaller parties.

The new coalition government faces many significant challenges, including considerable health workforce wage pressures, the need to replace or upgrade aging hospital infrastructure and pent-up dissatisfaction among primary care practitioners over funding models. Indigenous healthcare organizations have highlighted how the existing funding arrangements, particularly in primary care, systematically disadvantage Māori healthcare providers (Royal 2018). The incoming Health Minister commissioned a comprehensive review of the health system, due in early 2020 (Ministry of Health 2018c). This may lead to the opening of a new policy window for reform. However, no major policy changes are likely before the 2020 election. It remains to be seen whether the government will support the review's recommendations, and any proposed changes are likely to become issues in the 2020 electoral campaign.

Summary of Policy Reform

New Zealand stands out as a country that has been willing and able to make frequent and major changes to its health system. The framing and perception of health policy problems changed substantially over the past 30 years, from the need for greater efficiency in the 1980s and 1990s, to the need for improvements in population health and in equity of access in the 2000s. As problem definitions varied, so did the policy options of the day: from corporate governance and separation of policy, purchasing and provision in the 1990s, to devolved democratic governance in the early 2000s and to the greater emphasis on population health and regional collaboration in the 2010s. Experience since the early 2000s has also demonstrated that New Zealand health policy goes through sustained periods of slower, incremental change. With the 2017 change in government, a return to more far-reaching policy change is possible, but not guaranteed.

Still, no government, whatever its political complexion, has shown any desire to replace the tax base of healthcare by other sources of funding. Task forces appointed by government reviewed the existing arrangements in 1991 (Upton 1991) and in 2015 (Ministry of Health 2015), but neither recommended any fundamental change in healthcare financing.

The Drivers of Change

As in other nations, institutional enablers and constraints heavily shape New Zealand's health reforms, in particular: the political system, the path dependency of tax-based financing and the dynamics of the state-medical professional relationship. We argue that the confluence of these institutional features have dominated the shaping of the health policy agenda, the speed of change, the accommodation of contending interests and the final outcomes of the reform efforts.

New Zealand governments—like those of the United Kingdom—have more direct levers at their disposal than most other high-income countries. The concentrated constitutional power of the state, combined with its dominance over health funding and the fact that the most hospitals are (still) state-owned, means that governments play a very dominant role in the healthcare domain. The health financing out of taxation gives government hands-on controls. The highly concentrated constitutional powers in one house of Parliament (unitary system) provide the state with substantial autonomy. Consequently, governments dedicated to reform face few formal obstacles and veto points in the pursuit of major policy changes. This explains the comparative ease with which New Zealand's governments made significant legislative and structural changes in the 1990s and early 2000s. In contrast to some of the other countries featured in this book (like Israel, Switzerland or the Netherlands) where reforms faced numerous constraints, windows of opportunity for major policy reform occurred relatively frequently in New Zealand and tended to stay open for longer than elsewhere.

Such institutional capacity for reform would be the envy of many other high-income countries, yet it clearly has its downside. The concentrated power over policy easily results in reform hyperactivity and carries greater potential for reversal of reform measures (Weaver and Rockman 1993). While some commentators claimed that the move in 1996 to an electoral system based on proportional representation weakened the institutional power of the state, this shift only had a discernible effect on state capacity in the late 1990s. The main brake on hyperactivity since the early 2000s, however, was a general sense of reform fatigue and the growing realization of the limited impact of structural reform.

The high concentration of institutional power, and absence of veto points, also opens the door to novel policies. While this facilitates rapid innovation, it can also be problematic—a common feature of reforms discussed in this chapter has been a tendency to introduce new structures with little consideration of the practicalities for implementation (Gauld 2008). The waves of reforms indeed provoked considerable uncertainty and anxiety among service providers and others left with the responsibility of translating broad visions into concrete practice, with very little practical guidance.

The Medical Profession

The historical legacy of the dual system of user-paid primary care and publicly funded hospital care profoundly affected the relationship between the state and the medical profession. In effect, it has meant that New Zealand's policy arenas of primary care and hospitals have been largely separated since the early 1940s. State-doctor conflicts in the hospital sector tended to center on remuneration and the conditions of specialists working as salaried public employees. The parallel niche of private hospitals, together with an international labor market for their services, gave specialists a strong bargaining position over remuneration. The key interest group of medical professionals in the hospital sector, the Association of Salaried Medical Specialists (ASMS), essentially operates as a labor union. Specialists used their market power to resist managerialist pushes in the 1990s; nonetheless, they continue to feel significantly constrained by the level of resources in the public system (Ashton et al. 2013).

The policy territory in primary care is quite different. When the government lost the battle to prevent GPs from charging co-payments in the 1930s, primary care reverted to a predominantly private industry with limited state subsidy until the early 2000s. For primary care, one major legacy of the 1990s reforms was the establishment of networks of GPs and other primary health providers. At first, this occurred as GPs created Independent Practitioner Associations to offset the power of the RHAs as single purchasers. This set the scene for the establishment of PHOs in the 2000s, which in turn facilitated the Labour-led coalition's ambition to incorporate primary care into the public domain, with increased public subsidies.

Sensitive to the historical concerns of GPs losing their private business model, fee-for-service payment and the right to charge co-payments, the government initially opted for a voluntary arrangement sweetened by significant financial incentives. The government also excluded general practice interest groups from policy formulation in 2000.

Primary care doctors thus had little direct influence on the content of primary care policies. New Zealand does not have a tradition of corporatist interest bargaining in primary care (Tenbensel and Burau 2017). The primary care doctors were successful, however, in protecting their key interests in the control over fees and governance during the implementation of the Primary Health Care Strategy in the 2000s. The separation of policy terrains of primary and hospital care resulted in sector-specific interest group activity, and the New Zealand Medical Association (NZMA) has struggled to find a policy role that is relevant to both GPs and hospital specialists.

Summary

In applying Carolyn Tuohy's (1999) framework of structural and institutional dimensions, the New Zealand state has stronger structural power than most other high-income countries. There is a greater degree of hierarchical governance in New Zealand than in most of the other countries in this collection. Unlike countries such as the Netherlands and Israel (see the chapters in this volume), organized stakeholders do not generally play a major role in shaping health policy. Nevertheless, the medical profession is far from inconsequential. While it can be, and has been, largely side-lined from policy formulation, it still manages to exercise considerable influence over the operation of the system and implementation of reforms.

From an international perspective, the scale and frequency of changes to the New Zealand health system between 1991 and 2001 seem to indicate that changes to health reforms are easier to engineer than in most countries. However, did these reforms actually achieve their objectives?

Despite the rhetoric that accompanied the successive waves of reform over the decades, many of the key features of the health system remained unchanged (Gauld 2009; Ashton et al. 2005). Coverage remained universal, and public funding as a proportion of total expenditure has remained relatively constant (around 80 percent). Likewise, the mix of state-owned, publicly financed hospitals alongside privately owned primary care clinics that receive some state financing, has endured. While total health expenditure increased quite significantly (from 7.3 to over 9 percent of GDP between 1990 and 2017), the rate of increase is close to the OECD average (OECD 2018). Thus, the reality of reform often differed markedly from the rhetoric. Nonetheless, some real changes have occurred—and continue to occur—within the system.

Efficiency and Quality

The big bang reforms of the early 1990s aimed to improve the efficiency in healthcare—especially hospitals—by encouraging competition among providers. However, as noted earlier, there was no evidence of efficiency gains by 1996. None of the CHEs had returned dividends to their two shareholders, and many were in deficit. The agency charged with monitoring the performance of the CHEs concluded that: "performance seems, if anything, to have declined since the advent of the reforms" (Crown Company Monitoring and Advisory Unit 1996). Some critics argued that this lack of efficiency gains was due to the fact that some key features of the original proposals—such as competition between purchasers—had not been implemented (Finlayson 2001). In fact, the competition between providers, especially hospitals, remained extremely limited.

More recently, the MoH has set targets for each DHB to make "efficiency savings" by whatever means they can (Cowlishaw 2017). While at first this strategy met with some success, many DHBs were unable to realize further savings, and by 2018, 16 of the 20 DHBs were in deficit. The productivity in public hospitals has remained fairly constant in recent years, with case-weighted discharges increasing in line with funding levels between 2009 and 2016.

Alongside the attempts to reduce costs, the MoH spent much energy on developing quality indicators and data collection processes to enable quality monitoring. There have been some notable improvements in this field, for example, in reducing adverse events (e.g., hip fractures from falls) in public hospitals. Many other indicators show little or no change however. Patient satisfaction remained fairly constant with 90 percent of hospital patients reporting they were treated with dignity and respect. Other quality dimensions scored lower, however, such as communication and service integration (50–60 percent; Health Quality and Safety Commission 2016b).

Equity and Access

Reducing health inequalities has been an important policy goal for over 20 years, especially inequalities between Māori and non-Māori. Despite some notable improvements, for example, the near elimination of inequalities between immunization rates of Māori and non-Māori children in the early 2010s (Willing 2016), significant ethnic inequalities persist. Mortality rates and many indicators of morbidity are still higher for Māori than for non-Māori. Overall, Māori, Pacific people and those living in more socioeconomically deprived areas report poorer health and greater unmet health needs than other population groups (Ministry of Health 2016a; Ministry of Health 2018a).

Access to healthcare, especially primary care, is one factor contributing to these inequalities. The end of co-payments for GP consultations and pharmaceuticals for children aged under 14 years has removed the cost barrier for this group; however, in 2016, almost one-third of adults reported some unmet need for primary care, and the rate for Māori was 39 percent. The most common access barriers were cost, and the inability to get an appointment (Ministry of Health 2016b). Other barriers included access to transport, limited GP opening hours and cultural barriers (Sheridan et al. 2011).

Competition and Choice

As far as competition and patient choice were concerned, it is fair to say that the 1990s reforms had less impact than the government expected. While providers perceived that there was sometimes strong competition for contracts, in fact, most contracts were let to incumbent providers (Ashton and Press 1997). Most public hospitals continued to enjoy a monopoly in their areas, especially for the provision of acute services. While some private specialists and hospitals did win a few contracts for specified services, private hospitals only provided 1.5 percent of publicly funded case-mix adjusted discharges in 1999 (Ministry of Health 2000).

The expectation was that public hospitals would compete with each other for contracts. However, similar to the experience of other countries that introduced "purchaser-provider splits" (such as the United Kingdom and the Netherlands), the ability to compete was constrained by the need to continue to provide services to local populations. In sharp contrast to earlier reforms, one of the objectives of the 2001 reforms was to reduce competition between providers and "to avoid routine contestability for hospital services" (New Zealand Labour Party 1999). Patient choice of hospitals remained limited, and there does not appear to be much public demand for increased choice at this level of care.

In contrast, there has always been a fairly high degree of competition among GPs since most patients can chose their primary care provider. The 2001 reforms strengthened the power of patient exit because PHOs lose the capitation payment when a patient switches to another PHO. Some critics argue that switching providers opens up the possibility of risk selection by PHOs and this could dilute the power of exit.

Governance and Voice

A central feature of all four waves of reform has been a shift in the locus of decision-making, starting with increased centralization (from 14 Area Health Boards, to 4 RHAs, to 1 HFA) during the 1980s and 1990s, followed by a return to decentralized decision-making by the 21 DHBs in 2001. As the administrative structures changed, so too did the methods of governance. In 1993, commercial governance replaced the long-standing tradition of locally elected health boards. The expectation was that exit would replace voice as a mechanism to encourage good provider performance. In practice, however, as noted earlier, the degree of competition for hospital services was very limited.

The National–NZ First coalition government partially withdrew from the fully commercial model, appointing community representatives to the boards of public hospitals in the late 1990s. In 2001, its successor reintroduced governance arrangements that had prevailed prior to the 1990s, restoring both voice and decentralized decision-making. DHBs now comprise seven elected members plus up to four more members appointed by the Minister of Health.

Two questions arise from these changes. First, to what extent did the devolution of funds actually result in decentralized decision-making? Second, did elected boards lead to greater responsiveness to community preferences? In a decentralized system financed out of central taxes, there will inevitably be tension between the center responsible for raising the money, and the local or regional organizations responsible for spending it. Indeed, there has been little practical scope for effective incorporation of community voice into the DHB governance. DHBs needed to comply with national strategies under tight budget constraints, and faced difficulties of engaging with local communities in any meaningful way (Tenbensel et al. 2008; Laugesen and Gauld 2012).

Since 2009, there was a notable shift towards inter-organizational collaboration, formalized through DAs. Together with an increased emphasis on clinical governance in specific services (Gauld and Horsborough 2014), this indicated an acknowledgment by government of the role and legitimacy of clinicians in governing health services. That also reduced the scope for local voice and choice in the funding and planning of health services. At the same time, tight financial discipline exerted by governments constrained the scope for provider involvement and leadership.

Shifts over the last 30 years between local and central decision-making, together with the swings between corporate, community and clinical governance, illustrate the common difficulty of striking a balance between being responsive to community preferences, being responsive to clinicians, and being fiscally accountable.

Conclusion

New Zealand, more so than other countries represented in this book, underwent a series of fairly radical and rapid reforms to its public health system. Perhaps the most obvious explanation for this is the nature of the political institutions. Its unicameral parliament and the absence of federalism mean that governments can more easily bypass opposition from organized stakeholders and more quickly translate policy ideas into actual policy. Governments did not always engage in major reform; the period from the 1940s to the late 1980s, for example, was relatively stable, and the period since 2001 has also been characterized by stability and incremental change.

Nevertheless, the 1991–2001 period demonstrates New Zealand's institutional capacity to initiate radical reform. As a higher-income English speaking country, New Zealand felt the influence of neo-liberal policy prescriptions more strongly and earlier than continental European countries. The economic crisis of the 1980s prompted political parties to embrace more radical policy options. While they were fairly successful in realizing major economic and fiscal policy change, they faced strong resistance in the health sector against the neo-liberal prescriptions from professional stakeholders and the public. In effect, health policy became the key ideological battleground between the advocates of market signals and disciplines, and the defenders of a more social-democratic orientation.

Political ideology of the government of the day, rather than careful analysis of policy options, drove both rounds of health reforms. The shift to a contract model in the 1990s was based upon a belief in the power of markets to achieve efficiency gains. The underlying idea was that "exit" of patients or purchasers of health services would lead to better healthcare. In contrast, the shift back to a more integrated system that featured community governance in the 2000s was based on the notion that community "voice" would ensure responsiveness to the needs and preferences of the people.

New Zealand's experience illustrates that reform reality often differed from the rhetoric. Despite lofty ambitions and high hopes for the reforms, many of the defining elements of the system endured from its inception. Administrative structures and governance arrangements changed several times over, but the financing and the organization of service delivery remained largely unchanged. This indicates the remarkable resilience of the health system institutions, especially against top-down reform (Pierson 1994).

Despite fundamental differences in political ideology, neither major party has advocated for major health system changes in the 21st century. Incremental adjustments to the current structure, as well as on-going local innovations to service delivery, will be inevitable, however. While the reform efforts of the 1990s mostly entailed top-down whole-system structural change, local innovations appeared to have had a greater impact on system performance and patient outcomes.

New Zealand's experience demonstrates some important limits of health policy reform. It shows what can happen when the "irresistible force" of political institutions that facilitates major policy change meets the "immovable object" of the highly path-dependent health sector. The end result is that major changes may occur fast and frequently, but the effects of these changes tend to be far less than hoped for by the governments that initiate them. Disappointment with the results of major health policy reform led to a period of stability and incrementalism from 2002 to the late 2010s. However, at the turn of the new decade, government actors, and even some organized interests, may be developing an appetite for larger changes. If that is the case, then it is important that the lessons learnt about the potential and the limits of reform from the 1991–2001 period are not forgotten.

References

Ashton, T. 2002. "Running on the spot: lessons from a decade of health reform in New Zealand." *Applied Health Economics and Health Policy*, 1(2): 97–106.

Ashton, T., P.M. Brown, E. Sopina, et al. 2013. "Sources of satisfaction and dissatisfaction among specialists within the public and private health sectors." *N Z Med J*, 126(1383): 9–19.

Ashton, T., N. Mays, and N. Devlin. 2005. "Continuity through change: the rhetoric and reality of health reform in New Zealand." *Soc Sci Med*, 61(2): 253–262.

Ashton, T., and D. Press. 1997. "Market concentration in secondary health services under a purchaser-provider split: the New Zealand experience." *Health Econ*, 6(1): 13.

Boston, J., J. Martin, J. Pallot and P. Walsh (1996). Public Management, the New Zealand Model. Auckland: Oxford University Press.

Chalmers, L., T. Ashton and T. Tenbensel. 2017. "Measuring and managing health system performance: An update from New Zealand." *Health Policy*, 121(8): 831–835.

Cowlishaw, S. 2017. *DHBs Struggle under $200m Efficiency Plan.* https://www.newsroom.co.nz/2017/05/09/25736/dhbs-struggle-under-200m-efficiency-plan. Accessed April 4, 2019.

Crown Company Monitoring and Advisory Unit. 1996. *Crown Health Enterprises: Briefing to the Incoming Minister.* Wellington: Crown Company Monitoring and Advisory Unit.

Cumming, J. 2017. "Health policy." *Policy Quarterly*, 13(3): 12–17.

Cumming, J. and G. Salmond. 1998. "Reforming New Zealand Health Care." *Markets and Health Care.* W. Ranade (ed.). London and New York: Longman: 122–146.

Easton, B. 2002. "The New Zealand health reforms of the 1990s in context." *Appl Health Econ Health Policy*, 1(2): 107–112.

Finlayson, M. 2001. "Policy implementation and modification." *Health and Public Policy in New Zealand.* P. Davis and T. Ashton (eds). Auckland: Oxford University Press: 159–180.

Gauld, R. 2008. "The Unintended Consequences of New Zealand's Primary Health Care Reforms." *Journal of Health Politics Policy and Law* 33(1): 93–115.

Gauld, R. 2009. *Revolving Doors: New Zealand's Health Reforms* (2nd ed.). Wellington: Institute of Policy Studies.

Gauld, R. 2017. "The theory and practice of integrative health care governance: the case of New Zealand's alliances." *J Integrated Care*, 25(1): 61–72.

Gauld, R., and S. Horsburgh. 2014. "Measuring progress with clinical governance development in New Zealand: perceptions of senior doctors in 2010 and 2012." *BMC Health Services Research*, 14(1): 547.

Gwynne-Jones, D. and E. Iosua. 2016. "Rationing of hip and knee replacement: effect on the severity of patient-reported symptoms and the demand for surgery in Otago." *N Z Med J*, 129(1432): 59–66.

Health Quality and Safety Commission. 2016a. https://www.hqsc.govt.nz/about-us/. Accessed April 4, 2019.

Health Quality and Safety Commission. 2016b. *A Window on the Quality of New Zealand's Health Care.* https://www.hqsc.govt.nz/assets/Health-Quality-Evaluation/PR/window-on-quality-of-NZ-health-care-May-2016.pdf. Accessed April 4, 2019.

King, A. 2000. *The New Zealand National Health Strategy.* Wellington: Ministry of Health.

King, A. 2001. *The Primary Health Care Strategy.* Wellington: Ministry of Health.

Laugesen, M. and R. Gauld. 2012. *Democratic Governance and Health: Hospitals, Politics and Health Policy in New Zealand.* Dunedin, NZ: Otago University Press.

Malcolm, L., P. Barnett, and J. Nuthall. 1996. "Lost in the market? A survey of senior public health service managers in New Zealand's reforming health system." *Aust N Z J Public Health*, 20(6): 567–573.

Meier, C. 2017. "Cantabrians could face health service cuts of unprecedented scale." *Stuff.* https://i.stuff.co.nz/national/health/95996800/cantabrians-could-face-health-service-cuts-of-unprecedented-scale. Accessed April 4, 2019.

Ministerial Review Group. 2009. *Meeting the Challenge: Enhancing Sustainability and the Patient and Consumer Experience within the Current Legislative*

Framework for Health and Disability Services in New Zealand. https://www.beehive.govt.nz/sites/default/files/MRG%20Report%20Meeting%20the%20Challenge.pdf. Accessed April 4, 2019.

Ministry of Health. 2000. *Hospital Throughput Statistics 1998/99.* Wellington: Ministry of Health.

Ministry of Health. 2006. *The Annual Report 2005/06 Including the Health and Independence Report.* Wellington: Ministry of Health.

Ministry of Health. 2007a. *Health Expenditure Trends in New Zealand 1994–2004.* Wellington: Ministry of Health.

Ministry of Health. 2007b. *Primary Health Care: Implementation Programme 2006–2010: Primary Workings–Issue 3,* June 2007.

Ministry of Health. 2015. *From Cost to Sustainable Value.* An Independent Review of Health Funding in New Zealand. Commissioned by the Director General of Health on March 31, 2015. http://www.health.govt.nz/about-ministry/what-we-do/new-zealand-health-strategy-update/funding-review. Accessed April 4, 2019.

Ministry of Health. 2016a. *Annual Update of Key Results 2015/16 New Zealand Health Survey.* http://www.health.govt.nz/system/files/documents/publications/annual-update-key-results-2015-16-nzhs-dec16-v2.pdf. Accessed April 4, 2019.

Ministry of Health. 2016b. *New Zealand Health Strategy of Health: Future Direction.* Wellington: Ministry of Health.

Ministry of Health. 2016c. *The Structure of the New Zealand Health and Disability System.* Wellington: Ministry of Health. http://www.health.govt.nz/system/files/documents/pages/structure-nz-health-disability-sector-oct16.pdf. Accessed April 4, 2019.

Ministry of Health. 2018a. http://www.health.govt.nz/our-work/populations/maori-health/he-korowai-oranga/key-threads/equity. Accessed April 4, 2019.

Ministry of Health. 2018b. https://www.health.govt.nz/our-work/primary-health-care/about-primary-health-organisations. Accessed April 4, 2019.

Ministry of Health. 2018c. https://systemreview.health.govt.nz/overview/. Accessed January 17, 2019.

New Zealand Labour Party. 1999. *Focus on Patients: Labour on Health.* Wellington.

OECD. 2010. *Value for Money in Health Spending*. https://www.oecd.org/berlin/46201464.pdf. Accessed January 17, 2019.

OECD. 2017. *OECD Health Statistics 2017*. http://www.oecd.org/els/health-systems/health-data.htm. Accessed January 17, 2019.

Pollitt, C. and G. Bouckaert. 2000. *Public Management Reform: A Comparative Analysis*. Oxford: Oxford University Press.

Royal, S. 2018. "Brief of Evidence of Simon George Tiwai Royal concerning remedies." *Waitangi Tribunal Claim Wai 2575, #A75*. Wellington. https://forms.justice.govt.nz/search/Documents/WT/wt_DOC_144614759/Wai%20 2575%2C%20A075.pdf Accessed January 17, 2019.

Sheridan, N.F., T.W. Kenealy, M.J. Connolly, et al. 2011. "Health equity in the New Zealand health care system: a national survey." *Int J Equity Health*, 10(1): 45.

Statistics New Zealand. 2018. https://www.stats.govt.nz/infographics/major-ethnic-groups-in-new-zealand. Accessed April 4, 2019.

Tenbensel, T. and V. Burau. 2017. "Contrasting approaches to primary care performance governance in Denmark and New Zealand." *Health Policy*, 121(8): 853–861.

Tenbensel, T., L. Chalmers, and E. Willing. 2016. "Comparing the implementation consequences of the immunisation and emergency department health targets in New Zealand: A tale of two targets." *J Health Organ Manag*, 30(6): 1009–1024.

Tenbensel, T., J. Cumming, T. Ashton, et al. 2008. "Where there's a will, is there a way?: is New Zealand's publicly funded health sector able to steer towards population health?" *Soc Sci Med*, 67(7): 1143–1152.

Treasury. 2014. *2014 Briefings to Incoming Ministers Information Release*. https://treasury.govt.nz/publications/bim/briefing-incoming-minister-health-2014. Accessed April 4, 2019.

Tuohy, C. (1999). Accidental Logics: The Dynamics of Change in the Health Care Arena in the United States, Britain and Canada. New York: Oxford University Press.

Touhy, C (2018). Remaking Policy: Scale, Pace, and Political Strategy in Health Care Reform, Toronto, University of Toronto Press.

Upton, S. 1991. *Your Health and the Public Health*. Wellington: Ministry of Health: 1–153.

Weaver, R.K. and B. Rockman, Eds. 1993. *Do Institutions Matter? Government Capabilities in the United States and Abroad.* Washington, DC: Brookings Institute.

Willing, E. 2016. "Hitting the target without missing the point: New Zealand's immunisation health target for two year olds." *Policy Studies*, 37(6): 535–550.

Chapter 11

Healthcare Reforms in Singapore

Kee-Seng Chia and Meng-Kin Lim

Introduction

The Republic of Singapore is a tiny island-state of 721 km^2 and 5.6 million people, one of the most densely populated countries in the world. Founded in 1819 as a British colonial outpost, it gained self-rule in 1959 and independence from Malaysia in 1965. It is a parliamentary democracy. Its ruling People's Action Party (PAP) has been in power since 1959, providing the rare opportunity to be able to pursue its agenda without much opposition or undue interruption, supported by economic growth rates of 8–10 percent in the 1970s to 1990s and about 5 percent since.

Singapore inherited a largely tax-based public healthcare system with basic and rudimentary standards from the British. To fulfill an election pledge to "bring healthcare closer to the people," the government decentralized primary care in 1960. Primary care shifted from the main, overcrowded General Hospital to 26 satellite outpatient clinics and 46 maternal and child health clinics scattered throughout the island—a task that took four years to accomplish. Little else changed. As the health minister explained candidly in 1967: "Health would rank, at most, fifth in order of priority for funds—after national security, job creation, housing, and education, in that order" (Yong 1967). Health reform languished on the back burner for the next 20 years.

Only after emerging as one of Asia's miracle economies, when housing, education, job security and other basic needs had been met in good measure, did Singapore take on a major overhaul of the healthcare system in the mid-1980s. The principal driver for the reform was the rising level of people's aspirations, accompanying their new affluence. The government elected, on a democratic socialism platform in 1959, chose unorthodox themes as the centerpiece of its 1983 National Health Plan: individual responsibility and co-payment. It outlined an ambitious 20-year plan to modernize health facilities and raise medical standards. It applied the same no-nonsense, no-free lunch approach to healthcare that had underpinned Singapore's almost single-minded pursuit of economic growth. Welfarism, the government felt, was not a viable option, as it would breed dependency on the state. Co-payments were to encourage patients to assume personal responsibility for their own welfare. While using prices to curb demand, the government simultaneously softened financial consequences to protect lower-income groups.

Singapore indeed achieved a great deal within a short period of time. With low levels of health spending (about 5 percent of gross domestic product [GDP] as compared with 9 percent in other OECD nations; Registrar 2014), its health indicators rank among the best in the world. Infant mortality, now one of the lowest in the world, dropped from 34.9 to 2.4 per 1,000 live births between 1960 and 2017 (Registrar 2014). Average life expectancy increased from 63 to 85 years in that same period.

Private providers, some listed on the stock exchange, account for 20 percent of inpatient beds and 80 percent of outpatient visits. Patients have free choice of provider. To empower consumers, the government publishes selected quality indicators and comparative lists of procedure prices at different hospitals. The government encourages market competition. It also actively promoted health tourism in the 1990s and early 2000s.

Singapore offers an interesting example of policy-making by a government that combined the rhetoric of self-reliance and family responsibility with extensive welfare schemes and active social policies. Singapore's first Prime Minister, and co-founder of the PAP, Lee Kuan Yew, remained in power for 46 years (1954–1990). After that he continued on as a Senior Minister for another decade (1990–2004) and then remained politically active as Minister Mentor until his death in 2011. His successful economic policies and the establishment of a non-corrupt, effective government made him very popular in Singapore and drew admiration from abroad. Though he had many detractors, Lee's administration was able to deliver on its promises of economic growth and prosperity for the vast majority of the population, with universal access to housing, public transportation, education and health services.

This chapter illustrates the influence of ideas, interests and institutions on the shaping and outcome of public (health) policy-making (Klein and Marmor 2006). Singaporeans largely agree with the idea that they have individual responsibility for their own welfare and are therefore willing (and thanks to their very high income level, able) to pay for their own healthcare. At the same time, they feel strongly that government should support elderly and low-income families without the means to do so. This strong conviction has shaped the complicated mix of financing arrangements: on the one hand, individual savings accounts emphasize individual responsibility, on the other hand, a wide array of public schemes benefit vulnerable groups. This mix is not the most efficient way to finance healthcare but it serves different purposes.

The position of strong interest groups, such as self-employed physicians or specialized clinics, limited government efforts to establish an integrated provider network. Hospitals are also an example of institutions that, as Pierson (1994) once observed, tend to create their own constituencies. The government faced resistance when trying to absorb hospitals into greater provider units or change the range of services they were to offer.

Singapore's dominant political majority, as mentioned earlier, allowed shifts in policy-making and innovation at a rapid pace. This chapter shows how new challenges of changing demographics and epidemiology prompted a reorientation of Singapore's health policy.

Healthcare Financing: A Mixed, Multi-Layered System with Targeted Subsidies for the Elderly and Low-Income Families

Singapore offers universal healthcare coverage to its citizens. The mixed and multi-layered financing is anchored on the twin philosophies of individual responsibility and affordable healthcare for all (Lai 2016). It combines a mixed financing system: market-based mechanisms to promote competition and transparency and technological innovation to improve healthcare delivery. Underpinning the 1993 reform was the pledge by government that "no Singaporean will ever be denied needed health care because of lack of funds" (Thomas et al. 2016). The reform sought a gradual shift of the financial burden from the government to the private sector, at a pace and in a manner that the people could bear.

Total national health spending amounted to SG$14,919 million in 2011. The main financing sources of Singapore's healthcare are general taxation (about 25 percent), and out-of-pocket payments and compulsory savings from payroll deductions (together 60 percent). Other sources of financing include employer-provided benefits. The key elements of the reform are known as the three "M's": Medisave (1984), MediShield (1990), Medifund (1993) and MediShield Life (2015), while additional arrangements support vulnerable populations.

Medisave

Medisave was an extension of the Central Provident Fund (CPF), the pension savings scheme started by the British colonial government in 1955. Following independence, Singapore's government kept the plan that required high levels of savings and investment. CPF evolved into a tax-exempt, interest-yielding social security savings scheme. Six to eight percent of wages (depending on age) are sequestered into the individual's CPF Medisave account. It also covers retirement needs. Members can use their account to purchase homes and mortgage insurance or pay for their children's higher education. They can invest their CPF savings in blue chip stocks. The core features have not changed since its inception: it is compulsory for all employees, self-employed citizens and permanent residents. The government guarantees a minimum interest of 2.5 percent. The interest on CPF's Medisave accounts was 5 percent in 2018.

CPF includes three accounts: an ordinary account for buying a home or paying for CPF-approved insurance, investments and education; a special account for old age and investments in retirement-related financial products (e.g., life annuity); and Medisave for hospital costs, rehab and hospice care. Medisave expanded over the years to include outpatient management of chronic diseases, childhood and adult vaccinations, as well as selected health screenings. It covers certain expensive outpatient treatments (such as day surgery, radiation therapy, chemotherapy, renal dialysis and *in vitro* fertilization), and approved medical insurance. Account holders can use Medisave not only for themselves but also for their spouses, children, parents and grandparents. Any unspent balance is passed on to beneficiaries upon death (Lim 2004).

The combined Medisave accounts of all Singaporeans amounted to a stunning SG$42.4 billion, or $30.0 billion, in 2008, when one Singapore dollar equaled 0.7 US dollars—sixfold the total national health spending! Foreign commentators regularly mention Medisave as an effective instrument for cost control that give patients "skin in the game." In fact, Medisave payments only contributed 5 percent to total health expenditure.

The CPF model is not unique to Singapore. It was implemented elsewhere in Britain's colonies, too, including British Malaya and Africa, to avoid the social security needs of the aging populations draining British public funds. However, Medisave, the world's first medical savings account, is unique to Singapore.

MediShield and MediShield Life

MediShield was an optional catastrophic insurance for large hospital bills in case of serious illness or prolonged hospitalization. Over 90 percent of the population had MediShield coverage (Lai 2016). The compulsory scheme MediShield Life replaced MediShield in 2015. It offers higher payouts and lifelong protection to all citizens and permanent residents, including the very old and those with pre-existing conditions. The higher payouts resulted in higher premiums. Insured can pay those MediShield premiums out of their Medisave accounts, with additional government subsidies for those who cannot afford the premiums.

Medifund

Medifund, the third "M," is the public safety net for those without the means to pay, including people not covered by Medisave, or who have exhausted their quota. Medifund was set up as a large government-sponsored endowment fund. The government distributes its interest income to public hospitals and voluntary welfare organizations to cover hospital bills and other costs of patients who are genuinely unable to pay. Medifund committees within hospitals assess the inability to pay through means testing. The fund stood at SG$4 billion (or $2.95 billion) and the disbursement amounted to SG$155 million (or $114.4 million) in 2015 (Ministry of Health Singapore 2016).

Eldercare and ElderShield

The population share aged 65 and over was projected to double from 13 to 25 percent between 2017 and 2030. Concerned about rapid population aging, the government set up the Eldercare Fund in 2000 to support elderly care by voluntary welfare organizations. In addition, it created ElderShield funds in 2002 to cover the costs of severe disability and long-term care. The ElderShield300 scheme pays monthly cash amounts of $300 for a maximum of 60 months. Beneficiaries of ElderShield400 receive $400 for a maximum of 72 months. The latter scheme is for citizens and permanent residents who joined ElderShield after September 2007. They can pay their premiums out of their Medisave accounts. There were 1.2 million ElderShield policy-holders aged 40–83 by 2015.

Targeted Subsidies and Means Testing

The government periodically uses its budget surpluses to benefit lower-income families and the elderly. For example, it paid two years' worth of MediShield premiums for all Singaporeans aged 61 and above, while setting aside SG$19 million ($13.4 million) to help elderly pay for their ElderShield premiums in 2001. Likewise, it contributed SG$2.75 billion ($1.9 billion) to the Medisave and MediShield Top-Up schemes for the elderly. It also topped up the Medisave accounts of all those aged 51 and above to help pay for their increased MediShield premiums. The government added SG$400 million ($283 million) to the ElderCare Fund in 2008, increasing its size to SG$1.5 billion ($1.1 billion), and SG$200 million ($141 million) to Medifund, bringing the fund size to SG$1.7 billion ($1.2 billion). The government also created Medifund Silver for needy, elderly patients and the Community Health Assist Scheme (CHAS) that offers subsidized medical care and dental services to lower- and middle-income patients, and the Pioneer Generation benefits support the lifetime healthcare costs of the first generation of Singaporeans.

Another example of the targeting policies is the pricing of public hospital wards (Lim 1998). Subsidies are set according to the level of comfort and amenities, ranging from single bed rooms to open dormitories with eight or more beds. Patients in class-A beds pay full costs, while those in class C enjoy 80 percent subsidy. There is no difference in the standard of clinical care. The government feels that patients who can afford to pay should not occupy the subsidized beds (according to MoH estimates, over 90 percent of patients should be able to pay for their bills using their Medisave accounts). When the MoH found that many patients were crowding out lower-income patients, it decided to implement means testing for the subsidized wards. After several years of public dialogue and internal deliberation, the MoH started the program in January 2009, with a detailed sliding scale of declining subsidies ranging from 50 to 65 percent for class B-2, and up to 80 percent for class C. Subsidies for permanent residents were 10 percent lower than for citizens. Those without income, like housewives, retirees and children, and those living in government-subsidized housing continued to receive 80 percent subsidy for class C and 65 percent for class B-2 beds. The government estimated that the new payments would hardly affect 80 percent of the patients and promised that the changes would particularly benefit lower-income groups. To ensure non-contentious implementation, the government pledged to be flexible and "err on the side of generosity" (Lim 2008). Patients who could still not afford the subsidized wards would receive additional Medifund subsidy.

Healthcare Provision in Singapore

In 2015, there were 26 hospitals and specialty centers in Singapore. The 16 public facilities accounted for 80 percent of inpatient beds. The extensive primary care network (PCN) included private practitioners and public outpatient polyclinics. In addition, there was a wide array of traditional medicine (see below).

By 2016, the healthcare system employed 12,459 doctors, 7,909 of whom worked in the public sector and 4,788 as specialists; additionally 39,005 nurses and midwives, 24,000 in the public sector, plus a smaller number of allied health professionals (967 occupational therapists, 1550 physiotherapists and 474 speech therapists; Ministry of Health Singapore 2016).

Primary Care

Patients have free choice of primary care providers. Many go to their neighborhood family physician (general practitioner, GP) especially for acute conditions. In the 1980s, the MoH consolidated all public outpatient clinics (including maternal and child health clinics) into 16 polyclinics. These one-stop centers for all age groups provide immunizations, health screenings and health promotion, family planning, nutritional services, psychiatric counseling, dental care, pharmaceuticals, x-ray and laboratory services, as well as home nursing and rehabilitative services. Patients face modest charges to visit the polyclinic: SG$12 ($9) for adults and SG$6 ($4.50) for patients over 65 and children under 18 (Singhealth). The polyclinics tend to cater to patients with chronic conditions, as over the years the fees of private GPs have increased faster than those of the polyclinics.

The 2011 Primary Care Master Plan announced an expansion of the polyclinics and other steps to improve primary care. The plan included the CHAS to support lower-income patients at private GP and dental clinics, as well as the establishment of Community Health Centers (CHCs) to support GPs and provide screening and counseling services, in addition to the proliferation of Family Medicine Clinics (FMCs). FMCs follow a public–private partnership model to offer primary care to patients with complex chronic diseases. Additionally, in 2017, the MoH expanded the PCN. PCNs are virtual networks of (independent) GPs meant to deliver holistic and comprehensive care to patients via multi-disciplinary teams that include physicians, nurses, allied health professionals and care coordinators (MoH).

Secondary and Tertiary Care

Singapore's eight public hospitals and eight public specialty centers range in size between 185 and 2,010 beds. The 10 private hospitals tend to be smaller, with capacities ranging from 20 to 345 beds. The general hospitals provide acute inpatient and outpatient services and 24-hour emergency care. The national specialty centers offer medical care in their area: neuroscience, cancer, cardiac, eye, skin, dental and one multi-disciplinary medical center.

The government restructured all public acute hospitals and specialty centers into private (but fully state-owned) institutions. It gave management greater autonomy and flexibility to respond to patient needs. Hospitals installed new accounting systems to increase transparency of operating costs, financial discipline and accountability. Public hospitals were to be managed like non-profit organizations under the MoH's guidance. They received government subsidy for providing care to low-income patients.

In its 1993 White Paper, the government outlined a plan that restricted the range of specialty activities of secondary and community hospitals, while linking them to each other for referral services. This would give patients broader choices in hospitals when seeking less sophisticated care, while concentrating and thus restraining the cost of tertiary care. The national centers would offer specialized services for cancer, heart disease, skin and eye diseases. The White Paper highlighted concerns about spiraling healthcare costs, supplier-induced demand and moral hazard associated with free healthcare. It emphasized individual responsibility—but also, government assistance where needed.

Competition for patients, who were completely free to choose their healthcare provider, was strong. Competition for top talent in clinical specialists was even more intense. The loss of top specialists to the booming private sector was in fact one of the factors that led to the granting of hospital autonomy in 1985 (Lim 1998; MoH).

Freed from civil service constraints, the government argued that the public sector hospitals could compete with those of the private sector. This was a far cry from the situation in 1960, when fewer than 50 doctors in the whole country had specialist qualifications, almost all worked in public service. To develop the base for tertiary care, in the mid-1970s, the government sent top clinicians in the public sector to the best medical centers around the world for training. A decade later, private specialty clinics were mingling side by side with gleaming shopping malls on Singapore's fashionable Orchard Road, anchored by two private hospitals with tertiary capabilities. Many specialists left the public sector for the private sector as soon as they had made a name for themselves and served out their government bonds.

Traditional Medicine

Singapore has an ethnically and culturally diverse population. About 74 percent are Chinese, 13 percent Malay, 9 percent Indian and 4 percent other minority groups. Most originated from China, India, and the Malay Archipelago. Each subpopulation brought its own brand of traditional medicine. These medical practices remained popular as alternatives to conventional Western medicine. Traditional Chinese Medicine (TCM) is the most widely used form of complementary or alternative medicine (88 percent), followed by traditional Malay (Jamu) medicine (8 percent), and traditional Indian (Ayurvedic) medicine (3 percent). The MoH estimated that 12 percent of daily outpatient visits are with TCM practitioners. This fact, coupled with concern for patient safety, motivated the government to enact registration and licensing for TCM practitioners by a self-regulating body, under the supervision of the MoH's Chinese Proprietary Medicines Listing Unit.

Commercialization of Healthcare and Medical Tourism

The government actively encouraged the commercialization of medicine and medical tourism. The number of foreign patients doubled from 200,000 to 400,000 between 2002 and 2005. Four out of five were treated at private clinics and hospitals. To support this development, the government set up Singapore Medicine in 2003, a government industry partnership and other agencies. Private hospital chains (some listed on the stock exchange) expanded within the region, tapping into the booming multi-billion dollar Asian healthcare market.

The Economic Development Board supported investments in biomedical and high-tech healthcare innovation. International Enterprise Singapore (formerly the Singapore Trade Development Board) encouraged local healthcare players to collaborate on a regional level. In collaboration with the MoH, the Singapore Tourism Board looked after international marketing and promotion of biomedical research. Mandatory hospital quality committees and voluntary accreditation by the Joint Commission International (JCI) aimed to ensure that quality of clinical care and patient safety conformed to international standards. In recent years, however, the growth of foreign patients has leveled off, as medical tourism faced significant competition from lower cost regional rivals including Malaysia, Indonesia and Thailand (Newsweek 2007; Choo 2002; Strait Times 2016).

Hospital Restructuring

The most significant failed healthcare reform in Singapore's recent history was the attempt to privatize public hospitals in 1985. After the economic recession of the mid-1980s, the government sought to transfer the engine of economic growth from the public to the private sector. The Economic Committee (1986) had suggested healthcare as a prime candidate for deregulation and privatization. One stated goal was to attract and retain top medical talent in the public sector; once freed of civil service constraints, the Committee argued, hospitals could hire and fire at will, and pay handsome salaries if needed.

The government considered various models to reduce MoH control and grant hospitals greater autonomy, ranging from statutory boards to manage public hospitals, to wholesale privatization of hospitals and specialist centers. At first, the government chose the latter. Widespread public unhappiness over the planned privatization led to months of intense debate in public forums, media and Parliament. Facing that opposition, the government modified its original privatization plan. It opted instead for restructuring, or in World Bank parlance, corporatization (Phua 1991; Thomas et al. 2016; Our Singapore Conversation Survey), to improve the efficiency of hospitals and reduce public spending. Each hospital would become an independent entity, within the definition of Singapore's Companies Act. While completely government-owned, hospitals would be autonomous in fiduciary and operational matters.

The restructuring process took more than 20 years. The government created the Health Corporation of Singapore (HCS) Private Limited in 1987 as a state-owned company. HCS's task was to own and manage all corporatized hospitals and specialty centers. Thus, nominally private hospitals, each governed by its own board of directors, were ultimately public since they were 100 percent owned by HCS, which in turn was completely government owned. Every public hospital and specialty medical center had been restructured by 2000, even the largest 2,700-bed psychiatric hospital. Market mechanisms and structures replaced bureaucratic ones.

The reforms did lead to improved standards of care and reduced wait times—a far cry from the overcrowded wards and unresponsive outpatient clinics of yesteryear. By 2018, the average wait time for elective surgery was only 13 days (MoH).

After the restructuring, the hospitals were free to set their own directives and compete with each other. But, as each hospital focused on its own survival and bottom line, competition became counter-productive. They employed dysfunctional business tactics, like poaching staff from each by offering higher salaries. Non-cooperation between institutions resulted in missed opportunities for exploiting economies of scale, such as central drug purchasing or the development of a common information technology (IT) platform for electronic medical records. The hospitals vied to increase their market shares through high-tech acquisitions and other means, confident that the HCS or the MoH would eventually bail them out if they ran deficits. Doctors saw sharp pay rises. There was also concern over the over-treatment of patients and inappropriate care, as the new financial incentives designed to retain top specialists in the public sector rewarded doctors according to the volume of procedures they performed. Instead of cost control, the new model resulted in a sharp increase in hospital expenditures.

Clustering of Hospitals

In 1999, the Ministry of Health regrouped the hospitals into two competing healthcare clusters: the National Healthcare Group and the Singapore Health Services. These quasi-independent clusters, with MoH-appointed boards, still reported to the ministry. At the same time, the two clusters took control over all primary care polyclinics. Thus in one fell swoop, the government achieved horizontal and vertical integration of all public providers at the primary, secondary and tertiary levels. Shortly after it introduced case-based payment based on diagnostic-related groups (DRGs), followed by global budgeting, both aimed to curb supply-side moral hazard. However, the IT systems of the two clusters continued to go their separate ways. Only in 2004, under intense pressure from the MoH, did the two clusters finally accept the need to create an electronic medical exchange that enabled some degree of sharing of records.

There is no evidence that the splitting of Singapore's public healthcare institutions into two clusters resulted in the healthy competition that would have justified the increased overheads of maintaining two clusters, however. Nor did competition in price and quality between providers improve the overall efficiency or quality of the healthcare system. However, as a positive outcome, each cluster did create a Health Services Research unit to develop a stronger evidence-base for its medical practice.

The 1999 clustering of public polyclinics, community hospitals, general and specialized hospitals and other facilities aimed to develop economies of scale via horizontal integration and to encourage competition between the clusters. In practice, however, the acute hospitals tended to work in silos, without engaging the other healthcare providers in the community, leaving patients to navigate on their own.

A decade later, the MoH again re-organized the two clusters, by creating six regional clusters in 2009. This was the start of the concept for the regional health systems (RHSs). The acute general hospitals were to take the lead in developing integrated models of care.

The RHS is a broad and evolving concept. It aims to encourage collaboration between acute hospitals and other healthcare providers (community hospitals, nursing homes, home care and outpatient rehabilitation providers, as well as polyclinics and private GPs) within a geographical region "to deliver patient-centered care that is accessible, appropriate to patient need, affordable and sustainable" (Thomas et al. 2016). Other terms used were "seamless and holistic care," via referral channels and other organizational pathways that facilitate communication, cooperation and efficient transfer of patients between facilities.

The MoH supported the development of patient care plans to facilitate the transfer of care from hospital-based outpatient specialist clinics to GPs. In addition, it developed "integrated care plans" (ICPs) as nationwide treatment guidelines, accompanied by the monitoring and evaluation with explicit standards of care and treatment targets. ICPs are evidence-based recommendations to providers across the entire natural history of the disease. ICPs cover primary, secondary, tertiary and rehabilitative care.

These pathways recommend interventions but do not dictate where the care should be provided, thus allowing flexibility in implementation and consideration for cost-effectiveness. The ICPs are extensions of the clinical pathways used in hospitals to standardize care. Pioneer ICPs on stroke and coronary heart disease were developed in 2012.

To further develop the integrated care model, and lessen the pressure on public hospitals, the MoH also sought to strengthen intermediate and long-term care (ILTC). Together with the Ministry of Social and Family Development (MSF), the MoH announced plans to develop over 100 community-based elderly care facilities across the island. Many of these would be located within residential estates, close to the homes of the elderly patients' families to make it more convenient for visit.

In its broader reform plan of 2012, *Healthcare 2020*, the MoH emphasized the importance of good access, quality and affordability of Singapore's healthcare. Accessibility referred to both physical access (healthcare infrastructure) and financial access (through improvements in the safety net). Quality referred to good outcomes of personalized, holistic, integrated and patient-centered care. Finally, affordability ("better value") emphasized cost-effectiveness, value and long-term sustainability. During the 2016 budget debate, the Health Minister highlighted the need for a paradigm shift in the approach towards aging and health. He outlined Three Beyonds: (1) Beyond the hospital to the community: transforming healthcare delivery from hospital-centered to community-based care with greater reliance on primary healthcare; (2) Beyond quality to value: emphasizing care that is appropriate to the needs of patients; and (3) Beyond healthcare to health: the importance of primary prevention and health promotion to delay and prevent the onset of chronic diseases. To illustrate this point, the Health Minister declared a War on Diabetes (WoD).

Studies by the national School of Public Health had shown a dramatic rise in obese and overweight Singaporeans. With that growth, the number of diabetic patients was expected to grow from about 350,000 to over one million between 2010 and 2050, among the 5 million total residents. This was double the previous projection that only took aging into account. While being overweight or obese are risk factors for diabetes, this issue was not just a war on obesity because many Asians are not visibly obese as their fat distribution tends to be intra-abdominal.

The MoH undertook another reorganization of the six RHSs by merging them into three integrated clusters in 2017, to facilitate effective implementation of the Three Beyonds. Those three clusters are each to provide a broader range of healthcare services, with a larger pool of manpower and managerial resources. The integrated clusters can offer the healthcare workers greater development and training opportunities that enhance the competence of the workforce and improve quality of care.

Context of Healthcare Transformation

Political context

It is pertinent to point out that shortly after coming into power in 1959, the PAP took an ideological right turn in the early 1960s, leading to its eventual withdrawal (or perhaps expulsion) from the Socialist International in 1976. These were tumultuous years, characterized by worker strikes and racial riots. About 30 percent of the popular vote was left leaning. The majority of the Chinese immigrant population was emotionally attached to China. With Chairman Mao's propaganda targeting the Chinese diaspora, Singaporean leaders feared they could well become the Cuba of Southeast Asia. As it turned out, the right wing of the PAP party trumped the political left (from which it had openly split) in the battle for the hearts and minds of the people. Since then, Singapore has eschewed, at least rhetorically, egalitarian welfarism in favor of market mechanisms to allocate finite resources. Pragmatism, not ideology, would henceforth be the guiding principle.

What explains the people's ready acceptance of the government's hard-nosed policies with such heavy emphasis on individual responsibility? Again, it is necessary to understand the socio-politico-economic context. First of all, Singaporeans had started out as poor, hungry migrants escaping poverty and oppression in their original homelands: mainly China, India and the Malay Archipelago.

Under the 144 years of British colonial rule, the people had not benefitted from a comprehensive healthcare system. The British interest in the health of the locals was no different from that displayed by the Belgians in Africa, the French in Indochina or the Dutch in Indonesia: Western medicine on the heels of Western expansionism was principally concerned with the colonizers rather than the colonized. Local residents depended on traditional healers. Despite rampant poverty, malnutrition, overcrowding and disease, there were no hospitals and virtually no organized medical care for the low-income families in Singapore, until a wealthy businessman sponsored the first charity hospital (the Tan Tock Seng Hospital) in 1844, with funds raised by Chinese community leaders. Thus, the spirit of self-help is deeply ingrained in the Singaporean psyche. There is no tradition of state largesse.

Secondly, Singapore faced an uncertain future at its birth in 1965. It had not sought independence but was unceremoniously ejected after its two-year political union with Malaysia failed. Cut off from its vital hinterland, survival became the number one issue. Against all odds, Singapore not only survived but went on to become one of world's most prosperous countries, with a per capita income of over $81,000 in 2016 (adjusted for purchasing power parity, PPP). It was during those sink-or-swim years in the post-independence era that the government forged a strong bond with Singapore's population. The people placed their trust in a sagacious administration, which earned more trust as it proved reliable in delivering on its promises.

Re-examining the role of the state vis-à-vis social welfare, the government concluded that a welfare state based on heavy taxes would not only be unviable, but indeed disastrous. It resolved not to let an "entitlement culture" creep in to overburden public finances. At the same time, it sought to ensure that appropriate safety nets were in place at all times. Barely six months into office in 1960, the newly elected PAP government introduced user fees for the first time (50 cents per visit to a public outpatient clinic). This was a small step, but in hindsight a harbinger of larger things to come. Convinced that healthcare cost is inherently inflationary with infinite demand, the government adopted shared responsibility as the guiding philosophy of its 1983 National Health Plan. Government subsidy would make healthcare affordable, but Singaporeans had to contribute their share, too. The compulsory medical savings scheme provided the mechanism to mobilize private financial resources.

Singaporeans, grateful for a standard of living their parents or grandparents could only have dreamed of, understood that trade-offs were inevitable. Whether paid out of taxes, Medisave, employer benefits or insurance— ultimately citizens were facing the costs themselves, since taxpayers and insured pay taxes and insurance premiums, while employers contribute to benefits as part of wage costs. The people understood that overburdening the state or employers affects the competitiveness of the economy and, thus their own livelihoods. Singaporeans were, therefore, easily convinced that free healthcare in the face of potentially insatiable demand was illusory and possibly ruinous. They were also able to grasp that the opposite: fee-for-service, open-ended insurance-based healthcare, which only the rich can afford, would be too inequitable. Hence, it was almost inevitable that Singapore found a "third way." Interestingly, it became a path guided more by conscious avoidance of failed international models rather than a clear vision of what the perfect model might look like.

The 2011 General Elections provided an interesting turning point. The ruling party PAP won only 60 percent of the votes, the lowest since independence. It lost six seats, including the breakaway Group Representation Constituency (GRC), helmed by a cabinet minister. The prime minister said that the polls had "heightened [voters'] political consciousness and awareness," concluding that "many … desire to see more opposition voices in Parliament to check the PAP government" (Sunday Times 2011). The following year, the government launched a yearlong outreach program, Our Singapore Conversation. Over 47,000 Singaporeans participated in 660 dialogue sessions across the island. A survey during those sessions found that public healthcare was the top concern for those earning more than SG$5,000 per month and the second top concern for those earning less (Our Singapore Conversation Survey).

The abovementioned *Healthcare 2020* document already addressed some of the major healthcare concerns of the population. In addition, the government expanded MediShield to MediShield Life to offer lifelong protection, including those with pre-existing illnesses. It also sought to address longer-term strategic issues. The prime minister in his 2017 National Day Rally said "[while] immediate priorities are important … three longer term issues are important to the success and wellbeing of Singapore, for the current generation and also for future generations … Preschool (education), Diabetes, and Smart Nation—these are the things we must do now, work on now to build our future so that Singaporeans can start right, stay healthy and live smart at every age" (pmo.gov.sg).

Demographic and Epidemiologic Transitions

A second major context of Singapore's health transformation is the combination of the rapid demographic and epidemiological transitions and their impact on both healthcare financing and workforce productivity. Singapore's birthrate plunged, from six births per woman to below replacement level between 1960–1965 and 1980. This implied that the population would start to decline in 2025. In 2000, for every person aged 65 and above, there were 8.4 citizens of working age, but that number is projected to drop to 2.1 by 2030 (Thomas et al. 2016). By then, there will also be more people leaving the working age cohort than the number entering it.

At the same time, in line with the global pattern, the disease burden is shifting from infectious diseases to non-communicable diseases (NCDs). Excessive weight gain and obesity are relatively recent problems in Singapore, with especially high rates of increase among adolescents and young adults. The impact of these challenges has yet to be fully appreciated. NCDs including cancer, cardiovascular disease, type 2 diabetes and kidney disease all rank among the top 10 principal causes of death in Singapore (moh.gov.sg). Many suffer chronically from NCDs, contributing to years of life lost due to disability, in addition to lifetime expenditure on direct and indirect costs of healthcare and productivity losses at work.

The expected increase in healthcare expenditure associated with NCDs fueled the need to reform care financing and organization. The usual model of hospital-centered, volume-based subvention might have been appropriate for infectious diseases, but it is extremely costly for chronic diseases. This prompted government to shift focus to primary healthcare and create the RHS networks. As the GPs and other players in the primary care system remained private, however, those networks were limited to partnership alliances rather than fully integrated merger-and-acquisitions. Experiments are underway to develop bundled payments and some form of modified capitation, though this is politically challenging, given the geographically limited size, and a population used to free access to all providers in the public system.

The government has increasingly attached importance to primary prevention. It aligned the concept of primary prevention with the ethos of taking personal responsibility for health. The Health Promotion Board (HPB) is the responsible agency for primary prevention at the national level. The government seeks different ways to enact its prevention agenda. For example, it introduced legislation and fiscal measures for tobacco control. In other areas, like healthy eating and increasing physical activity, it adopted a more promotional approach: increasing health literacy, implementation of community-level programs, behavioral nudges and reminders to encourage healthy behaviors.

Organizational and Governance Context

The governance of the public healthcare system evolved from central state control to corporatized clusters with high degree of autonomy. This came with a generation of independent, innovative and highly competitive healthcare leaders. One unintended consequence was a proliferation of clusters from the original two to six, perhaps fragmenting even further into eight clusters. In this way, Singapore's healthcare system was moving rapidly towards a one-country-six-or-more-systems. The government therefore decided to, again, reorganize the six RHSs into three integrated clusters to more effectively implement the "Three Beyonds."

Conclusions

Overall, Singapore has a high-functioning healthcare system. Its health indicators rank among the best in the world. There have been tremendous improvements in health outcomes such as infant mortality, under-five mortality rates and life expectancy. Other indicators like childhood vaccination coverage, breast cancer survival or recovery from acute myocardial infarction are often superior relative to other developed countries. At the same time, Singapore's health spending has remained relatively low in comparison to other high-income countries.

There is strong public support for the principle of individual responsibility for health and healthcare among Singapore's population. However, there have also been concerns that this principle, coupled with the quasi-free market can disproportionately affect vulnerable groups such as the elderly or lower socio-economic groups. This is further compounded by rapid changes in demographics and epidemiology, with both an aging population and an increase in chronic diseases. In response, Singapore's government actively broadened its financial safety nets in healthcare. It also announced that it would take on a larger proportion of the national health budget, from the current 30 percent in 2018 to 40 percent or more by 2030. The safety net expansion, however, has led to a proliferation of new schemes beyond the original 3M plus subsidy framework. The result has been increasing complexity for citizens to navigate the system, administrative redundancy and higher costs. Simplification would enable citizens to better understand the availability of programs.

There is also increasing recognition for the need to integrate primary, secondary and tertiary healthcare services, as well as ILTC. Additionally, the government has acknowledged the importance of primary prevention, as reflected in its anti-tobacco legislation, and public statements, such as Beyond Healthcare to Health and the War on Diabetes. The achievement of all these health policy goals will require effective government programs and successful coordination and cooperation between government and other actors and stakeholders.

References

Choo, V. September 28, 2002. "Southeast Asian countries vie with each other to woo foreign patients." *Lancet,* 360: 1004. https://www.moh.gov.sg/content/moh_web/home/statistics/Health_Facts_Singapore/*Principal_Causes_of_Death*.html. Accessed December 12, 2018.

Klein, R. and T. Marmor. 2006. "Reflections on Policy Analysis: Putting It Together Again." *The Oxford Handbook of Political Science*. R. Goodin (ed). Oxford: Oxford University Press: 982–912.

Lai, W.L. 2016. "Paying for Healthcare." *Singapore's Health System: What 50 Years Have Achieved*, Chap. 4. L.C. Earn and K. Satku (eds.). Singapore: World Scientific.

Lim, M.K. 1998. "Healthcare systems in transition II. Singapore, Part I. An overview of the healthcare system in Singapore." *Journal of Public Health Medicine*, 20(1): 16–22.

Lim, M.K. 2004. "Shifting the burden of health care finance: case study of public-private partnership in Singapore." *Health Policy*, 69(1): 83–92.

Lim, M.K. 2008. "Implementation of means testing." *Health Policy Monitor Survey*, 11.

Ministry of Health. https://www.moh.gov.sg/content/moh_web/home/our_health-care_system/Healthcare_Services/Primary_Care/primary-care-networks.html. Accessed December 12, 2018.

Ministry of Health. https://www.moh.gov.sg/content/moh_web/home/press-Room/Media_Forums/2012/about-bill-sizes-doctor-exodus.html. Accessed December 12, 2018.

Ministry of Health. https://www.moh.gov.sg/content/moh_web/home/press-Room/Parliamentary_QA/2014/ admission-waiting-time-for-subsidised-patients-for-operation.html. Accessed December 12, 2018.

Ministry of Health Singapore. 2016a. *Costs and Financing Singapore 2016* [updated April 4, 2016.] https://www.moh.gov.sg/content/moh_web/home/costs_and_financing.html.

Ministry of Health Singapore. 2016b. *Health Manpower Singapore* [updated May 20, 2016] https://www.moh. gov.sg/content/moh web/home/ statistics/Health Facts Singapore/Health Manpower.html.

Our Singapore Conversation Survey. https://www.reach.gov.sg/read/our-sg-conversation. http://www.pmo.gov.sg/national-day-rally-2017. Accessed December 12, 2018.

Phua, K.H. 1991. *Privatization and Restructuring of Health Services in Singapore*. Institute Policy Studies. Occasional Paper No. 5. Singapore: Time Academic Press.

Pierson, P. 1994. *Dismantling the Welfare State? Reagan, Thatcher and the Politics of Retrenchment*. Cambridge: Cambridge University Press.

Registrar-General of Births and Deaths. 2014. *Report on Registration of Births and Deaths 2013*. Singapore: Registry of Births and Deaths, Immigration and Checkpoints Authority.

"Singapore Medicine, Singapore-A Global Affair." *Newsweek,* October 5, 2007.

Strait Times. 2016. http://www.straitstimes.com/singapore/health/spore-tops-for-medical-tourism-but-rivals-catching-up-quickly. Accessed December 12, 2018.

Sunday Times. 2011. "Pledge to serve responsibly and humbly." *Sunday Times*, May 8.

Thomas, J.S., S.E. Ong, H.P. Lee, et al. 2016. "A brief history of public health in Singapore." *Singapore's Health Care System: What 50 Years Have Achieved.* C.E. Lee and K. Satku (eds.). Singapore: World Scientific: 45.

Yong, Y.L. November 21, 1967. *Speech by the Minister of Health at the Opening of the WHO Seminar on Health Planning in Urban Development.* Singapore.

Chapter 12

Taiwan's Single-Payer National Health Insurance: Recent Reforms and Future Challenges

Tsung-Mei Cheng

Introduction

Taiwan is a high-income democracy of 23.4 million citizens and approximately 800,000 foreign nationals, with a per capita income of $49,827 (in PPP international dollars) in 2017, slightly below that of Germany and Australia, but above that of Denmark, Austria and Canada (IMF 2018). Since 1995, Taiwan has had a government-run, single-payer, universal health insurance, the National Health Insurance (NHI).[1] As of 2018, the NHI covered 99.9 percent of the population at a cost of 6.3 percent of gross domestic product (GDP) (MOHW 2016).

Taiwan's health policy pursues three major social goals: social solidarity and equity in access to healthcare; high-quality healthcare; and cost-effectiveness, that is, the greatest benefit for a given outlay of resources, or alternatively, minimizing the cost of a given outcome (Cheng

---

[1] It is important to note that the term "single payer" can refer to different arrangements. It includes systems where one (governmental) agency is the sole channel for the stream of public money to healthcare providers; in other systems, there may be multiple agencies that all work under common rules (e.g., the Canadian system where the provinces act as the insurers on behalf of their provincial populations).

2008). The NHI has proven to be an efficient, cost-effective universal health insurance system, able to deliver a comprehensive package of benefits at a low cost, with short or negligible wait times for patients. This is a significant difference between Taiwan's single-payer system and those of other single-payer health systems such as Canada and the United Kingdom. NHI benefits include inpatient and outpatient care, dental care, prescription drugs, traditional Chinese medicine, renal dialysis, prenatal care and obstetrics, physiotherapy and rehabilitation, home health care and chronic mental health care (NHIA 2017–2018). It is thus more comprehensive than that of Canada's medicare, which does not include outpatient prescription drugs, dental care or long-term care (LTC).

The NHI shares features with the traditional European social health insurance arrangements mentioned in the introduction to this book. The most important common feature is universal access to health insurance as guaranteed by law. The contribution rate a person pays is not influenced by their health status or pre-existing conditions, and health insurance coverage is guaranteed from the cradle to the grave. In fact, as in other social health insurance systems, enrollment in the NHI is mandated for all citizens and legal residents.

This chapter walks the reader through the experience of the NHI from its inception in 1995. It begins with an overview of its genesis and the factors leading to its establishment. This is followed by an account of the government's decision to adopt a single-payer system and NHI's legislation and implementation—all of which were notable for their elements of surprise, speed and positive outcomes. This chapter shows how a strong and determined government can implement key new social policy and additionally, how sound policy advice at the right time—in Taiwan's case during the NHI's planning stage in the late 1980s—can play a major role in shaping reform initiatives. This chapter then provides an overview of the NHI's modus operandi, the changing role of stakeholders, recent reforms and challenges the health system faces today. This chapter ends with some general conclusions and a call for higher health spending in Taiwan despite its apparent success to date.

History of Taiwan's NHI

Before the establishment of the NHI in 1995, Taiwan had 13 different social health insurance schemes, each covering a subset of the population. For example, the Labor Insurance covered private sector workers, the Government Employees Insurance covered public sector workers including teachers, and Farmers Insurance covered farmers, and so on. Together, those insurance schemes covered almost 59 percent of the population (Cheng 2003). The remaining 41 percent of the population, however, did not have any health insurance and had to pay out-of-pocket or forego needed care. The uninsured were often the groups who had the greatest need for health insurance: largely vulnerable populations like children under 14, women, the elderly and disabled. Medical bills frequently impoverished patients and their families, and resulted in significant health disparities.

By the 1980s, things began to change. The confluence of several factors created a window of opportunity for major health reform, which gave birth to Taiwan's much-treasured NHI (Cheng 2003).

First, buoyed by robust economic growth, averaging more than 8 percent a year from the early 1950s to the 1980s, the public expected and demanded a higher quality of life, which included better healthcare and financial protection from the cost of illness. Second, in 1987, the long-ruling Nationalist Party (Kuomintang, or KMT) lifted the martial law that it had imposed in 1949. That ushered in a period of political liberalization with the emergence of an increasingly vocal, influential and well-organized political opposition. The Democratic Progressive Party (DPP) began to compete openly for political power with the KMT, which had been in power since the Chinese government retreated from the mainland to Taiwan in 1949, after losing the civil war to the Chinese Communist Party.

In reaction, Taiwan's then KMT President, Lee Ten-Hui, announced plans to create a NHI plan that followed the advanced, industrialized nations of the time. Lee personally orchestrated the massive undertaking implemented by successive premiers under his leadership. This episode parallels the establishment of the social health insurance in Germany during the late nineteenth century: the conservative Chancellor Otto von Bismarck introduced social insurance in 1883 for industrial workers as a pre-emptive strike against the rise of the labor movement and the growing political power of socialism. In Taiwan, it was a pre-emptive strike against the growing political power of the opposition party DPP. In both cases, one may think of it as a mixture of paternalistic concern for the welfare of the people and self-serving political interests. In addition, Taiwan's top policy-makers were eager to learn from health systems around the world (Cheng 2003).

Planning for the NHI

The planning for the NHI began in the mid-1980s. The government sought advice from foreign experts, and sent officials and researchers abroad to study foreign healthcare systems and experiences (Cheng 2003). The government therefore had the opportunity to consider a range of policy options and alternative models of health systems, including Germany's Bismarckian social insurance, the United Kingdom's Beveridgean, tax-financed National Health Service (NHS), Canada's medicare and the United States' mixed system of public and private insurance.

In the end, Taiwan decided to adopt a single-payer model in June 1990. The decision followed the recommendation of Princeton University economist Uwe Reinhardt, who was a high-level adviser to Taiwan's Council of Economic Planning and Development at the time (Council of Economic Planning and Development 1990). It was based on the following considerations: first, a single-payer system is equitable as it can impose uniform benefits and payments to providers regardless of ability to pay; second, a single-payer system can control costs effectively with standardized administrative rules; and third, a single-payer system is simple and easy for all stakeholders, including the public, to understand (Cheng 2018). Reinhardt also urged the government to keep the existing mixed public–private delivery system instead of going for a government takeover of the delivery of all health and medical services (Cheng 2018). NHI's almost quarter-century-long existence has shown that its single-payer design largely achieved the intended policy goals: equity, cost control and administrative efficiency.

Legislation and Implementation

The government submitted the NHI bill to Parliament in early 1993. Following 18 months of extensive debate, Parliament passed the NHI Law on July 19, 1994 (Cheng 2003). The Law originally envisioned a five-year phase-in period for the NHI, with full implementation by 2000. Impatient with that long of a wait, however, President Lee decreed that the NHI be implemented as of March 1, 1995—five years ahead of schedule. This announcement came, perhaps not incidentally, just a year before the first direct-vote presidential election in the history of the Republic of China (Taiwan), in March 1996. The decision created great uncertainty, confusion and opposition among some stakeholders, including physicians, as no one knew how or whether the new system would work out. Many felt such premature implementation of the plan would surely lead to its failure.

President Lee and his government did not waver. After allowing healthcare providers a mere three days to give feedback, from February 26 to 28, 1995, they went ahead with the implementation of the NHI as scheduled on March 1, 1995. Chaos followed and providers were in shock. Despite this rush, the NHI covered 90 percent of the population by the end of 1995 and 99 percent by 2003 (Yeh 2002; Chang 2005).

History may well show that this rapid implementation was a smart move. In 1997, the Asian financial crisis struck. While Taiwan was not directly hit by that crisis, its economic growth slowed down between 1998 and the late 2000s. It even had a negative growth rate of negative 2.2 percent in 2001 after the dot-com bubble burst in 2000 (DoH 2005). Had the government waited until 2000 to implement the health insurance, as stipulated by law, the NHI might never have seen daylight because of concerns over fiscal affordability and sustainability (Cheng 2003).

Modus Operandi of Taiwan's NHI

Governance

Taiwan's central government serves as a single-payer for the NHI. Under the Ministry of Health and Welfare (MOHW), the National Health Insurance Administration (NHIA) is responsible for administering the NHI. The NHIA works through six regional offices. A powerful information technology (IT) system helps keep administrative costs down—less than 1 percent of the total NHI budget in 2018 (NHIA 2017–2018).

NHIA's administrative functions include the collection of contributions, claims processing and payment to healthcare providers. It conducts medical reviews, monitors utilization, sponsors research and development. Under the direction of the MOHW, the NHIA also manages relationships with care providers, patient advocacy groups, individual patients, the media and lobbying groups, including the US Trade Representative (USTR), which fronts US business interests under the mantle of the World Trade Organization (WTO). An example of the roles of the USTR and WTO on national health policy in Taiwan concerned anti-tobacco policy in Taiwan, where the USTR objected to the government policy to impose higher tobacco taxes on imported US cigarettes (Cheng 2002).

Financing

The major source of NHI financing consists of contributions (see Figure 1). Payroll-based contributions accounted for 92 percent of total NHI revenues in 2018, levied as 4.69 percent of wages or salaries. These are shared between households (36 percent), employers (30 percent) and government (34 percent; NHIA 2018–2019).

To assess the taxable incomes and contributions, the NHIA divides the population into six categories: employed, self-employed, union workers, farmers, fishermen, the indigent, veterans and others (see Table 1). Varying amounts of government subsidies—from 0 to 100 percent—apply to the contributions for these six categories.

In contrast to the German sick funds that charge contributions on a household basis, the NHIA collects the NHI contributions on a per capita

Table 1. Payment Shares of Taiwan National Health Insurance Contributions, by Population Category (Percent)

Category	Insured	Employer	Government
1 Private sector employees	30	60	30
Government employees	30	70	—
Self-employed/employers	100		
2 Occupational union members	60	—	40
3 Farmers/fishermen	30	—	70
4 Conscripted military	—	—	100
Prisoners	—	—	100
5 Low-income households	—	—	100
6 Veterans	—	—	100
Community groups	60	—	40

Source: National Health Insurance Administration 2018–2019.

basis. Larger households consequently pay more, but only up to four members. Any additional household member is insured free of charge. Employers contribute to the premiums of their employees and their dependents. The healthcare for the 1.5 percent of Taiwan's residents who live in remote, mountainous areas or on islands falls under a separate system. This arrangement is organized as an integrated delivery system with providers paid on a capitation basis to safeguard optimal access to care. It is highly popular.

The government instituted a "supplementary premium" to broaden the NHI revenue base and ensure the long-term financial stability of the NHI in 2013 (see under Recent Reforms). The supplementary premium, based on non-payroll incomes, accounted for 8 percent of the total NHI revenues in 2019 (NHIA 1018–1019).

Cost Sharing by Patients

Patients in Taiwan face co-payments and co-insurance for all services: inpatient and outpatient care, dental care, traditional Chinese medicine and prescription drugs. There are ceilings for total annual co-payments and co-insurance, however, to limit the impact of medical costs on a household's finances. The NHI law also exempts 30 major diseases and conditions from co-payments and co-insurance to safeguard access to essential care. Patients with one or more of those 30 diseases or conditions receive first-dollar coverage for necessary medical services and medicines (NHIA 2017–2018).

Out-of-pocket spending (OOPs) in Taiwan amounted to 34 percent of all health spending in 2016 (MOHW 2018). That level seemed high by OECD standards, but according to a former director general of the NHIA, only about one-third of the reported OOPs (or 12.1 percent of total health spending) was actually co-payments or co-insurance for office visits and inpatient care (Cheng 2015a).

Patients also pay a small registration fee each time they visit their physician or hospital (not unlike the cover charges in European restaurants). This has been a government-approved practice since the NHI's inception.

Healthcare Delivery in Taiwan

The NHI serves as the sole population-wide health insurer. The provision of health services is largely private, however—as in several European nations. Two-thirds of hospital beds are private (not-for-profit) and 53 percent of physicians work in their own private clinics. For-profit hospitals are not allowed, but—as in some other OECD nations (see, e.g., the Netherlands), many non-profit hospitals behave directly or indirectly like for-profits. All hospitals, private or public, engage in fierce competition for patients in order to maximize revenues.

Taiwan had about the same bed-population ratio as the OECD median for countries in 2015: 3.4 beds per 1,000 habitants (OECD 2017; MOHW 2018). Bed occupancy in Taiwan averaged 66.3 percent, indicating overcapacity. The larger medical centers had higher occupancy rates than small and medium-sized hospitals, following an accelerated trend of hospital mergers. Increasingly, market share and resources for health services and high-tech medical devices have become concentrated in large hospitals, apparently reflecting patients' preferences.

Taiwan has low physician- and nurse-population ratios (of 1.9 and 6.3 per 1,000 population, respectively) compared to OECD countries (3.2 and 8.8, respectively; MOHW 2018; OECD 2017). In fact, the utilization of medical services in Taiwan is among the highest in the world. The average number of visits to doctors, per person per year, in Taiwan was 11.9 in 2015, far higher than the OECD average (6.3 per year) and only lower than that of Japan (12.7) and South Korea (16; MOHW 2018). Still, this has not resulted in long wait times. For example, the average wait time for cataract surgery in Taiwan was 11 days (NHIA 2015), compared to 58 (median) in Canada and 72 (mean) in the United Kingdom (OECD 2018). Taiwanese patients regularly complain that visits with providers are too short, however (Cheng 2015b).

There is no gatekeeping. Patients enjoy complete free choice of doctors, hospitals and other healthcare professionals. The government has tried to establish a referral system to improve the rational use of resources, with financial incentives like higher co-payments for patients who access tertiary facilities without a referral (NHIA 2017–2018). So far, results have been mixed.

Paying Healthcare Providers

Over 93 percent of all healthcare providers had a contract with the NHIA (NHIA 2017–2018). NHIA payments were their largest source of income. With few exceptions, providers are not allowed to charge more than the NHI fee schedule. In recent years, the NHIA has allowed patients to buy more expensive versions of certain devices and pay the difference in cost themselves. Other sources of provider revenues were patient registration fees, co-payments and co-insurance, and services and products not covered by the NHI, like cosmetic surgery or orthodontia.

The dominant payment method of the NHI has been fee-for-service (FFS). The fees vary by the level of provider. For example, the fees for tertiary medical centers are higher than those for local or regional hospitals. Within the same level, however, the fees are the same for all providers. The government sets the fee schedule after consultation with providers, but there are no formal negotiations between the government and associations of providers like in Canada, Germany or Switzerland.

The NHIA introduced additional payment methods to improve the efficiency and quality of healthcare. It implemented case-based payment (diagnostic-related groups [DRG]) for inpatient services in 2010. Full implementation of the DRG system for the hospital sector, however, has met with stubborn provider resistance. It has not proceeded according to plan, an experience similar to other nations (see e.g., the chapters on Chile, Israel and The Netherlands in this volume). The NHIA also introduced pay-for-performance (P4P), with payments based on the quality and outcomes of treatments. For residents living in remote mountainous areas and islands, the NHIA pays providers on a capitation basis through an integrated delivery system.

Cost Containment through Global Budgets

The original design of the NHI included global budgeting as a way to contain costs (Cheng 2003). The NHIA started to implement global budgets, sector by sector, beginning with dental care in 1999, followed by traditional Chinese medicine in 2000, primary care in 2001, hospitals in 2002 and renal dialysis in 2003. The global budget for hospitals met with considerable opposition from the powerful hospital sector.

Although global budgets are not the ideal long-term solution to financial problems of health systems, they appear to be a pragmatic and effective solution for reining in overall health spending, especially the large global hospital budget. Total health expenditure in Taiwan stood at 6.1 percent of GDP in 2017 (Cheng 2019).

The NHI's Health Information System

The organizers of the NHI recognized the importance of a strong IT system to enable the entire NHI to efficiently perform its core functions. They invested heavily in IT to allow the system to hit the ground running (Cheng 2009). Every resident in Taiwan received a credit card–sized NHI card in 2002, which enabled patients to access care. This allows the NHIA to collect data about the card carrier's medical history (limited to the last six visits). This data collection provides the NHIA with a bird's-eye view of service utilization, provision and total costs on an almost real-time basis. The IT system further supports early detection of public health emergencies like influenza or the bird flu in real time. In addition, it provides the basis for medical reviews and detection of fraud and abuse.

The NHIA next introduced the IT application PharmaCloud in 2013, which allowed providers to see their patients' prescription drug history for the previous three months via a VPN connection to the PharmaCloud database. This system aimed to enhance efficiency and patient safety as it helped prevent potential adverse drug reactions due to prescriptions from multiple doctors, and reduce duplications of prescriptions. Next, the NHIA introduced the electronic personal health record, My-Health-Bank, in 2014. Patients can download their complete medical history from the past year and enter the data into a small personal health bankbook. This way, patients can keep track of their healthcare usage and better manage their own health.

NHIA's latest and perhaps most ambitious IT initiative was its 2016 MediCloud. Providers upload medical records to the MediCloud, and with the patient's consent, providers anywhere in Taiwan can easily download the data when he or she seeks a second or third opinion. Using big data analysis, this system also traces duplications of high-tech examinations such as computed tomography (CT) and magnetic resonance imaging (MRI) scans, lab testing, as well as expensive prescriptions that account for significant costs and waste within the NHI.

Beginning in January 2018, the NHIA encouraged all hospitals to upload their CT and MRI images and reports in real time, to enable easy referral and immediate access by local primary care facilities (NHIA 2017–2018). The NHIA expects that, once fully implemented, MediCloud will improve the quality of services as well as patient safety by reducing unnecessary duplications of imaging and tests. It can also help reduce waste and save out-of-pocket expenses for unnecessary imaging and tests.

The Role of the State and Organized Stakeholders in Taiwan's Health Policy

As a single payer, Taiwan's government exercises monopsonistic power over providers. The government has used effective cost control measures like the uniform national fee schedule, global budgets, medical reviews and provider contracting.

At the same time, the government is facing mounting constraint from growing voices and activism by stakeholders and interest groups, like any other society that has become more democratic and pluralistic, Taiwan is no exception. Furthermore, provider groups like associations of physicians and hospitals participate in elaborate annual consultations with the NHI over global budgets, fee schedules or the coverage of new benefits. Patient groups increasingly make demands on the government for coverage of new drugs or procedures. The media channels the public's views on proposed premium rate increases, usually a loud and clear "No."

The considerable involvement of organized interest groups and lobbyists, however, is not always in the best interests of patients. Nor does it result in the most efficient utilization of resources. An illustration of effective lobbying by interest groups came to light a decade ago in a Superior Court case involving alleged political contributions made by the Taiwan Dentist Association (TDA) to numerous members of Parliament, both past and present, in its attempt to influence decision-making. TDA's objective was to make sure oral hygiene services (a profitable part of dentists' practices and closely guarded dental professionals' turf) would not be delisted in the proposed oral hygiene bill (Tien and Chen, 2007).

In recent years, doctors in Taiwan, especially hospital-based doctors, have become increasingly vocal in demanding change, complaining about being overworked and underpaid. There is evidence of high incidence of burnout and occurrences of malpractice (Cheng 2015). In October 2018, primary care providers and labor organizations complained to the MOHW about being left out of consultations and planning for their working conditions, which they repeatedly criticized as "blood and sweat working conditions." In response, the MOHW agreed to invite primary care providers to the meetings.

The Parliament, generally sympathetic with labor and concerned that its voice be heard, next called for the MOHW to invite all healthcare labor organizations to any government planning meetings relating to issues of accreditation, facilities standards and NHI payments (Luo 2018). Other physician groups are actively engaged in dialogue to gain better terms with the MOHW and protection of their rights under the Labor Standards Act. The Taipei Doctors' Union, for example, is in the process of negotiating better protection for resident physicians in their standard employment contract (Lee 2018).

Public satisfaction with the NHI, meanwhile, has been consistently high since its inception in 1995 (see Figure 1). Satisfaction dipped each time the government raised the contribution rates (as in 2002 and 2010), but recovered quickly afterwards. Like Britain's NHS and Canada's medicare, within a few decades, the NHI had become a treasured and highly

Figure 1. Public Satisfaction with Taiwan's National Health Insurance.

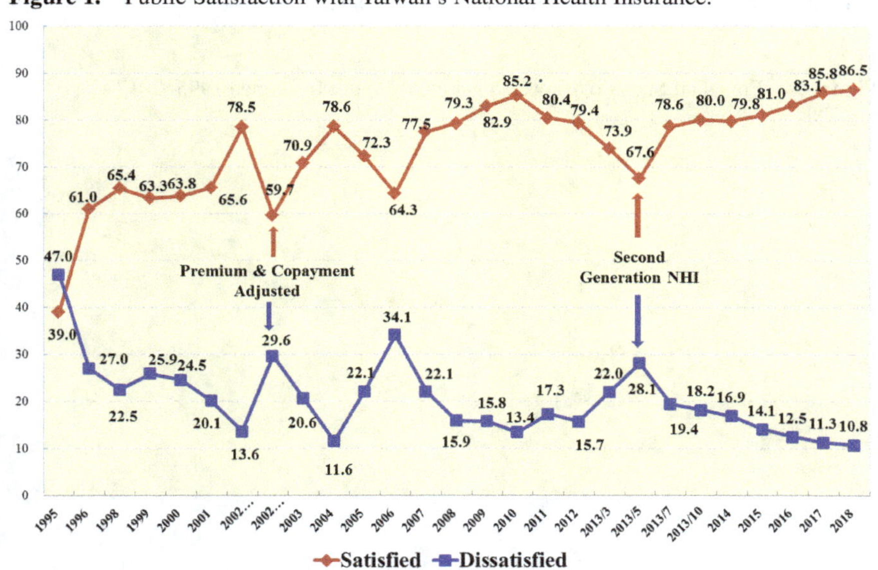

Source: National Health Insurance Administration 2018–2019.

valued public institution. In fact, many Taiwanese Americans return to Taiwan to seek medical care.

Recent Reforms

Financial instability has dogged the NHI since its inception in 1995. For most years, expenditures outpaced revenues by one to two percent points. That resulted in continuous deficits, except during a brief period (2002–2004), after modest contribution increases (see Figure 2). NHI's cumulative deficits reached 15.1 percent of its annual revenue in 2009 (Cheng 2015a). This led the government to again raise contribution rates in 2010. Understandably, the reform debates regularly turn to the NHI's finances. Figure 2 shows the history of NHI's financial status since inception in 1995–2017.

The NHI contribution rates increased on September 1, 2002 from 4.25 to 4.55 percent, and on April 1, 2010 to 5.17 percent. On Jan 1, 2013, the contribution rate decreased from 5.17 to 4.91 percent, but at the same time, insured faced a supplemental contribution of 2 percent. On January 1, 2016, the contribution rate went down further from 4.91 to 4.69 percent and the supplemental contribution from 2 to 1.91.

Figure 2. Financial Status of Taiwan's National Health Insurance 1995–2017.

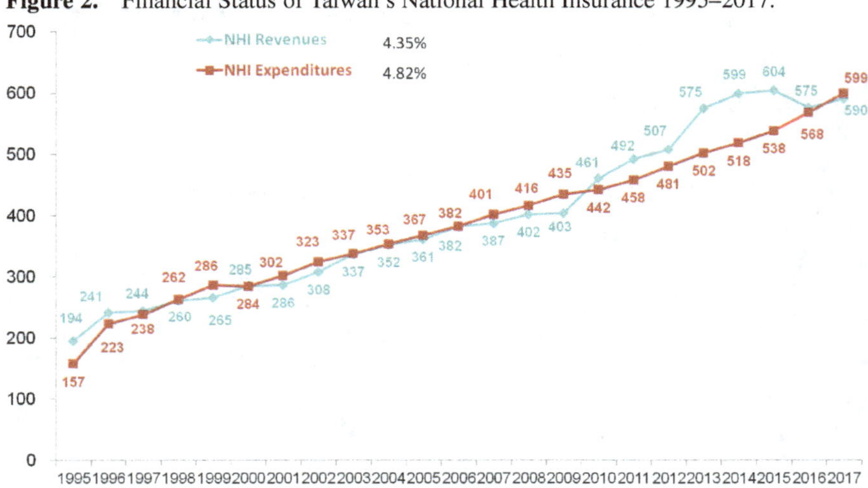

Source: National Health Insurance Administration 2018–2019.

The NHI law permits increases in contribution rates every two years, if needed. Facing persistent public resistance, however, the government has time and again postponed hikes in contributions, thus aggravating the deficits and raising concerns that the NHI might go bankrupt. The only NHI contribution rate increases took two determined health ministers, Lee Ming-Liang (in 2002) and Yaung Chih-Liang (in 2010), who were willing to face down public opposition. They both carried out their decisions, but resigned from their posts afterwards.

The increase in contribution rates in 2010 eliminated NHI's large deficits and restored its financial balance. It enabled the NHIA to accumulate a surplus by January 2013, which it banked as reserve funds. As of October 2014, the surplus amounted to 27 percent of the NHI expenditures for the first 10 months in 2014 (Cheng 2015a).

Despite the buildup of surpluses from increased contributions in 2010, the government deemed the payroll-based payments insufficient to meet future expenditure growth. Moreover, it regarded purely payroll-based financing as inequitable. To address these concerns, it decided to broaden the tax base for healthcare financing. It introduced a supplementary premium scheme in January 2013, in what is known as the Second-Generation NHI reform. The supplementary contributions were levied on six non-payroll income sources: large bonuses, income from second and third jobs, rent, interest, dividends and professional fees. The initial rate was 2 percent of supplementary income. Low-income households were exempt.

With the supplementary contributions, the total tax base included over 90 percent of Taiwan's national income, compared to the payroll base that drew on approximately 60 percent of national income. It thus represented a significant improvement in the fairness of financial contributions based on people's ability to pay (Cheng 2015a).

The government next lowered the regular, payroll-based premium rate from 4.91 to 4.69 percent, and the supplementary rate from 2 to 1.9 percent in January 2016 (NHIA 2017–2018). At the same time, it raised the income threshold for the collection of supplementary contributions. As a result of those changes, NHI's revenues declined, but the resulting deficits were absorbed by the large surpluses NHI had built up between 2012 and

2016. The shrinking surpluses raised new concerns for NHI's future financial stability, however.

Challenges

As noted earlier, the NHI has served Taiwan's population well. It provides universal coverage with comprehensive benefits and equity in access for all its citizens and foreign residents at an affordable cost, 6.1 percent of GDP in 2019. Like the United Kingdom's NHS or Canada's medicare, Taiwan's NHI is a treasured public institution. Nevertheless, like the health systems of many other nations, it faces a number of challenges.

Demographic Transition

Taiwan is still young relative to most OECD countries, but its population is aging more rapidly than many other countries. In 2016, 13.2 percent of Taiwanese were 65 or older, one of the lowest rates in the industrialized world (MOHW 2018). However, the population over 65 is expected to grow to 20 percent by 2020, 24 percent by 2030, and 37 percent by 2050 (Cheng 2015a). This poses an urgent challenge for the NHI in two ways: the high healthcare costs associated with the elderly population and the as-yet limited scope of LTC.

Aging is a major factor in the increasing prevalence of non-communicable diseases (NCDs) and associated medical costs. Medical costs for Taiwan's elderly have been high; as in other nations, there is a large difference in average medical costs between young and elderly population groups, with a ratio of about 1 to 4.6 (NHIA 2015). This ratio will increase as population aging accelerates. In 2014, the group 65 and over already accounted for 35.4 percent of total NHI expenditure (NHIA 2015).

The Burden of NCDs

NCDs, including cancer, now increasingly affect younger people in Taiwan, as well. NCDs accounted for almost 80 percent of all deaths in

Taiwan in 2013 and nearly 70 percent of all deaths among those over 65 (Cheng 2015b). This has serious implications for both growing utilization of medical services and associated medical costs, and the potentially increased demand for a larger healthcare workforce. It also requires new forms of LTC and LTC financing (see below).

Quality of Care

The relatively modest level of health spending in Taiwan comes with remarkable health outcomes. Life expectancy in 2015 was 80.2 years, 1.1 years lower than the OECD median, and lower than that of Japan (83.9), Australia (82.5), Canada (81.7) and Germany (80.7), but higher than that of the United States (78.8), which spends almost three times what Taiwan spends on healthcare.[2] The NHI has been associated with a reduction in amenable mortality, with fewer deaths due to improved access to timely and effective care (Cheng 2015b). Yet, some studies suggest that the quality of care in Taiwan leaves room for improvement, both in its clinical quality and cost-effectiveness (Cheng 2015b).

Parallel Private System Evolving

Taiwan appears to be developing a de facto private sector for self-paying wealthy patients. Physicians dissatisfied with the NHI's tight budget and fee restrictions have resorted to selling new products and services to earn higher incomes. For example, Taiwan's leading medical centers operate private VIP clinics staffed with senior physicians who see patients willing and able to pay the facilities' much higher registration fees. The non-governmental Federation of NHI Public Oversight alleges that this practice has created access barriers (Wei 2007). It deprives patients of lesser

---

[2] There is, of course, the issue of attribution: the rise of life expectancy cannot be attributed to improved access to healthcare or higher healthcare spending (see also the introduction to this volume). As in Singapore, the rapid rise of income levels and improved living conditions were perhaps more important factors. So, it is important to separate the "amendable" versus "non-amendable" changes in mortality.

means the opportunity to be seen by the best and brightest senior doctors. Patients often perceive the care provided by these senior physicians to be superior to that of more junior doctors. There are several examples of similar "parallel privatization" in other countries, see, for example, the Netherlands or Israel in this volume.

The impact of supplier-induced-demand on the cost and quality of healthcare is another concern that may become significant in the long term.

Workforce Shortages

As discussed earlier, Taiwan has fewer doctors and nurses than most other industrialized nations. Those low workforce ratios seem inadequate, especially in view of the high per capita utilization. Some studies predict a shortfall of up to 7,000 doctors across five specialties that currently appear to struggle with shortages: internal medicine, surgery, pediatrics, obstetrics and gynecology and emergency medicine (Cheng 2015b). Likewise, adequate nursing staff is important to safeguard the quality of care and patient safety.

Long-Term Care

Taiwan's rapidly aging population makes LTC a top priority. There is, as of yet, no LTC insurance. The government launched the "Long-Term Care 2.0 Plan" in January 2017, to be financed by taxes on tobacco, large gifts and inheritances. This replaced its predecessor's contribution-based "Long-Term Care 1.0 Plan" (Taiwan's Business Weekly 2018). One year after the launch of the plan, just 10 percent of those who needed LTC were actually receiving services, due to various supply capacity constraints. Satisfaction was low, both amongst LTC workers and users, who faced an increase in financial burden under the government's new rules and regulations (Huang 2018). For example, in December 2017, the government suddenly changed the payment rules for LTC providers, effective January 2018, from hourly payments to a fee schedule consisting of 152 service items such as bathing or hair washing.

Long-Term Financial Sustainability

The rapid development of expensive medical technology, new drugs and rising public expectations all pose challenges for the NHI's long-term financial sustainability. As noted earlier, while the financial reforms were initially successful in wiping out deficits and restoring NHI's financial balance, this only lasted through 2017. The NHIA continued to draw down its reserve funds in 2018, and policy-makers face renewed pressures to increase revenues.

Conclusions

Taiwan's NHI has made remarkable progress. It provides universal health coverage at an affordable cost to all citizens and foreign residents, and enjoys consistently high public satisfaction.

NHI's history and experience in administering the program provides useful potential lessons for other countries aspiring to equitable and affordable universal healthcare. It also provides important lessons going forward for Taiwan's own health policy-makers and the public.

Taiwan's government rejected the idea of consumer choice or exit (Hirschman 1970) in health insurance, but—after carefully considering options—decided that mandatory social health insurance would be the best model to realize the policy goals of universal access, quality, efficiency and cost control. Within three decades, the NHI has succeeded in realizing those policy goals to a large extent, and has become very popular. This experience confirmed that, in general, (as we have seen in other chapters in this volume) citizens seem more concerned with their choice of general practitioner, local hospital or other healthcare provider than with the choice of health plan.

Taiwan provides an interesting case of a shift from exclusionary policy-making (Labra 2007) by the authoritarian KMT regime that, over time, became more inclusionary in its consultations with major stakeholders in healthcare. This chapter showed how rising income levels and public expectations also resulted in a more democratic and pluralistic society where healthcare providers, patients and other stakeholders increasingly—and effectively—voiced their demands.

This chapter also shows the importance of ideas, interests and institutions (Klein and Marmor 2006) in the shaping and outcome of health policy-making. While during the first decades of its rein, the KMT government had enough power to impose policy change without much opposition, over time (particularly after the end of martial law in 1987 and the growth of the opposition party, DPP), it realized that it needed the support of the population and organized interest groups. Gaining popular support requires a widely shared understanding in society. In many countries, the majority of the population feels that everyone should have access to healthcare, regardless of his or her ability to pay. Taiwan was no exception. The universal coverage of the NHI, and its very rapid implementation, made the NHI very popular.

Finally, this chapter leads to a conclusion about both the success and shortcoming of NHI's cost control. Relative to its high per capita income ($48,535 PPP in 2016 and $49,827 in 2017), Taiwan's total health spending (6 percent of GDP and $2,897 in 2016) is considerably lower than that of rich OECD countries ($41,649 on average per capita income, health spending of 8.8 percent of GDP, $4,033 per capita health spending in 2016). The large discrepancy in health spending between Taiwan and other industrialized nations reflects the NHI's high overall system efficiency, but it also suggests underfunding for certain healthcare services.

Taiwan—given its high income—is in the enviable position of having the means to pay for higher health spending than it currently does. Higher health spending would enable, for example, faster adoption of new medical technologies; increases in health workforce—doctors, nurses, and allied health workers; strengthening of health technology assessment capabilities to increase both the cost- and clinical effectiveness of covered treatments; better payment for providers; implementation of a LTC program for Taiwan's rapidly aging population; and more health services research. Whether it will actually increase its healthcare spending depends on the political willingness to do so and the ability to convince the public that payments will need to go up.

References

Chang, H.I. 2005. *Taiwan's National Health Insurance: Current Development and Performance.* Proceedings of Taiwan NHI's 10th Anniversary International Symposium. Taipei: Bureau of National Health Insurance, Department of Health. The Executive Yuan.

Cheng, T.M. June 4, 2018. *Author's Email Communication with Cheng-Hua Lee,* Vice Director-General, National Health Insurance Administration. Taiwan: Ministry of Health and Welfare.

Cheng, T.M. 2002a. *Meeting with Minister of Health Ming-Liang Lee of Taiwan and Uwe E. Reinhardt regarding the NHI's Financial Crisis.* Princeton, NJ.

Cheng, T.M. 2002b. *Author's Personal Communication with Minister of Health Ming-Liang Lee of Taiwan.* Taipei, Taiwan.

Cheng, T.M. 2003. "Taiwan's new national health insurance program: genesis and experience so far. *Health Affairs,* 22(3): 61–76.

Cheng, T.M. 2008. *Taiwan's National Health Insurance: Lessons for the United States.* Washington, DC: Congressional Briefing, U.S. Congress.

Cheng, T.M. 2009. "Lessons from Taiwan's Universal National Health Insurance: A Conversation with Taiwan's Health Minister Ching-Chuan Yeh." *Health Affairs,* 28(4): 1035–1044.

Cheng, T.M. 2015a. "Reflections on the 20th anniversary of Taiwan's single-payer National Health Insurance System." *Health Affairs,* 34(3): 502–510.

Cheng, T.M. May 14, 2015b. *Taiwan's Health Care System: The Next 20 Years.* Washington, DC: Brookings Institution.

Cheng, T.M. February 1, 2018. Presentation to the Ministry of Health and Welfare of Taiwan on the occasion of the award of the Ministry of Health and Welfare of Taiwan Health Services Medal of the First Order and the Professional Excellence Medal to Uwe E. Reinhardt of Princeton University, Taipei.

Cheng, T.M. January 23, 2019. *Author's Personal Communication with Official of the National Health Insurance Administration,* Ministry of Health and Welfare.

Council of Economic Planning and Development. June 25, 1990. Prepared by Hsiao, W.C.L. *A Summary of the National Health Insurance (NHI) Plan Adopted by the Republic of China (Taiwan).* Taipei, Taiwan.

Department of Health. 2005. *2004 Health Statistics and Trends.* Taipei: Department of Health, The Executive Yuan.

Huang, T.R. 2018. "Long term care fictitious: long term care 2.0 only serves 10 percent of those who need it." *Business Weekly*, April 3.

Hirschman, A.O. 1970. *Exit, Voice and Loyalty. Responses to Decline in Firms, Organizations, and States.* Cambridge: Harvard University Press.

Kingdon, J. 1984. *Agendas, Alternatives, and Public Policies.* New York: Longman.

Labra, M.E. 2007. Modes of Health Policy Making and Medical Interests in Chile in the 20th Century. Updated English version of M.E. Labra. 2000. Padrões de Formulação de Políticas de Saúde no Chile no Século XX. Rio de Janeiro: *DADOS-Revista de Ciências Sociais*, 43(1): 153–182.

Klein, R., and T.R. Marmor. 2006. "Reflections on Policy Analysis: Putting It Together Again." *The Oxford Handbook of Political Science.* R. Goodin (ed.). Oxford: Oxford University Press: 982–912.

International Monetary Fund. 2017. *World Economic Outlook Database*, January 2018. Accessed September 2, 2018.

Lee, I.C. 2018. "Resident physicians urge improvements to contract." *Taipei Times*, August 12.

Luo, Z. 2018. Discussing hospital and nursing working conditions without inviting primary care participation: ministry of health and welfare says it will invite if their wish were made known. *United Daily News*, October 4.

Ministry of Health and Welfare (MOHW). 2018. *Health Statistics and Trends 2016.* Taipei: MOHW.

National Health Insurance Administration (NHIA). *2017–2018 National Health Insurance Annual Report.* Taipei: NHIA, MOHW.

National Health Insurance Administration (NHIA). *2018–2019 National Health Insurance Annual Report.* Taipei: NHIA, MOHW.

National Health Insurance Administration, Ministry of Health and Welfare. 2015 data.

OECD. 2018. *Health Statistics 2017.*

Tien, S.M., and S. T. Chen. 2007. "Interest groups shuttling back and forth parliament brazenly." *Liberty Times*, July 18.

Wei, L.W. 2007. "Tiering of patient access: rich receive VIP—and poor poor treatments." *United Daily News*, July 27.

Yeh, C.C. 2002. *The Legend of the National Health Insurance.* Taipei: The Tung Foundation.

Conclusions

Kieke Okma and Tim Tenbensel

This volume presents a description and analysis of the health reform experiences of 12 small and medium-sized nations across the world during the last quarter of the 20th century and the early decades of the 21st century. As mentioned in the introduction, the countries vary in population size, ethnic composition, income levels, healthcare arrangements, cultural backgrounds and styles of policy-making. In that sense, the volume represents a "most different system design" under a broad, common analytical approach. Still, the nations have some important elements in common. They share the overall policy goal of providing universal health coverage (UHC)—access to healthcare for all—with financing that protects families against catastrophic costs of medical care. They seek to safeguard the availability of decent healthcare services, at affordable costs and without insurmountable financial barriers. They faced similar challenges: fiscal and budgetary pressures, demographic and epidemiological transitions, changing consumer preferences and changing views on the proper role of the state.

The countries discussed in this volume considered a markedly similar set of policy options, ranging from full nationalization of healthcare financing and provision to mixed systems, and the privatization of services and finance. Moreover, they did not just discuss reform options for their health systems, but actually engaged in major restructuring efforts in the last three or four decades. The concurrence of widespread discontent with existing arrangements, combined with seemingly feasible policy options and political leaders able and willing to act, created windows of opportunity for change.

In the end, however, despite those similarities, we found no convergence in the pace, direction or outcomes of the health reform processes. In fact, there was wide variation in national experiences, ranging from efforts to return to the social insurance model of the earlier 20th century in the Eastern European countries after the fall of communism, to programs in sub-Saharan African countries aimed at transforming local community schemes and insurance for specific population groups into universal health insurance. The consumer-driven healthcare of Switzerland and Holland (that, a decade later, mainly seemed to have driven up costs) and new procedures for establishing the entitlements of Israel's social health insurance were quite different from the complicated transformations of the healthcare systems of Chile and Ecuador after the return to democracy and dismantling of the legacies of military dictatorships. Similarly, the pragmatic policies of two of Asia's tiger economies, Taiwan and Singapore, in setting up two vastly different models of universal coverage contrasted with New Zealand, where ideology appeared to be the main driving force of rapid changes in regional governance, but with striking stability of its tax-based financing.

So, the central question of this volume has been: What explains the divergence in the health reform experience of 12 nations that shared policy goals, faced similar challenges and discussed similar policy options? Why did we not see a pattern of convergence in their healthcare systems?

To address that puzzle, we used economic terms to describe the healthcare arrangements, largely relying on earlier publications of the Organization of Economic Co-Operation and Development (OECD) to describe the financing, contracting and ownership of healthcare services (OECD 1992; 1994; see the Appendix for the "house model"). We also found Hirschman's (1970) terms "voice" and "exit" useful to show how healthcare programs position and channel the influence of patients, insured and citizens. Did they exercise their democratic voice as citizens by electing political representatives on the federal, regional and local levels and, for example, board members of hospitals or regional health boards, or does the program allow for the exit of dissatisfied insured or patients by offering choice of health plan and providers? In addition, all healthcare systems require arrangements for administering healthcare and health insurance, as well as (government) regulation.

Describing healthcare systems in those terms, however, does not explain the patterns of change and non-change. We therefore combined these economic terms with vocabulary from political science to *analyze* the shaping of health reforms in the diverse nations of this book.

Divergent processes of healthcare reforms did not mean we couldn't draw lessons from the 12 cases. In fact, we found that the experience of the 12 nations can be seen as a rich laboratory of change, which provides important information to other nations, too. Health reform debates often tend to be parochial (perhaps more so in the Unites States than in other nations) and policy ideas travel swiftly around the world, without time for much scrutiny of their accuracy or applicability in either the country of origin or destination. Serious study of international experience can help to broaden the horizon, serve as a mirror for one's own experience and as an inspirational source for policy ideas—but only when taken seriously and done in a way that allows for drawing conclusions. This study aims to serve exactly that purpose.

Our study resulted in two main categories of conclusions: empirical and theoretical. The first concerns the actual changes we found in very different nations from across the globe; the second regard the use of theoretical models or analytical approaches to analyze national fiscal and social policy-making. The following list summarizes first these empirical findings, followed by our theoretical conclusions.

Empirical Findings

Our first, perhaps most important, finding was that ambitions for major policy change rarely translated into lasting, big bang health reforms. In several cases, pressure for change (widespread discontent with existing arrangements, fiscal and budgetary pressure and demographic change), the availability of policy options that seemed to fit the current situation and political willingness to act upon opened windows of opportunity. Health ministers eager to be seen as policy entrepreneurs (Kingdon 1984) announced ambitious transformations for the financing and provision of healthcare. In practice, however, those ambitious big bang reforms often turned into processes of incremental change that would be more appropriately characterized by Lindblom's term "muddling through" (Lindblom 1959).

Second, while the group of smaller and mid-sized nations in this volume is understudied in comparative research (as noted in the Introduction, they are somewhat "under the radar"), they did indeed, as mentioned earlier, provide a rich, interesting laboratory of change.

Third, several of the cases showed (large) gaps between the policy rhetoric, policy expectations and reality. For example, the ambitions to create universal coverage in the sub-Saharan nations, or competing health funds in the Czech Republic clearly failed to meet expectations. Likewise, the rhetoric of consumer-driven healthcare in Switzerland and Holland did not match the reality of accelerating market concentration, rapidly rising health expenditure and declining consumer trust in both nations.

Fourth, the statistical Appendix shows how population growth in all 12 nations of this volume leveled off, but in different degrees. Continued population growth in relatively poorer nations aggravated the pressure on land, as illustrated by the very high population density (especially per arable land surface) in Tanzania and Chile. Income levels, too, rose everywhere, but at different growth rates. That led to growing income gaps between the wealthiest and the poorest nations (there is also growing income disparity within nations). The data further showed a close association between income levels and health status—wealthier people are generally healthier than poorer ones, and with rising income levels, the overall health of population generally improves. There is also a close association between income and health spending: wealthier people spend a higher proportion of their income on healthcare (even while they are healthier). Moreover, a higher share of their health spending runs though collective (or prepaid) financing: taxation or social health insurance. The poorest families in the poorest nations, as a result, pay most out-of-pocket. The gap in health financing also reflects in available resources. In the last three decades, the majority of wealthier nations sought to reduce hospital capacity and shift patient care to outpatient settings (and substitute highly skilled for lower skilled workers). By contrast, poor nations are still building new hospitals (and, facing mounting shortages aggravated by brain drain, struggle to expand their health workforce). Finally, despite the abovementioned problems, there have been major improvements in health outcomes everywhere. For example, the data show a dramatic drop in child and maternal mortality in all nations studied in this volume, even in those with very low levels of health spending.

Fifth, conflicts between central (or federal governments) and regional or local authorities proved to be common, entailing shifts in both financial responsibilities and decision-making powers downwards, and sometimes upwards (also shifting the blame for failure or claiming success, if any). The clearest examples of such disputes are found in Chile, Switzerland and Tanzania.

Sixth, reforms in how to pay healthcare providers proved hard to implement, time-consuming and expensive, with little or no evidence of success, illustrated by the experiences of Ecuador, Taiwan and the Netherlands.

Seventh, since the mid-20th century, social health insurance had become the major source of health financing in several European and Latin American nations. The histories of those systems, especially in Germany, show how they are very difficult to realize overnight. They require administrative capacity, experience, a long actuarial time horizon, public trust, active membership, effective control of fraud, and a non-inflationary environment. The chapters about the Czech Republic, Slovenia, Ghana, Tanzania, Chile and Ecuador illustrate this point. The African cases, in particular, show the problem of too much dependence on external donor aid and government subsidies.

Eighth, user fees are unpopular everywhere. In many cases—for example, in Ghana, the Netherlands, Taiwan, Tanzania and Singapore—governments softened the consequences by exempting certain groups of users like the elderly, low-income families or chronically ill, thus defeating the very purpose of user fees.

Ninth, in several cases, non-government organizations and international organizations like the World Bank and the World Health Organization (WHO) and the European Union (EU) appear to have been stronger with slogans and theoretical models than with realistic policy advice. For example, the World Bank, together with the International Monetary Fund, pushed for the Washington Consensus in the 1980s as the recipe for economic growth and supposed anti-poverty policy (in later stages the Bank abandoned this course). This advice led to sharp reductions in government spending, while failing to bring the promised economic growth. The WHO, supported by other international agencies, gained fame with the promise of health as a fundamental human right in the 1960s and promoting UHC in the early 2000s (see e.g., Economist 2018). According to a 2018 WHO fact sheet, "UHC means that all individuals and communities receive the health services they need without suffering financial hardship. It includes the full spectrum of essential, quality health services, from health promotion to prevention, treatment, rehabilitation, and palliative care" and "UHC enables everyone to access the services that address the most significant causes of disease and death, and ensures that the quality of those services is good enough to improve the health of the people who receive them" (WHO 2019). UHC is example of an expression more aspirational than descriptive or operational, however. The case studies in this volume illustrate how embracing the idea of UHC does not easily translate into operational policies. None of the countries that announced their ambition to replace existing arrangements with universal coverage were able to do so.

Theoretical Findings

Our study illustrated the need to combine the description of healthcare arrangements with the analysis of the healthcare reform experiences across nations. It also showed that combining economic terms with vocabulary from political science allowed for a wider and richer comparison of health policy-making than many studies that rely solely on only one particular approach (say, studies based on aggregate statistical data, or efforts to categorize nations based on their perceived welfare state model as a base for predicting policies).

Second, we found striking similarities in the basic elements of the health systems (the financing, provision and contracting of healthcare combined with administration and government regulation, see the Appendix) as well as in the basic nature of the policy issues (the appropriate mixes of financing, provision and governance arrangements). That similarity allowed for systematic cross-examination of their health reform experiences. While we found no clear patterns of convergence in the overall direction or pace of the healthcare reforms across the nations in this study, as noted earlier—we found many similar experiences at the level of specific programs and policies. Thus the *level of analysis* matters.

Third, as widely noted by political scientists (e.g., Klein and Marmor 2006): ideas, institutions and interests are the main factors shaping the processes and results of fiscal and social policy-making. So ideas matter, as illustrated by the strong popular support for solidarity, which limited the options for what governments could change, or forced governments to soften certain measures, for example, in the Czech Republic, Holland, New Zealand and Singapore. Likewise, institutions matter—defined not only as political arrangements for decision-making but also as long-lasting traditions and health facilities with old historical roots. For example, in Chile, the Czech Republic, Israel, Holland, New Zealand, Slovenia and Switzerland, institutional legacies created barriers for major change in the existing arrangements. Next, interests matter, too. In many counties, the national associations of physicians, hospitals or insurers turned out to be powerful veto players in the health policy arena, for example, in Chile, the Czech Republic, Israel, Holland and New Zealand. In several cases, national organizations of patients gained influence as well. Thus, government agencies and departments no longer (if ever) remained the dominant players in the policy arena, even in nations with autocratic regimes.

Fourth, as noted earlier, big bang reforms tended to fizzle out and become more incremental, as in the case, for example, of the healthcare reforms of the Czech Republic, Israel and the Netherlands. Incoming health ministers often have high ambitions for sweeping change. After announcing major reforms, however, they faced the reality of fiscal and budgetary constraints, popular opposition against higher user charges or budget cuts and powerful stakeholders opposing certain measures. Announcing universal coverage is one thing, but actually making sure the entire population signs up with a new plan (and pays their contributions) is quite another, as we have seen. In fact, health policy-making is more often incremental than big bang, and often somewhat incoherent, rather than following any logic of a clear-cut blueprint. However, announcing a course of "muddling through" (as Lindblom found in 1959, the most common policy direction) sounds less heroic than major reform or universal coverage or consumer-driven healthcare.

Fifth, things change over time. Exclusionary regimes may become more inclusionary as seen in the cases of Chile, Singapore and Taiwan. As another example, the composition of healthcare financing changed in Chile, Ghana, Holland and Tanzania. Those arrangements became more hybridized, combining elements of (universal) tax-financed schemes with employment-based social insurance. With that hybridization, it has also become harder to group nations into clear categories.

Finally, how do we locate this study? As we have noted elsewhere, there has been a dramatic growth of the body of international comparative studies of healthcare reforms since the late 1970s (Okma and Marmor 2003). The vast majority of those comparative studies are largely descriptive. Few actually pay attention to what it is, conceptually, that they compare (Rose 1993). There are, in fact, four categories of comparative studies: (1) studies based on aggregate statistical data (this category started with the OECD health data and expanded to include non-OECD nations over time); (2) collections of mostly descriptive, individual case studies hardly related by common analytical frameworks; (3) thematic case studies that seek to address specific policy issues, for example, competition in healthcare or manpower research of healthcare reforms; (4) theoretical comparative research applied to a limited number of cases.

This study broadens the scope of the third category abovementioned by including 12 very different smaller and mid-sized countries across the globe that are not usually included in international comparative research, and by applying a wide range of theoretical approaches to describe and analyze the healthcare reforms across those nations.

We hope that this volume will contribute to the next generation of comparative studies.

References

Economist. April 28–May 4, 2018. Universal health care. Special report. *Economist,* 427(9089): 3–12.

Hirschman, A.O. 1970. *Exit, Voice and Loyalty: Responses to Decline in Firms, Organizations, and States* Cambridge: Harvard University Press.

Kingdon, J.W. 1984. *Agendas, Alternatives, and Public Policies.* Boston, MA: Little, Brown and Company.

Klein, R. and T.R. Marmor. 2006. "Reflections on Policy Analysis: Putting It Together Again." *The Oxford Handbook of Political Science.* R. Goodin (ed.). Oxford: Oxford University Press: 982–1001.

Lindblom, C.E. 1959. "The Science of 'Muddling Through'." *Public Administration,* XIX(2): 79–89.

OECD. 1992. *The Reform of Health Care: A Comparative Analysis of Seven OECD Countries.* Paris: Organisation for Economic Co-operation and Development.

OECD. 1994. *The Reform of Health Care: A Comparative Analysis of Seven OECD Countries.* Paris: Organisation for Economic Co-operation and Development.

Okma, K.G.H. and T.R. Marmor. 2003. "Health Care Systems in Transition of the World Health Organisation." (Book review essay). *Health Policies Politics and Law,* 28(4): 747–755.

Rose, R. 1993. *Lesson-Drawing in Public Policy. A Guide to Learning Across Time and Space.* Chatham, NJ: Chatham House Publisher.

WHO. 2019. *Universal Health Coverage* (Fact Sheet). January 24, 2019.

Appendix

Kieke Okma and Tim Tenbensel

This Appendix presents selected data on the population, area, income level and composition of health spending and the health status of the population for the 12 countries discussed in this volume. As we have argued elsewhere, many international comparative studies are based on such aggregated statistical data (see the Introduction to this volume). While those data illustrate a certain association or statistical correlation between phenomena, they do not directly provide the base for drawing causal inferences. That is why this Appendix serves to illustrate some general patterns across the nations, not as the main source of information or for drawing lessons from our case studies, as we have done in the main text of this volume. The data support seven general conclusions, already familiar to most experts in the domain of public health.

The first two general conclusions regard population growth and population density (see Tables 1–3). All 12 cases of this study belong to the category of smaller or mid-sized nations, with populations of about 10 million or (much) less by 1950. The population growth rates leveled off almost everywhere, but to different degrees. The population density of the 12 nations ranged from 9.0 per km^2 in New Zealand to 2,333 per km^2 in Singapore in 1960, but went up to 17.5 and 7,908, respectively, in those two nations in 2015.

It is important to note the total land area is not the same as land available for agricultural cultivation, however. Table 4 shows that not only the total land area, but also the share of arable land (basically the potential land available for food production) varies widely across nations.

Table 1. Population, 1960–2015 (Thousands of Persons)

Country	Year						
	1960	1970	1980	1990	2000	2010	2015
Chile	7,717	9,564	11,266	13,242	15,263	16,993	17,763
Czech Republic	9,590	9,818	10,349	10,341	10,290	10,536	10,604
Ecuador	4,546	6,073	7,976	10,218	12,629	14,935	16,144
Ghana	6,652	8,597	10,802	14,628	18,939	24,512	27,583
Israel	2,090	2,850	3,745	4,500	6,014	7,426	8,065
Netherlands	11,449	13,002	14,148	14,965	15,926	16,683	16,938
New Zealand	2,373	2,818	3,147	3,398	3,859	4,370	4,615
Singapore	1,633	2,072	2,412	3,013	3,914	5,074	5,535
Slovenia	1,587	1,670	1,836	2,006	1,988	2,045	2,075
Switzerland	5,296	6,169	6,304	6,675	7,167	7,832	8,320
Taiwan	10,702	14,693	17,472	20,293	21,840	23,102	23,486
Republic of Tanzania	10,075	13,606	18,683	25,460	34,178	46,099	53,880

Source: UN 2018a.

Table 2. Population Growth, 1960–2015 (Annual Growth Rates per Five-Year Periods)

Country	Year					
	1960–65	1970–75	1980–85	1990–95	2000–05	2010–15
Chile	2.21	1.74	1.56	1.53	1.13	0.89
Czech Republic	0.46	0.51	−0.04	0.03	−0.06	0.13
Ecuador	2.88	2.81	2.52	2.26	1.68	1.56
Ghana	2.95	2.68	3.26	2.72	2.58	2.36
Israel	3.76	3.16	1.73	3.40	1.87	1.65
Netherlands	1.35	1.02	0.51	0.66	0.55	0.30
New Zealand	2.03	1.79	0.76	1.57	1.38	1.09
Singapore	2.79	1.73	2.30	2.88	2.75	1.74
Slovenia	0.53	0.86	1.16	−0.15	0.08	0.29
Switzerland	1.92	0.60	0.48	1.00	0.67	1.21
Taiwan	3.35	1.99	1.53	0.88	0.69	0.33
Republic of Tanzania	2.96	3.22	3.12	3.26	2.85	3.12

Source: UN 2018a.

Table 3.   Population Density, 1960–2015 (Persons per Square Kilometer)

				Year			
Country	**1960**	**1970**	**1980**	**1990**	**2000**	**2010**	**2015**
Chile	10.4	12.9	15.2	17.8	20.5	22.9	23.9
Czech Republic	124.2	127.1	134.0	133.9	133.2	136.2	137.3
Ecuador	18.3	24.5	32.1	41.1	50.8	60.1	65.0
Ghana	29.2	37.8	47.5	64.3	83.2	107.7	121.2
Israel	96.6	131.7	173.0	208.0	277.9	343.2	372.7
Netherlands	339.5	385.6	419.6	443.8	472.3	494.7	502.3
New Zealand	9.0	10.7	12.0	12.9	14.7	16.6	17.5
Singapore	2333.0	2960.4	3445.3	4304.2	5591.4	7248.9	7907.5
Slovenia	78.8	82.2	91.2	99.6	98.7	101.5	103.0
Switzerland	134.0	156.1	159.5	168.9	181.4	198.2	210.5
Taiwan	302.2	414.9	500.3	573.6	616.8	652.4	663.3
Republic of Tanzania	11.4	15.4	21.1	28.7	38.6	52.0	60.8

Source: UN 2018a.

Table 4.   Area, Arable Land and Population Density, 1960–2010 (Population and Population per Square Kilometer)

	Area 2016 (km^2)	**Arable Land (percent of Total Area)**		**Arable Land per Person (Hectare per Person)**	
Country		**2000**	**2006**	**2000**	**2006**
Chile	743.500	2.4	1.7	0.11	0.07
Czech Republic	77.200	42.0	32.3	0.32	0.24
Ecuador	248.400	6.5	3.9	0.13	0.06
Ghana	227.500	6.5	3.9	0.21	0.17
Israel	21.600	15.6	13.6	0.05	0.03
Netherlands	33.700	27.0	30.5	0.06	0.06
New Zealand	263.300	5.7	2.2	0.39	0.12
Singapore	700	1.5	0.3	0.00	0.00
Slovenia	20.100	8.6	9.1	0.09	0.09
Switzerland	39.500	10.3	9.1	0.06	0.05
Taiwan	36.000	—	10.2	—	0.03
Rep. Tanzania	885.800	9.7	15.2	0.25	0.24

Source: UN 2018b; Taiwan: CIA 2018.
1 km^2 = 100 hectares.

Arable land or food availability is usually not taken into account as a main concern in health policy studies, but obviously, access to affordable food is crucial to the health of the population. Chile, for example, seemed very sparsely populated, with only 8.2 people per km^2 in 1960, doubling to 16.9 in 2010. However, according to the data of the UN Department of Economic and Social Affairs, measured as the number of people per square kilometer of arable land, that ratio went up from 161 to 1,013 between 1960 and 2010 due to the combination of population growth and loss of arable land (or as seen in Table 4, e.g., in Chile, the available land area per habitant dropped from 0.11 to 0.07 hectares between 2000 and 2006). Countries with a small or declining share of arable land face the need to increase food imports, with fiscal and budgetary consequences, or ensure that agricultural productivity at least keeps up with their population growth. Only a few nations, for example, Tanzania, were able to expand their arable land in the last decades. Still, its population density, measured by arable land, increased from 1,776 to 4,520 between 1960 and 2010.

Third, average incomes in all countries of this study have risen since the 1960s, both in nominal terms and measured in purchasing power parity (see Tables 5a and 5b). However, the income growth rates showed major divergence, resulting in growing income gaps. In 1970, there was a 20-fold difference between the lowest (Tanzania) and the highest (Switzerland) incomes; that gap had risen to a 100-fold difference by 2015. Moreover, what the tables do not show is the growing income disparity within nations (see e.g., the World Inequality Report 2018).

The fourth general point is that there is a close association between both income levels and spending for healthcare, and income levels and health. In general, as shown in Tables 6a and 6b, the higher the country's income, the higher the level of its healthcare spending. That is true not only across countries, but also within countries. Higher income nations, and higher income groups, are generally healthier than poorer ones, but they still spend larger amounts on healthcare. Moreover, higher income levels generally go hand in hand with a higher share of collective (or public) financing out of general taxation or mandatory social health insurance (see Tables 7a–7c).

Table 5a. Income per Capita, 1960–2015 (Current US Dollars per Capita)

	Year						
Country	**1960**	**1970**	**1980**	**1990**	**2000**	**2010**	**2015**
Chile	532.6	954.2	2,577.3	2,500.6	5,101.4	12,860.1	13,736.6
Czech Republic	—	—	—	3,917.2	6,011.6	19,808.1	17,715.6
Ecuador	455.3	471.4	2,241.8	1,491.4	1,451.3	4,657.3	6,150.2
Ghana	183.0	257.7	411.5	402.6	263.1	1,312.6	1,783.1
Israel	1,229.2	2,369.1	6,228.6	12,658.2	21,043.0	30,642.9	35,691.0
Netherlands	1,068.8	2,889.7	13,615.8	21,019,1	25,921.1	50,338.3	44,746.3
New Zealand	2,312.9	2,356.5	7,436.8	13,670.2	13,641.0	33,692.0	38,649.4
Singapore	427.9	925.3	4,927.0	11,864.3	23,792.6	46,569.7	54,940.9
Slovenia	—	—	—	—	10,227.8	23,437.5	20,873.2
Switzerland	1,788.4	—	18,832.2	38,428.4	37,868.3	74,605.7	82,016.0
Taiwan	—	—	2,367.0	8,178.0	14,877.0	19,262.0	22,358.0
Republic of Tanzania	—	—	—	172.0	306.7	701.6	872.3

Source: World Bank 2019. Data Taiwan: Website Ministry of Health and Welfare.

Table 5b. Income per Capita, 1960–2015 (Constant 2011 PPP Dollars)

	Year			
Country	**1990**	**2000**	**2010**	**2015**
Chile	8,991.8	14,315.4	19,442.1	22,516.6
Czech Republic	20,023.1	21,193.9	28,352.9	30605.4
Ecuador	7,472.0	7,387.6	9,352.3	10,749.1
Ghana	1,919.0	2,259.1	3,059.4	3,823.5
Israel	20,520.4	26,824.7	29,743.0	32,024.5
Netherlands	32,090.2	41,721.7	45,524.7	46,494.4
New Zealand	23,671.3	27,620.5	32,119.2	35,309.8
Singapore	34,344.7	51,706.4	72,115.8	81,741.1
Slovenia	—	22,723.3	28,678.4	29,037.7
Switzerland	48,181.8	50,776.0	55,866.3	57,264.2
Taiwan	10,048.0	21,591.0	38,593.0	46,915.0
Rep. of Tanzania	1,472.6	1,481.5	2,090.6	2,491.0

Source: World Bank 2018; Taiwan data: MoH Taiwan 2018.

Table 6a. Health Expenditure, 1990–2015 (percent gross domestic product (GDP)

Country	1990	2000	2010	2015
Chile	4.7	7.0	6.8	8.1
Czech Republic	5.9	5.7	6.9	7.3
Ecuador	4.1	3.3	7.5	8.5
Ghana	3.5	5.1	6.5	5.9
Israel	4.8	6.8	7.1	7.4
Netherlands	7.9	7.1	10.4	10.7
New Zealand	7.2	7.5	9.7	9.3
Singapore	1.9	3.4	3.2	4.3
Slovenia	3	7.8	8.6	8.5
Switzerland	7.5	9.3	10.7	12.1
Taiwan	—	—	6.3	6.2
Republic of Tanzania	4.7	—	—	6.1

The header "Year" spans the four year columns.

Source: 1990: World Bank 1993; 1990 data for the Czech Republic as Czechoslovakia; 1990 data for Slovenia as Yugoslavia; 2000–2015: World Development Indicators; Taiwan: Website Ministry of Health and Welfare.

Table 6b. Health Expenditure, 2000–2015 (Current US Dollars and PPP Dollars)

Country	2000 Current US\$	2000 PPP US\$	2010 Current US\$	2010 PPP US\$	2015 Current US\$	2015 PPP US\$
Chile	358.8	614	871.3	1,195	1,102.0	1,677
Czech Republic	342.9	982	1,373.9	1,930	1,284.1	2,146
Ecuador	48.1	198	350.2	541	530.1	797
Ghana	21.9	83	85.5	161	79.6	145
Israel	1,496.9	1,762	2,218.4	2,116	2,756.1	2,599
Netherlands	1,836.2	2,350	5,249.4	4,699	4,746.0	5,202
New Zealand	1,053.9	1,614	3,239.9	3,477	3,553.6	4,018
Singapore	820.7	1,139	1,503.0	2,792	2,280.3	4,047
Slovenia	796.6	1,453	2,008.2	2,452	1,771.6	2,698
Switzerland	3,540.8	3,232	8,018.8	5,395	9,817.0	6,468
Taiwan	—	—	—	—	—	—
Republic of Tanzania	12.6	39	36.1	106	31.7	137

The header "Year" spans the six data columns; each year groups a "Current US\$" and a "PPP US\$" sub-column.

Source: World Bank 2018.

Table 7a. Public Health Spending (Taxes and Social Health Contributions as Percent of Total Health Expenditure)

Country	Year			
	2000	**2005**	**2010**	**2014**
Chile	53.3	37.9	47.3	49.5
Czech Republic	90.3	87.3	83.8	85.5
Ecuador	26.5	22.3	41.7	49.2
Ghana	50.0	64.9	71.8	59.8
Israel	62.6	59.3	62.7	60.9
Netherlands	63.1	69.5	86.7	87.0
New Zealand	78.0	79.7	83.1	82.3
Singapore	45.0	26.8	34.7	41.7
Slovenia	74.0	73.1	74.2	71.7
Switzerland	55.4	59.5	64.1	66.0
Taiwan	60.6	62.5	—	—
Republic of Tanzania	43.4	63.6	39.1	46.0

World Bank 2018; Taiwan: Lu and Chiang 2011.

Table 7b. Social Health Insurance, 2000–2015 (Percent of Total Health Expenditure)

Country	Year			
	2000	**2005**	**2010**	**2015**
Chile	33.2	37.1	44.1	47.5
Czech Republic	—	81.3	77.9	70.4
Ecuador	12.7	25.1	18.1	21.1
Ghana	0.0	16.0	17.7	9.1
Israel	—	—	46.0	—
Netherlands	—	62.6	25.4	19.4
New Zealand	—	8.1	8.6	7.8
Singapore	1.8	5.6	3.7	5.2
Slovenia	—	70.0	69.9	68.7
Switzerland	—	—	3.9	3.5
Taiwan	3.5	4.1	1.8	7.1
Republic of Tanzania	—	—	—	—

World Bank 2018.

Table 7c.   Out-of-Pocket Spending (Percent of total health spending)

Country	Year		
	2000	**2010**	**2015**
Chile	42.8	34.5	32.2
Czech Republic	10.2	15.2	14.8
Ecuador	63.8	49.8	43.7
Ghana	64.2	43.9	36.1
Israel	29.5	23.7	24.4
Netherlands	9.4	9.8	12.2
New Zealand	15.4	12.6	11.0
Singapore	48.2	47.5	36.7
Slovenia	11.5	12.6	12.5
Switzerland	33.0	28.0	28.3
Taiwan	33.6	34.3	—
Republic of Tanzania	37.7	31.9	26.1

Source: World Bank 2018; Taiwan: data Lu and Chiang 2011.

Table 7d.   Foreign Development Aid, 1990–2015 (Percent of Total Health Spending)

Country	Year			
	1990	**2000**	**2010**	**2015**
Ecuador	4.1	2.8	1.4	0.4
Ghana	14.2	9.3	10.2	25.6
Israel	—	—	1.3	—
Republic of Tanzania	48.2	38.8	39.4	36.6

Source: World Bank 2018, 1990: WDR 1993.

Thus, wealthier people generally have better protection against high costs of medical care than poorer families; the latter face higher out-of-pocket expenditures (OOPs). In short, the poorest groups in the poorest countries pay for most of their healthcare themselves.

Fifth, there have been some important changes in the inputs of the healthcare systems (Tables 8a–8c). The major categories of health spending concern manpower, infrastructure (buildings), medical technology and pharmaceuticals.

Table 8a. Number of Hospital Beds, 1960–2015 (per '000 Population)

	Year						
Country	1960	1970	1980	1990	2000	2010	2015
Chile	3.6	3.8	3.4	3.2	2.3	2.3	2.1
Czech Republic	—	—	11.3	11.4	8.8	8.4	7.0
Ecuador	1.9	2.3	1.9	1.6	1.7	—	1.6
Ghana	0.8	1.3	—	1.5	0.9	0.9	—
Israel	6.7	—	6.8	6.2	6.1	6.3	3.5
Netherlands	—	—	—	5.8	4.8	4.8	—
New Zealand	11.7	10.8	10.2	8.5	6.6	6.7	—
Singapore	4.4	3.7	4.0	3.6	3.2	3.2	—
Slovenia	—	—	7.0	6.0	5.4	4.8	4.6
Switzerland	—	—	—	—	5.5	5.5	5.0
Taiwan	0.7	2.4	3.2	4.1	5.1	5.7	—
Republic of Tanzania	1.5	—	1.4	1.0	1.1	1.7	0.7

Source: World Bank 2018; data Taiwan: Lu and Chiang 2011; WHO 2009.
Data from different sources are not entirely compatible.

Table 8b. Number of Physicians, 1960–2015 (per '000 Population)

	Year						
Country	1960	1970	1980	1990	2000	2010	2015
Chile	0.6	0.5	—	1.1	1.1	—	—
Czech Republic	—	1.8	2.3	2.7	3.4	3.6	—
Ecuador	0.4	0.3	—	1.04	1.5	1.7	—
Ghana	0.05	0.08	—	0.04	0.2	0.1	—
Israel	2.5	2.9	3.1	3.2	3.8	—	3.5
Netherlands	1.1	1.2	1.9	2.5	3.2	—	3.5
New Zealand	—	—	1.6	1.9	2.1	2.6	3.1
Singapore	0.4	0.7	0.9	1.3	1.5	1.7	2.2
Slovenia	—	—	1.7	2.0	2.2	2.4	2.8
Switzerland	1.4	1.5	2.5	3.0	3.5	3.8	4.2
Taiwan	0.5	0.4	0.7	1.0	1.3	1.5	—
Republic of Tanzania	0.06	0.05	0.04	0.03	0.01	0.008	—

Source: World Bank 2018; data Taiwan: Lu and Chiang 2011; WDR 1993; WHO 2009.
Data from different sources are not entirely compatible.

Table 8c. Nurses and Midwives, 1990–2015 (per '000 Population)

Country	Year			
	1990	**2000**	**2010**	**2015**
Chile	4.542	0.115	0.145	0.6
Czech Republic	—	—	8.493	8.385
Ecuador	0.926	1.63	2.084	—
Ghana	—	0.946	0.926	—
Israel	—	8.138	4.838	5.072
Netherlands	—	—	—	10.542
New Zealand	—	8.51	10.579	10.997
Singapore	—	4.324	5.777	7.12
Slovenia	—	—	8.22	8.84
Switzerland	—	—	16.303	18.23
Taiwan	—	—	—	—
Republic of Tanzania	—	0.371	0.428	0.416

Source: WHO 2018; OECD 2018.

The tables show large variations in the level of inputs across the 12 nations, with big changes over time. In the last three decades, facing excess hospital capacity and realizing that new medical technology allowed for much of the treatment in outpatient settings, many higher income nations reduced their hospital capacity and shifted medical care from inpatient to outpatient settings. In contrast, in some of the poorer nations, there was still the need to expand hospital capacity and medical technology. The wide variation in the composition of the healthcare workforce suggests that there is no obvious "best mix" of health professionals. Health manpower studies have shown that there are no clear borders between professional domains; in fact, those lines are shifting over time and there is increasing overlap between the activities of different groups of health professionals (see e.g., Okma et al. 2014). In high-income nations, manpower policies commonly focus on cost control and efforts to substitute other health professionals (e.g., physician assistants or nurse practitioners) for physicians. Low- and medium-income nations commonly face different problems: how to educate and retain health professionals and prevent brain drain. In both Ghana and Tanzania, for example, even the very low physician/population rates went down, mostly due to emigration. Likewise, while wealthier nations struggled to restrain market access of new drugs and equipment, poorer nations struggled with dire shortages of basic inputs.

Sixth, the lifestyle behaviors that (negatively) affect smoking, alcohol consumption, lack of physical activity, and high caloric diets associated with obesity are all changing, but not evenly (see Tables 9a–9c). Behaviors that (negatively) affect health are also closely associated with socio-economic status (Evans et al. 1994). In New Zealand, for example, the share of all adults who smoked went down from 24 to 15 percent between 1996 and 2015 (Ball et al. 2016). Within that average, the Māori population smoked more than any other group (its rate went down from about 42–32 percent between 2006 and 2014). The smoking rate of those of Asian descent dropped from about 10–8, followed by a drop in the smoking rate of those of European descent, from 25 to 22, and that of the Pacific population from 30 to about 22 percent in those years. That pattern in not unique to New Zealand.

Table 9a. Smoking Prevalence Adults, 2000–2015 (Percentage)

	Year			
Country	**2000**	**2005**	**2010**	**2015**
Chile	46.6	44.1	42.8	40.0
Czech Republic	40.7	39.5	38.5	37.4
Ecuador	21.4	18.4	15.9	14.0
Ghana	9.2	10.3	11.6	13.1
Israel	43.6	42.5	41.8	41.2
Netherlands	36.7	32.4	29.4	26.2
New Zealand	—	—	—	—
Singapore	27.4	27.5	27.6	28.0
Slovenia	29.9	27.0	24.6	22.3
Switzerland	35.0	31.8	29.2	26.9
Taiwan	—	—	—	—
Republic of Tanzania	27.7	24.7	22.0	19.5

Source: World Bank 2019.

Table 9b.   Alcohol Consumption (Liters of Pure Alcohol per Head Over 15)

Country	Year					
	1970	1980	1990	2000	2010	2015
Chile	9.2	10.2	8.61	6.24	7.93	—
Czech Republic	—	10.2	12.98	13.22	12.69	—
Ecuador	—	—	2.10	3.99	3.95	—
Ghana	—	—	1.30	1.60	1.69	—
Israel	4.6	2.9	1.84	2.53	2.63	—
Netherlands	7.8	11.5	9.91	10.06	9.33	—
New Zealand	9.8	11.8	11.31	8.91	9.62	8.70
Singapore	—	—	1.61	2.03	1.84	1.79
Slovenia	—	15.2 (3)	13.79	11.90	10.32	—
Switzerland	14.2	13.5	12.99	11.26	10.01	—
Taiwan	—	—	—	—	—	—
Republic of Tanzania	—	—	4.98	3.89	4.19	—

Source: 1970–1980 OECD Health Data; 1990–2015 WHO; WHO 1985.

Table 9c.   Overweight Prevalence, 1980–2015 (Percent of Adults)

Country	Year				
	1980	1990	2000	2010	2015
Chile	43.1	48.9	54.5	60.0	62.6
Czech Republic	49.9	54.0	56.8	60.2	62.0
Ecuador	31.8	39.3	46.4	52.5	55.4
Ghana	12.6	16.5	21.9	28.3	31.4
Israel	49.1	54.2	58.6	62.3	64.0
Netherlands	36.0	42.3	48.9	55.0	57.4
New Zealand	45.1	51.1	57.3	62.7	65.1
Singapore	23.5	25.5	27.7	30.2	31.5
Slovenia	39.2	44.7	49.0	53.5	55.7
Switzerland	33.0	41.7	48.0	52.0	53.9
Taiwan	—	—	—	—	—
Republic of Tanzania	10.3	14.1	18.4	23.8	27.0

Source: World Bank 2018.

On average, 15.5 percent of US adults were smokers in 2016 (CDC 2018). Only 9 percent of Asian Americans and 10.6 percent of Hispanics were listed as smokers, 16.5 of non-Hispanic Blacks, 16.5 percent of Whites, but 31.8 percent of American Indians. Thus, in both countries, the smoking rate of indigenous populations or "first nations" remained much higher than any other group.

Finally, despite all the issues mentioned earlier, there have been major improvements in some crucial health outcomes (see Tables 10–12). For example, child and maternal mortality rates fell dramatically in all countries. Even in the poorest countries of this study, progress was impressive in Tanzania and in Ghana, for example, the infant mortality dropped by about 75 and 50 percent, respectively (the absolute level is still high compared with other countries). With those improvements, average life expectancy rose everywhere (see Table 15). Importantly, those improvements took place even in nations with very low amounts of health spending. As many studies have shown, health outcomes are rarely directly attributable to national health expenditure.

Table 10. Maternal Mortality Rate (Modeled Estimate, per 100,000 Live Births)

Country	Year			
	1990	2000	2010	2015
Chile	57.0	31.0	26.0	22.0
Czech Republic	14.0	7.0	5.0	4.0
Ecuador	185.0	103.0	75.0	64.0
Ghana	634.0	467.0	325.0	319.0
Israel	11.0	8.0	6.0	5.0
Netherlands	12.0	14.0	8.0	7.0
New Zealand	18.0	12.0	13.0	11.0
Singapore	12.0	18.0	11.0	10.0
Slovenia	12.0	12.0	9.0	9.0
Switzerland	8.0	7.0	6.0	5.0
Taiwan	—	—	—	—
Republic of Tanzania	997.0	842.0	514.0	398.0

Source: World Bank 2019.

Table 11.   Infant Mortality Rate (per '000 Live Births)

Country	1960	1970	1980	1990	2000	2010	2015
				Year			
Chile	131.3	66.5	27.9	16.1	9.2	7.5	6.7
Czech Republic	—	—	—	10.3	4.5	2.7	2.5
Ecuador	119.8	95.8	67.1	42.4	24.3	15.7	13.0
Ghana	124.2	120.1	100.8	79.3	64.1	48.9	38.9
Israel	—	—	15.5	9.7	5.6	3.7	3.0
Netherlands	16.5	12.4	8.8	6.8	5.1	3.7	3.4
New Zealand	22.6	16.9	12.7	9.2	6.1	5.1	4.6
Singapore	35.6	22.0	12.0	6.2	3.0	2.2	2.1
Slovenia	—	—	—	8.8	4.6	2.6	1.9
Switzerland	21.7	15.0	8.4	6.6	4.7	3.9	3.8
Taiwan	—	—	—	—	—	—	—
Republic of Tanzania	143.2	126.0	106.6	100.3	79.5	48.1	41.0

Source: World Bank 2019.

Table 12.   Life Expectancy 1960–65 to 2010–15 (Years at Birth)

Country	1960–65	1970–75	1980–85	1990–95	2000–05	2010–15
			Year			
Chile	57.3	62.3	69.1	73.7	77.4	78.8
Czech Republic	70.4	70.0	70.1	72.5	75.5	78.2
Ecuador	54.8	58.9	64.6	70.2	73.6	75.5
Ghana	46.9	50.0	53.1	57.8	57.5	61.7
Israel	71.0	72.6	74.6	77.2	79.6	81.9
Netherlands	73.5	74.1	76.1	77.3	78.7	81.3
New Zealand	71.2	71.8	73.8	76.4	79.1	81.3
Singapore	66.4	69.1	72.9	77.0	79.2	82.3
Slovenia	69.2	69.8	71.2	73.7	76.7	80.3
Switzerland	71.6	73.7	76.1	77.9	80.5	82.7
Taiwan	65.0	69.4	72.1	74.4	76.9	79.3
Republic of Tanzania	44.3	47.7	50.6	49.6	53.7	62.8

Source: UN 2018a.

The "House Model" of Healthcare Systems

Any given healthcare system can be described in terms of the financing, contracting and provision of health services (OECD 1992; OECD 1994). Other important elements are the administration and regulation of healthcare and insurance, as well as underlying cultural values that contribute to the shaping of government policy. Together, we can depict those elements as a "house model" (see Diagram 1).

Values or dominant cultural orientations in societies—depicted as the foundation of the abovementioned house model—provide the moral base and popular support for much of social policy. Values are subjective views about what has worth or is important (Marmor et al. 2002). In politics, these are views about the ends to which social institutions ought to advance, and virtues they ought to embody. Values compete with one another, but they are general: they do not express preferences for one particular arrangement, or one particular policy course over another. Shared value orientations exist side by side with substantial variations in public and private administrative arrangements, policies and rules.

Diagram 1.   Core Elements of Healthcare Systems.

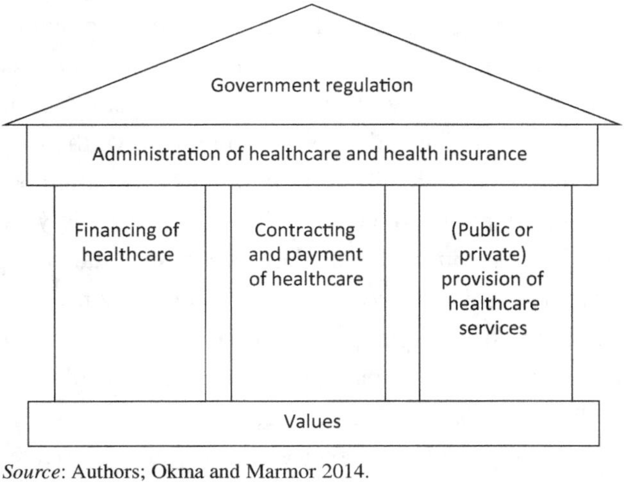

Source: Authors; Okma and Marmor 2014.

The main *financing sources* for healthcare are general taxation, earmarked taxes and social insurance contributions, private insurance premiums, direct out-of-pocket spending by patients, charitable contributions and, for some developing countries, external aid. All countries of the world combine at least two different funding sources. There is a strong correlation between income level and the degree of collective (or prepaid) financing of healthcare: higher income nations usually have a much higher prepaid share of their health expenditures, financed out of general taxation or (social) health insurance, than low-income countries. Second, within nations, on average, low-income families pay a much higher share of their incomes on out-of-pocket medical expenses than wealthier families.

There are three basic models for *contracting* medical care. The first is the "integrated model," with funding and provision of healthcare under the same (public or private) authority. The best-known example of a public integrated model was the British National Health Service (NHS) of 1948. Examples of a private integrated model are the original health maintenance organizations (HMOs) that took off in the United States in the early 1970s. The second contracting model, typical for social health insurance, is exemplified by the long-term contracts between third payers (governments or social health insurance carriers) and independent healthcare providers. The third model is that of reimbursement, common in private insurance: the patient first pays for his medical care and then seeks full or partial reimbursement from his health insurer. The contracting mode is closely related to the way healthcare providers receive their incomes: as employees, as independent health professionals or as a member of a particular group who bargain collectively. There are a variety of payment modes for medical care in physicians' offices or hospitals: employment-based, per treatment episode, per day or per hour, per patient registered with a particular practice (capitation), by case-based amounts (diagnosis-related group based, DRG) or payments for specific activities including bonus for quality care (pay-for-performance).

The *ownership* of healthcare services can be public, private (both for-profit and non-profit), or—as in most countries—a mix of those. Moreover, there are country-specific mixes of formal and informal care,

346

traditional and modern medicine, acute medical care and long-term social care. Definitions and borderlines of all those categories can differ according to country-specific traditions.

The *administration* of health insurance and healthcare concerns the arrangement for the managing and dispensing of health insurance and healthcare that reflects public and private responsibilities for allocating scarce resources, for example, in the composition of elected or appointed hospital boards of directors or governors.

Finally, *government regulation* affects healthcare in a variety of ways in all nations, ranging from the licensing of medical professionals, accreditation of hospitals, market access of pharmaceutical products and medical devices, mandated health insurance and other rules that aim to safeguard access to healthcare, to quality control, patient safety, labor market concerns and direct consumer marketing of prescription drugs. Still other regulatory concerns are medical school enrollment and the planning of hospital capacity. At the same time, healthcare is an important economic activity and as such, subject to industrial policy and antitrust law. Regulation also includes self-regulation by industry or professional groups, for example, accreditation of hospitals or physicians.

References

Ball, J., J. Stanley, N. Wilson, et al. August 4, 2016. "Smoking Prevalence in New Zealand from 1996–2015: A critical view of national data sources to inform progress towards the Smokefree 2025 goal." *New Engl J Med,* 129(1439): 6958.

CDC. 2018. *Burden of Tobacco Use in the U.S.* Centers for Disease Control and Prevention, Office on Smoking and Health, tobacco/about/osh/idex.htm. Accessed February 1, 2019.

Evans, R.E., M.L. Barer, and T.R. Marmor (eds). 1994. *Why Are Some People Healthy and Others Not? The Determinants of Health of Populations.* New York: Aldine de Gruyter.

Lu, J-F.R. and T-L. Chiang. 2011. "Evolution of Taiwan's healthcare system." *Health Econ Policy Law,* 6(1): 85–107.

Marmor, T.R., K.G.H. Okma, and S.R. Latham. 2002. *National Values, Institutions and Health Policies: What Do They Imply for Medicare Reform?* Discussion paper for the Commission on the Future of Health Care in Canada.

OECD Health Data. 2018.

Okma, K.G.H. and T.R. Marmor. 2014. "Health Risks and Health Care Reforms in Western Europe and North Americas." *Int Rev Public Admin,* 19(3): 274–285.

Okma, K.G.H., J. Rojas, and N. Edelman. 2014. "The Changing World of Health Care Professionals in North America and Western Europe." *Le Revenu des Professions de Santé.* J. De Kervasdoué (ed). Paris: Mutualité française/ Economica.

MoH Taiwan. 2018. Website Ministry of Health and Welfare Taiwan.

UN. 2018a. UN Population Division, *World Population Prospects: The 2017 Revision.* POP/DB/WWP/REV.2017/POP/F06. Accessed April 10, 2018.

UN. 2018b. Department of Economic and Social Affairs, *World Population Prospects the 2017 Revision,* File POP/6 Population Density by Region, 1950-2100. Accessed April 10, 2018.

WHO. 2018. *Global health observatory date repository.* World Health Organization.

World Bank. 1993. *World Development Report 1993.* Washington, DC: World Bank.

World Bank. 2018. *Health, Nutrition and Population Statistics.* Washington, DC: World Bank.

World Bank. 2019. *World Bank World Development Indicators.* Accessed January 20, 2019.

Contributors' Biographies

Toni Ashton, PhD, is an honorary professor of Health Economics at the University of Auckland. Her research interests have focused primarily on the funding and organization of health systems and healthcare reforms. She has co-authored a book on health policy in New Zealand and has published many papers in peer-reviewed journals. Toni has served on the editorial boards of several international journals including *Health Policy* and the *Journal of Health Services Research and Policy*. She has been a member of a number of government working parties and task forces, and has undertaken a range of consultancies, including two for the World Health Organization.

Erika Billick, MD, PhD, worked as a medical scientist for 15 years (publishing and presenting her research on prostate cancer, HIV and melanoma) before turning to editing. She received her PhD in biology from Rockefeller University and MD from Weill Cornell Medical College. She has developed an expertise in editing work written by non-native English speakers, and has worked on everything from Science Fiction books to Chemistry blogs.

Tsung-Mei Cheng is health policy research analyst at the Woodrow Wilson School of Public and International Affairs, Princeton University, New Jersey. Cheng's current research focuses on cross-national comparisons of healthcare systems in the United States, Canada, Europe and Asia; healthcare reforms in the United States, Canada, China and Taiwan; health technology assessment and comparative effectiveness research; and healthcare systems change in East Asian healthcare systems. She is co-founder of the Princeton Conference, an annual national conference on health policy that brings together government, the private sector and the US research community on issues affecting healthcare and health policy in the United States. Cheng serves as a member of the editorial board of Health Affairs, the leading health policy journal in the United States. Cheng also serves as an adviser to the China National Health Development Research Center (CNHDRC), the Chinese government think tank for health policy under China's National Commission of Health (formerly Ministry of Health).

Kee-Seng Chia is the founding dean of Singapore's only School of Public Health at the National University of Singapore. He set the school on a mission to translate research into public health programs and policies. During his tenure, he has been instrumental in phasing in several initiatives in Singapore, including tobacco control policies, "Singapore's War on Diabetes," as well as the "Total Workplace Safety and Health" (Total WSH) as an integrated approach to managing employee safety, health and well-being in the workplace. Kee-Seng was trained in occupational medicine and epidemiology, and is now actively involved in teaching and research of health systems and policies.

David Chinitz holds a PhD in Public Policy Analysis from the University of Pennsylvania and is professor of health policy and management at the School of Public Health at the Hebrew University and Hadassah in Jerusalem. His research and publications are in the areas of comparative health system reform, healthcare priority setting, management of cancer services, mental health policy and the impact of quality improvement programs at the level of frontline staff in community and hospital settings. David has consulted for the World Health Organization, and served as president of the International Society for Priority Setting in Health Care and as Chair of the Scientific Advisory Board of the European Health Management Association. He has served on the editorial boards of *Health Economics, Policy and Law* and the *Israel Journal of Health Policy Research*. Chinitz has been a Visiting Scholar at several universities in Europe and the United States.

Santiago Illescas Correa received his PhD from the University of Madrid and is professor of Public Management in the School of Government and Public Administration at the National Institute of Advanced Studies, and principal of the Sucre Institute of Technology in Ecuador. His research interests are the study of public policy, decentralization and deconcentration, governance models and social policy. His articles have appeared in *Comparative Political Studies* and other journals, as well as textbooks in Ecuador and Spain.

Luca Crivelli, PhD, is an economist specialized in public health policy, health insurance, as well as social policy research. He is professor and head of the department at the University of Applied Sciences and Arts of Southern Switzerland, titular professor at the Università della Svizzera Italiana and deputy director of the Swiss School of Public Health+ (SSPH+). Since 2004, Crivelli has been active as a policy analyst within the international health policy and reform network; since 2011 he has participated in the activities of the Health Systems and Policies Monitor led by the European Observatory of Health Systems and Policies. Luca served as consultant for the advisory committee of the Swiss conference of cantonal health ministers, covering the ongoing reforms of Swiss health insurance from 2004 to 2007. He has been a member of the expert committee of the national health policy strategy "Gesundheit2020" since 2003. He serves on the editorial boards of *Health Policy*, *Politiche Sanitarie*, *International Review of Economics/Journal of Civil Economy* and the *International Journal of Public Health*.

Carlo De Pietro is professor of healthcare management and policy at the Department of Business Economics, Health and Social Care of the University of Applied Sciences and Arts of Southern Switzerland (SUPSI). Before moving to Switzerland in 2008, he was a SDA Professor and CERGAS researcher at Bocconi University in Milan (1998–2008). de Pietro regularly lectures at several universities, including those in Ancona, Aosta, Bergamo, Bologna, Bozen, Geneva, Lausanne, Lugano, Milan and Saõ Paulo FGV. Carlo also participates in competitive research projects and research commissioned by government agencies. His areas of expertise and publications include the regulation of health professions, healthcare management, evaluation of health policy, comparative health system analysis and private health insurance.

Aad de Roo is professor emeritus of healthcare management and co-founder of the TRANZO Scientific Center for Health and Welfare at Tilburg University. His research and consultancy work has been focused on strategic responses of healthcare providers to changing market conditions in the sector. He was director of the Master of Health Administration program of the TIAS business school at Tilburg from 1992 to 2002. He founded the Erasmus Master of Health Business Administration in 2002, and was director of that program until 2017. Aad was chairman of the Dutch Association of Nursing Homes and president of the European Health Management Association. He is a member of the national committee that evaluates health sector laws for the Dutch government, and he has lectured and published widely on issues of health management and healthcare reforms in the Netherlands.

Igor Francetic is a doctoral fellow at the Swiss Tropical and Public Health Institute of the University of Basel and at the University of Applied Sciences and Arts of Southern Switzerland. He holds a master's degree in Economics from the University of Lausanne (Switzerland). His research interests include the economic analysis of health systems governance in low- and middle-income countries (with a specific focus on Tanzania), global health, health economics and behavioral economics applications to health and health policy in Switzerland.

Adam Fusheini, PhD, is a lecturer at the Department of Preventive and Social Medicine, the University of Otago in New Zealand. Before that, he worked as a lecturer at the University of Health and Allied Sciences (2015–2018) in Ho, Ghana. He also served as a postdoctoral research fellow at the Centre for Health Policy, University of the Witwatersrand (2014–2015). Between 2010 and 2013, he was a PhD researcher at Ulster

University in Jordanstown, Northern Ireland, United Kingdom, where he worked on the implementation of Ghana' National Health Insurance Scheme leading to the award of the PhD degree in Social Policy and Administration in 2014. Adam has since been publishing in the area of health policy, health insurance, universal health coverage (UHC) and health systems reforms and governance in lower and upper middle-income countries of sub-Saharan Africa.

Floor Grootenhuis is a Dutch/Kenyan artist and consultant. She has lived and worked across the world including Kenya, the Netherlands, Spain, Indonesia and New York, and worked with UN organizations including UNFAO and UNWFP, as well as non-governmental organizations (NGOs) like Action against Hunger (ACF), Save the Children, Oxfam, Cash Learning Partnership (CaLP) and the International Federation of the Red Cross (IFRC). Her main focus has been on participatory evaluation, training, grant writing, monitoring, program management support, strategic planning related to food security and cash-based programming. She is a household economy approach (HEA) practitioner, and with a degree in Human Geography of developing countries, she brings in a holistic lens to her approaches. Floor also completed a master's in art and social practice at Queens College, New York, New York in 2018. In 2017, she was a More Art Engaging Artist Fellow. She has received grants from Social Practice Queens and Queens Art Intervention and a NYFA immigrant artist mentorship grant. The Queens Museum, the Godwin-Ternbach Museum and Five Myles Gallery in New York have exhibited her work, as well as the Centro de Cultura Contemporánia in Barcelona, Spain. Floor is fluent in English and Dutch and speaks French, Spanish and Kiswahili.

Zuzana Kotherová has worked as academic in the Czech Republic for over 15 years. She presently teaches at the Charles University in Prague and the Czech Technical University in Prague. Her teaching included post as Professeur Invitée at Rennes I University (2010 and 2018). Zuzana has lectured and published on a broad range of health system reform issues, health politics and policy.

Meng-Kin Lim, our colleague and friend Meng-Kin Lim, sadly passed away on January 31, 2013. He had contributed the chapter about Singapore to the publication "Six Countries, Six Reform Models, The Healthcare Reform Experience of Israel, the Netherlands, New Zealand, Singapore, Switzerland and Taiwan" published in 2010. Meng-Kin had had a long and distinguished career in the military, starting with his specialty in aviation medicine and ending as a Brigadier-General. Meng-Kin was awarded the Public Service Star for his heroic role in saving many lives in the aftermath of the Hotel New World collapse, when he did not give up trying to find people buried in the rubble. After obtaining his degree in Public Health at Harvard, he became associate professor at the Saw Swee Hock School of Public Health of the National University of Singapore in the fields of health policy and management. He published many articles, served on the editorial board of several academic journals and gave advice to international organizations like the World Bank and the World Health Organization.

Kieke Okma received her PhD at the medical faculty of the University of Utrecht in the Netherlands. She has worked with a variety of government agencies in the Netherlands and with international organizations including the World Bank, the World Health Organization and OECD for over 25 years. Since 2004, she has lived in New York and worked as an international health consultant and academic. Her teaching included posts as associate or visiting professor at the Mailman School of Public Health of Columbia University; the Wagner School of Public Services of New York University; Cornell University; Catholic University Leuven, Belgium; McGill University, Montreal; Queen's University, Kingston, Ontario, Canada; the University of British Columbia, Vancouver; and Professeur Invitée at the Conservatoire National des Arts et Métiers in Paris; in addition to Research Fellowships in Montreal, Canada; Bremen, Germany and Canberra, Australia and the University of Amsterdam. Kieke has served on several editorial boards including *Zorg & Verzekering [Healthcare and Insurance]*, *Health Policy*, the *Journal of Health Politics, Policy and Law* and the *Journal of Health Services Research and Policy*. Kieke Okma has lectured and published widely on a broad range of issues of international comparison, health policy, health politics, health manpower and the changing role of international organizations.

Hans Maarse is professor Emeritus in Health Policy and Administration at the Faculty of Health, Medicine and Life Sciences of Maastricht University, in the Netherlands. His professional background is political science. He has authored books and articles on a variety of topics including solidarity in health insurance, cross-border healthcare, privatization in healthcare, the market-oriented reforms in Dutch healthcare, the reform of long-term care and low popular trust in Dutch health insurance. In 2018, he co-authored a book (in Dutch) on affordable healthcare. Currently, he is working on a book with the provisional title *Health Policy Analysis: Five Analytical Perspectives*. He is a regular reviewer of articles for *Health Policy, Health Economics, Politics and Law* and the *Journal of Health Politics, Policy and Law*.

Guillermo Paraje is professor of economics at the Business School of the Universidad Adolfo Ibáñez, Chile. He specializes in topics such as health equity, health systems and the economics of NCDs (tobacco, alcohol and unhealthy diet). He is one of the recipients of the 2018 WHO World No Tobacco Day Award for the America Region. Paraje has been consultant for the World Bank, the World Health Organization, the United Nations Development Program, UNICEF, the Economic Commission for Latin America and the Caribbean, the Inter-American Development Bank and other organizations. Guillermo was a member of the 2014 Presidential Commission to Reform Health Insurance in Chile and has been recently appointed to the Ministry of Health Advisory Committee on Universal Health Guarantees. He was a member of the International Advisory Board of the Program for Research, Advocacy and Capacity Building on Tobacco Taxation (ACS/CRUK) and is a Global Fellow of the American Cancer Society. He received his bachelor's degree in Economics from the National University of Córdoba, Argentina and a PhD in economics from the University of Cambridge, United Kingdom.

Marek Pavlík is an assistant professor at the Faculty of Economics and Administration of Masaryk University, Prague. His research is focused on health policy, politics and economics, primarily on the problem of health policy implementation. His teaching included post as Professeur Invitée at Rennes I University (2017). Marek is also involved in the research of sport policy and economics with a special interest in the role of municipalities. He uses both practical and theoretical experiences in the field of sport research. He was a member of advisory committees and a member of municipality body (2007–2010).

Staniskava Setnikar Cankar, PhD, is a professor at the University of Ljubljana, Faculty of Administration. She was a dean of faculty and a minister for education, science and sport. She dealt with the economics of the public sector, the assessment of efficiency and effectiveness in the public sector, the entrepreneur functions in the public sector, centralization and decentralization of public sector services, public procurement, transfer of good practices with cross-border cooperation, innovation and creativity in the public sector and education. For 15 years, Stanka was the editor of the *International Journal for Public Administration*. She led and coordinated research projects about the reform of the public sector, the measurement of efficiency, health and cross-border integration. She was a member of the Senate of the University of Ljubljana for a decade and a member of the Administrative board of the international network of institutes and schools of public administration in Central and Eastern Europe NISPAcee.

Dalibor Stanimirovic is the head of the Centre for Health Care Informatics at the National Institute of Public Health of the Republic of Slovenia. He is an assistant professor of Informatics at the University of Ljubljana. He serves on the editorial board of several international academic journals. He has published in high-ranking scientific journals and presented his research at numerous conferences and seminars. His general research interests include ICT policies and projects in healthcare, evaluation metrics and models, government enterprise architectures and health information systems.

Tim Tenbensel is an associate professor in health policy at the School of Population Health, University of Auckland, New Zealand, where he has been based since 2005. He obtained his PhD at the Australian National University in 1995 in Political Science, and he lectured in political science at the University of Auckland from 1997 to 2004. Tim has researched and published extensively in the areas of health and public policy, comparative health policy, health policy implementation and New Zealand health services research since the late 1990s. From 2005 to 2012, he served as a handling editor for health policy–related manuscripts for the journal *Social Science & Medicine.* His current research focuses on primary healthcare policy and performance management in New Zealand in comparative perspective.

Index

F

facilities owned by the central state, 210

failed international models, 292

faith-based and private hospitals, 58

faith-based providers, 28

fall of communism, 322

Family Medicine Clinics (FMCs), 282

family physician, 282

family responsibility, 276

farmers, 301

federal health insurance (FHI) Act, 152

federalist political structure, 154

fee-for-service, 32, 123, 239, 307

fee-for-service payments, 235

fee schedule, 307

fees for outpatient services, 153

fertility rates, 86

financial accountability, 242

financial barriers, 22

financial burden of long-term care, 122

financial conditions, 4

financial instability, 231

financial protection from the cost of illness, 301

financial reserves, 136

financial risks of illness, 119

financial safety nets, 295

financial shortages, 199

financial sustainability, 47

financing, 120

financing, contracting and ownership of healthcare, 322

National Health Insurance Institute
(NHII), 235
National Health Insurance (NHI), 299
National Health Insurance Scheme
(NHIS), 25
national health policies, 89, 103
National Health Policy, 61, 103
National Health Policy in 1990, 57
National Institute of Public Health,
212, 219
national insurance scheme, 59
national IT projects, 212
national priorities, 101
national, regional, provincial and
municipal authorities, 104
national standard basket of services,
236
nearly universal coverage, 231
need to integrate primary, secondary
and tertiary healthcare, 295
neglect prevention, 175
neo-corporatism, 117
neo-corporatist, 234
neo-corporatist policy-making, 14,
124
neo-corporatist structures, 128
neo-corporatist style of social
policy-making, 121, 235
neo-corporatist tradition, 123
neo-liberal economic policies, 37
neo-liberal policy prescriptions, 252
neo-neo-corporatism, 129
network of providers, 196
new agencies, 130
new entrants, 134
new health financing options, 58

new investments, 85
New providers, 118
new public hospitals and clinics, 107
New Public Management, 232
new public management ideas, 252
New Zealand Health Strategy of
2016, 257
New Zealand Medical Association
(NZMA), 262
Non-governmental organizations, 28,
212, 326
non-government provision, 121
non-profit organizations, 283
non-profits, 100, 119
non-state healthcare provision, 117
non-state provision of services, 122
not-for-profit healthcare, 123
number of beds, 218
nurses and auxiliary nurses, 122
nurses and midwives, 86
nurses and other health workers, 222
nursing homes, 120

O

obese and overweight, 289
obesity, 184
Okma, Kieke, 354
older physicians, 200
one mandatory NHI under a central
administration, 38
one of the health insurance
companies, 188
one-party state, 55
open enrollment, 237
operating deficits, 47
opposition from physicians, 82

R